Disaster and Trauma

Editors

STEPHEN J. COZZA
JUDITH A. COHEN
JOSEPH G. DOUGHERTY

CHILD AND ADOLESCENT PSYCHIATRIC CLINICS OF NORTH AMERICA

www.childpsych.theclinics.com

Consulting Editor
HARSH K. TRIVEDI

April 2014 • Volume 23 • Number 2

ELSEVIER

1600 John F. Kennedy Boulevard • Suite 1800 • Philadelphia, Pennsylvania, 19103-2899

http://www.theclinics.com

CHILD AND ADOLESCENT PSYCHIATRIC CLINICS OF NORTH AMERICA Volume 23, Number 2
April 2014 ISSN 1056–4993, ISBN-13: 978-0-323-28991-7

Editor: Joanne Husovski
Developmental Editor: Stephanie Carter

Child and Adolescent Psychiatric Clinics of North America (ISSN 1056-4993) is published quarterly by Elsevier Inc., 360 Park Avenue South, New York, NY 10010-1710. Months of issue are January, April, July, and October. Business and Editorial Offices: 1600 John F. Kennedy Boulevard, Suite 1800, Philadelphia, PA 19103-2899. Periodicals postage paid at New York, NY and additional mailing offices. Subscription prices are $310.00 per year (US individuals), $491.00 per year (US institutions), $155.00 per year (US students), $360.00 per year (Canadian individuals), $598.00 per year (Canadian institutions), $200.00 per year (Canadian students), $430.00 per year (international individuals), $598.00 per year (international institutions), and $200.00 per year (international students). International air speed delivery is included in all *Clinics* subscription prices. All prices are subject to change without notice. **POSTMASTER:** Send address changes to *Child and Adolescent Psychiatric Clinics of North America*, Elsevier Health Sciences Division, Subscription Customer Service, 3251 Riverport Lane, Maryland Heights, MO 63043. **Customer Service: 1-800-654-2452 (U.S. and Canada); 314-447-8871 (outside U.S. and Canada). Fax: 314-447-8029. E-mail: JournalsCustomer Service-usa@elsevier.com (for print support) or journalsonlinesupport-usa@elsevier.com (for online support).**

Reprints. For copies of 100 or more of articles in this publication, please contact the Commercial Reprints Department, Elsevier Inc., 360 Park Avenue South, New York, New York 10010-1710 Tel.: 212-633-3874; Fax: 212-633-3820, E-mail: reprints@elsevier.com.

Child and Adolescent Psychiatric Clinics of North America is covered in *MEDLINE/PubMed (Index Medicus), ISI, SSCI, Research Alert, Social Search, Current Contents,* and *EMBASE/Excerpta Medica.*

Printed and bound by CPI Group (UK) Ltd, Croydon, CR0 4YY

Contributors

CONSULTING EDITOR

HARSH K. TRIVEDI, MD
Associate Professor of Psychiatry, Vanderbilt University School of Medicine; Executive Medical Director, Chief of Staff, Vanderbilt Psychiatric Hospital, Nashville, Tennessee

CONSULTING EDITOR EMERITUS

ANDRÉS MARTIN, MD, MPH

FOUNDING CONSULTING EDITOR

MELVIN LEWIS, MBBS, FRCPSYCH, DCH

EDITORS

STEPHEN J. COZZA, MD
Professor of Psychiatry, Associate Director, Center for the Study of Traumatic Stress, Uniformed Services University of the Health Sciences, Bethesda, Maryland

JUDITH A. COHEN, MD
Professor of Psychiatry, Medical Director, Center for Traumatic Stress in Children and Adolescents, Allegheny General Hospital, Drexel University College of Medicine, Pittsburgh, Pennsylvania

JOSEPH G. DOUGHERTY, MD
Program Director, Training Director, National Capital Consortium, Child and Adolescent Psychiatry Fellowship, Uniformed Services University of the Health Sciences School of Medicine; Staff Psychiatrist, Walter Reed National Military Medical Center, Bethesda, Maryland

AUTHORS

ZACHARY W. ADAMS, PhD
Postdoctoral Fellow, Department of Psychiatry and Behavioral Sciences, National Crime Victims Research and Treatment Center, Medical University of South Carolina, Charleston, South Carolina

STEVEN BERKOWITZ, MD
Associate Professor of Clinical Psychiatry, Department of Psychiatry, Perelman School of Medicine, University of Pennsylvania, Philadelphia, Pennsylvania

ERNESTINE C. BRIGGS, PhD
Assistant Professor, Department of Psychiatry and the Behavioral Sciences,
Duke University School of Medicine, Center for Child and Family Health; NCCTS Program
Director, UCLA-Duke University National Center for Child Traumatic Stress, Durham,
North Carolina

ALLAN K. CHRISMAN, MD
Associate Professor, Division of Child and Adolescent Psychiatry, Department of
Psychiatry and Behavioral Sciences, Duke University Medical Center; Duke Child and
Family Study Center; Staff Psychiatrist, Mental Health Service Line, Department of
Veterans Affairs Medical Center, Durham, North Carolina

CINDY W. CHRISTIAN, MD
Chair, Child Abuse and Neglect Prevention, The Children's Hospital of Philadelphia;
Professor, Pediatrics, The Perelman School of Medicine, The University of Pennsylvania,
Philadelphia, Pennsylvania

JUDITH A. COHEN, MD
Professor of Psychiatry, Medical Director, Center for Traumatic Stress in Children and
Adolescents, Allegheny General Hospital, Drexel University College of Medicine,
Pittsburgh, Pennsylvania

LISA CONRADI, PsyD
Rady Children's Hospital, San Diego–Chadwick Center for Children and Families,
San Diego, California

MICHAEL D. DE BELLIS, MD, MPH
Professor of Psychiatry and Behavioral Sciences, Director, Healthy Childhood Brain
Development and Developmental Traumatology Research Program, Department of
Psychiatry and Behavioral Sciences, Duke University Medical Center, Durham,
North Carolina

KATHARINE DONLON, MS
Virginia Polytechnic Institute and State University, Blacksburg, Virginia

JOSEPH G. DOUGHERTY, MD
Program Director, Training Director, National Capital Consortium, Child and Adolescent
Psychiatry Fellowship, Uniformed Services University of the Health Sciences School of
Medicine; Staff Psychiatrist, Walter Reed National Military Medical Center, Bethesda,
Maryland

KATE DREWRY, MSW, LCSW
Children's Advocacy Services of Greater St Louis, Department of Psychology, University
of Missouri–St Louis, St Louis, Missouri

TRACY FEHRENBACH, PhD
Assistant Professor, Department of Psychiatry and Behavioral Sciences, Northwestern
University Feinberg School of Medicine, Chicago, Illinois

LISA H. JAYCOX, PhD
RAND Corporation, Arlington, Virginia

BROOKS R. KEESHIN, MD
Assistant Professor of Pediatrics, Mayerson Center for Safe and Healthy Children,
Cincinnati Children's Hospital Medical Center; Division of Child and Adolescent
Psychiatry, Department of Pediatrics, Cincinnati Children's Hospital Medical Center,
Cincinnati, Ohio

CASSANDRA KISIEL, PhD
Research Associate Professor, Department of Psychiatry and Behavioral Sciences,
Northwestern University Feinberg School of Medicine, Chicago, Illinois

MATTHEW KLIETHERMES, PhD
Associate Clinical Professor, Children's Advocacy Services of Greater St Louis,
Department of Psychology, University of Missouri–St Louis, St Louis, Missouri

HARRIET L. MACMILLAN, MD, MSc, FRCPC
Professor, Departments of Psychiatry and Behavioural Neurosciences and of Pediatrics,
Chedoke Health Chair in Child Psychiatry, Offord Centre for Child Studies, McMaster
Children's Hospital, Hamilton Health Sciences, McMaster University, Hamilton, Ontario,
Canada

MEGHAN L. MARSAC, PhD
Research Assistant Professor of Clinical Psychology, Center for Injury Research and
Prevention, The Children's Hospital of Philadelphia; Department of Psychiatry, Perelman
School of Medicine, University of Pennsylvania, Philadelphia, Pennsylvania

LAURA K. MURRAY, PhD
Associate Scientist, Department of Mental Health, Johns Hopkins University School of
Public Health, Baltimore, Maryland

ELANA NEWMAN, PhD
McFarlin Professor of Psychology and Co-Director, Department of Psychology,
Tulsa Institute of Trauma, Abuse and Neglect, University of Tulsa, Tulsa, Oklahoma

AMANDA NGUYEN, MA
Doctoral Student, Department of Mental Health, Johns Hopkins University School of
Public Health, Baltimore, Maryland

PASCAL NITIÉMA, MD, MPH, MS
Research Biostatistician, Terrorism and Disaster Center, Department of Psychiatry and
Behavioral Sciences, College of Medicine, University of Oklahoma Health Sciences
Center, Oklahoma City, Oklahoma

BETTY PFEFFERBAUM, MD, JD
George Lynn Cross Research Professor, Paul and Ruth Jonas Chair, Professor and
Chairman and Director, Department of Psychiatry and Behavioral Sciences, Terrorism
and Disaster Center, College of Medicine, University of Oklahoma Health Sciences
Center, Oklahoma City, Oklahoma

BENJAMIN E. SAUNDERS, PhD
Professor and Associate Director, Department of Psychiatry and Behavioral Sciences,
National Crime Victims Research and Treatment Center, Medical University of South
Carolina, Charleston, South Carolina

MEGAN SCHACHT, PhD
Assistant Clinical Professor, Children's Advocacy Services of Greater St Louis, Department of Psychology, University of Missouri–St Louis, St Louis, Missouri

SAMANTHA SCHILLING, MD
Fellow, Child Abuse Pediatrics, The Children's Hospital of Philadelphia, Philadelphia, Pennsylvania

BRADLEY D. STEIN, MD, PhD
RAND Corporation, Pittsburgh, Pennsylvania

FREDERICK J. STODDARD Jr, MD
Clinical Professor, Department of Psychiatry, Harvard Medical School, Massachusetts General Hospital, Boston, Massachusetts

JEFFREY R. STRAWN, MD
Assistant Professor of Psychiatry and Pediatrics, Division of Child and Adolescent Psychiatry, Department of Pediatrics, Cincinnati Children's Hospital Medical Center; Department of Psychiatry and Behavioral Neuroscience, College of Medicine, University of Cincinnati, Cincinnati, Ohio

ELIZABETH TORGERSEN, BA
Department of Psychiatry and Behavioral Sciences, Northwestern University Feinberg School of Medicine, Chicago, Illinois

VANDANA VARMA, MBBS
Associate Research Scholar, Department of Psychiatry and Behavioral Sciences, Terrorism and Disaster Center, College of Medicine, University of Oklahoma Health Sciences Center, Oklahoma City, Oklahoma

C. NADINE WATHEN, PhD
Associate Professor, Faculty of Information & Media Studies, The University of Western Ontario, London, Ontario, Canada

MARLEEN WONG, PhD
School of Social Work University of Southern California, MRF 214-MC0411, Los Angeles, California

ABIGAIL ZISK, AB
Research Staff Member, Healthy Childhood Brain Development and Developmental Traumatology Research Program, Department of Psychiatry and Behavioral Sciences, Duke University Medical Center, Durham, North Carolina

Contents

> The epidemiology of traumatic experiences in childhood is a key context for research, clinical treatment, program management, and policy development. This article discusses the conceptual, methodological, and programmatic challenges in precisely answering even relatively simple questions concerning the basic prevalence and incidence of important trauma types among American youth. Findings from studies using nationally representative samples and directly interviewing youth about their trauma histories are reviewed, and lifetime prevalence rates for various types of traumatic experience presented. Clinical application of this information and future directions are discussed.

> Trauma in childhood is a psychosocial, medical, and public policy problem with serious consequences for its victims and for society. Chronic interpersonal violence in children is common worldwide. Developmental traumatology, the systemic investigation of the psychiatric and psychobiological effects of chronic overwhelming stress on the developing child, provides a framework and principles when empirically examining the neurobiological effects of pediatric trauma. This article focuses on peer-reviewed literature on the neurobiological sequelae of childhood trauma in children and in adults with histories of childhood trauma.

> Assessment is a critical part of understanding and addressing the needs of children and adolescents exposed to trauma. A comprehensive approach to assessment that measures a range of traumatic exposures and domains of impact and uses multiple informants and techniques over time is needed to best capture the complexity of needs and presentations of traumatized youth. This approach provides a pathway to effective treatment planning. The purpose of this article is to offer a comprehensive overview of the assessment of childhood trauma, with a focus on specific tools and techniques, and the use of assessment information in practice settings.

> There is a great need to recognize, prevent, reduce, or treat the immediate and long-term effects of childhood trauma. Most children affected by trauma will not develop long-term posttraumatic sequelae due to their resilience, but comorbid psychopathological outcomes occur and are more common after exposure to severe traumatic events. Factors influencing posttraumatic outcomes are numerous. Young dependent children tend to be more susceptible than older children; children with pain or injury are also more susceptible. Psychopathological effects may not be evident until adulthood. Awareness of the range of adverse outcomes underscores the importance of preventive interventions, accurate assessment, diagnosis and where possible, treatment. Advocacy and public policy initiatives are essential to improving outcomes.

Section 2: Disaster and Trauma Exposure Types

> Disasters, war, and terrorism expose millions of children globally to mass trauma with increasing frequency and severity. The clinical impact of such exposure is influenced by a child's social ecology, which is understood in a risk and resilience framework. Research findings informed by developmental systems theory and the related core principles of contemporary developmental psychopathology are reviewed. Their application to the recent recommendations for interventions based on evolving public health models of community resilience are discussed along with practical clinical tools for individual response.

> Schools are well positioned to facilitate recovery for students exposed to community or school violence or other traumatic life events affecting populations of youth. This article describes how schools can circumvent several key barriers to mental health service provision, outcomes that school interventions target, and the role of the family in school-based services. It includes a description of the history of schools in facilitating recovery for students exposed to traumatic events, particularly related to crisis intervention, and the current status of early intervention and strategies for long-term recovery in the school setting. Challenges and future directions are also discussed.

> Children's exposure to intimate partner violence (IPV) is now recognized as a form of child maltreatment associated with significant mental health impairment. This article provides an overview of the epidemiology of children's exposure to IPV, including prevalence, risk, and protective factors and associated impairment, and a summary of assessment and

interventions aimed at preventing its occurrence and responding to children and families. Information about evidence-based approaches to responding to children who present with impairment after exposure to IPV, such as posttraumatic-stress disorder symptoms, is discussed. Some of the challenges in understanding children's needs with regard to safety and protection are outlined with recommendations for future directions.

This article provides an overview of child physical abuse and neglect, and describes the magnitude of the problem and the triggers and factors that place children at risk for abuse and neglect. After examining the legal and clinical definitions of child abuse and neglect, common clinical outcomes and therapeutic strategies are reviewed, including the lifelong poor physical and mental health of victims and evidence-supported treatment interventions. Mandated reporting laws, and facilitating collaboration among child welfare, judicial, and health care systems are considered. Important tools and resources for addressing child maltreatment in clinical practice are discussed, and future approaches posited.

This article begins by defining sexual abuse, and reviews the literature on the epidemiology of child sexual abuse (CSA). Clinical outcomes of CSA are described, including health and mental health. An outline is given of all the services often involved after an incident of CSA, and the need for coordination among them. Treatment strategies and evidence-based recommendations are reviewed. Challenges around dissemination and implementation, cultural considerations, and familial dynamics are described. Possible future directions are discussed.

Complex trauma refers to traumatic events that are chronic, interpersonal, and occur within the context of caregiving relationships; the term also describes the pattern of symptoms associated with such experiences. This article explores the prevalence, causes, and phenomenology of complex trauma in children and adolescents. The investigators also describe family-related and system-related issues, assessment strategies, diagnostic challenges, and clinical intervention options.

This review addresses universal disaster and terrorism services and preventive interventions delivered to children before and after an event. The article describes the organization and structure of services used to meet

CHILD AND ADOLESCENT PSYCHIATRIC CLINICS

Preface

Disaster and Trauma

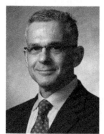 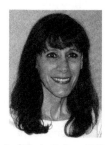 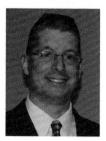

Stephen J. Cozza, MD   Judith A. Cohen, MD   Joseph G. Dougherty, MD
Editors

Stress comes in many forms and can vary in intensity, from everyday stress to life-threatening experiences. In addition, it can be acute or chronic in nature. When a stressor overwhelms a child's capacity to integrate the experience, adversely impacting development or leading to significant distress or symptoms of disorder, we refer to it as a **trauma.** Over the last few decades, researchers and clinicians have become increasingly aware of the widespread, diverse, and complex nature of trauma experienced during childhood (defined here as occurring from birth until 18 years old). Exposure to trauma negatively shapes children's development, biologically, psychologically, and interpersonally, and has been linked to elevated risk for adolescent and adult psychiatric disorders, behavioral and interpersonal problems, and high-risk behaviors.

Children's traumatic exposure risks, outcomes, and therapeutic needs must be understood within a developmental context. Typically, children do not have the capacity to fend for themselves, care for themselves, or communicate fully their complex emotional needs to others. Given their dependent position in families and communities, they face greater risk, particularly related to predatory, coercive, or aggressive behavior on the part of adults, whether caregivers or others. Trauma can, and often does, occur in silence or in secret, and children often possess limited capacity to alert others to their plight. In the aftermath of trauma, children must also rely on caring adults in their lives to help them recover from traumatic sequelae and those adults and systems of care must be sensitive to, ready, and able to respond to those needs.

The complexity of childhood traumatic exposure defies our ability to categorize these experiences neatly. Single-episode traumas (eg, an animal attack, motor vehicle accident, or house fire) may seem relatively simple for children to overcome but these are also complex experiences (eg, they frequently involve maladaptive cognitions, loss of function, property, and/or life). Children may be victims of physical abuse and/or sexual abuse perpetrated by a parent, a sibling, neighbor, or other family friend, teacher, and/or strangers. Within their homes, many children observe intimate partner

Child Adolesc Psychiatric Clin N Am 23 (2014) xiii–xvi
http://dx.doi.org/10.1016/j.chc.2014.01.005
1056-4993/14/$ – see front matter Published by Elsevier Inc.

violence between parents or other adults, or violence perpetrated toward siblings. An unfortunate few have witnessed a parent's murder, sometimes perpetrated by the other parent. Children may be exposed to physical, supervisory, emotional, medical, or educational neglect, among other forms of child neglect. Children sometimes are victims of chronic deprivation and abuse, leading to profound impairment in development, health, and functioning. Too many children live in dangerous communities where they witness repeated violence (eg, threatened or actual beating, shooting, or stabbing that results in severe injury or death). Increasingly, mass violence events, including wars and disasters such as hurricanes, earthquakes, and terrorist acts, also impact large numbers of children. Far too frequently, children become victims to a combination of these adversities.

Traumatic exposures result in outcomes that depend on the type, severity, and chronicity of the event(s), a child's developmental age, pre-existing individual and family risk factors, as well as peri-exposure and post-exposure experiences. Clinicians immediately tend to think of posttraumatic stress disorder (PTSD) as the likely result of traumatic exposure, but even significantly stressful events do not always result in traumatic outcomes. While it is the signature traumatic disorder, PTSD is only one of several outcomes that range from resilience to severe illness in exposed children. An understanding of the complexity of types of exposures and resultant outcomes in children can best inform clinical practice, including screening, assessment, and intervention (whether preventive or evidence-based clinical treatments). All clinical efforts should be **trauma-informed**, incorporating science into practice.

This issue cannot review all relevant information related to disaster and trauma and their impact on children. Together, these articles provide a broad overview of some of the most salient areas for clinicians who work with children. Each group of authors provides a summary of the most important topical information, identifies key points, offers an abbreviated review of the pertinent literature, and discusses application for clinical practice, tools for practice, and areas where future work is needed.

This issue of *Child and Adolescent Psychiatric Clinics of North America* is broken down into three sections. In Section 1, "Fundamentals of Child Disaster and Trauma," Benjamin Saunders and Zachary Adams open the volume by reviewing the "Epidemiology of Traumatic Experiences in Childhood" and highlight some of the challenges to the science of epidemiology of childhood trauma. They also point out the high prevalence of traumatic exposure of children within the US population, necessitating that clinicians working with children be knowledgeable. In "The Biological Effects of Childhood Trauma," Michael DeBellis and Abigail Zisk describe developmental traumatology as the construct within which to examine the biological effects of childhood trauma. While acknowledging the limitations of the field, they summarize our current understanding of the dysregulating effect of trauma on anatomical and neuroreceptor stress response systems, as well as its impact on neuropsychological functioning and brain development. In "Assessing the Effects of Trauma in Children and Adolescent in Practice Settings," Cassandra Kisiel and colleagues underscore the critical role of assessment in evaluating and addressing the needs of traumatized children. The authors review the components of comprehensive trauma assessment, highlighting that it should be conducted with flexibility and compassion. Practical assessment tools are also included. Finally, Frederick Stoddard discusses the "Outcomes of Traumatic Exposure," noting a range of outcomes, from resilience to severe PTSD and other psychiatric disorders, and the likelihood of comorbidity when illness is present.

Section 2 of this volume reviews different "Disaster and Trauma Exposure Types," beginning with Allan Chrisman and Joseph Dougherty's article on "Mass Trauma: Disaster, Terrorism, and War." These authors contrast mass trauma from other forms of childhood trauma and describe how such events are increasing in frequency and severity around the world. They highlight the unique impact of mass trauma on children, particularly since mass trauma can undermine the societal supports that typically sustain children and keep them safe. Lisa Jaycox, Bradley Stein, and Marleen Wong discuss "School Intervention Related to School and Community Violence," emphasizing the large numbers of children exposed to community and school violence and the important role that school-based intervention can have in their recovery. In their article, "Children's Exposure to Intimate Partner Violence," Harriet MacMillan and Nadine Wathen review the epidemiology of intimate partner violence, define exposure to such aggression as a form of child maltreatment, and outline the need for skilled assessment and intervention. Samantha Schilling and Cindy Christian provide an overview of "Child Physical Abuse and Neglect." They review legal and clinical definitions, mandated reporting laws, common clinical outcomes, and appropriate therapeutic strategies. Laura Murray, Amanda Nguyen, and Judith Cohen discuss "Child Sexual Abuse," reviewing its epidemiology, health, and mental health outcomes. These authors highlight the importance of cultural considerations, family dynamics, and coordination of the multiple systems/services (eg, pediatric, mental health, legal, and child protective services) in providing effective intervention. In the final article of this section, Matthew Kliethermes, Megan Schacht, and Kate Drewry discuss "Complex Trauma," a developing construct within the field of pediatric traumatology, which results from chronic, multiple traumatic exposures during developmentally vulnerable periods within the context of important caregiving relationships. The authors emphasize the uniquely negative outcomes resulting from complex trauma, which include emotional, behavioral, somatic, and cognitive dysregulation.

Finally, Section 3 includes three articles describing "Prevention and Clinical Interventions." Since trauma typically leads to vulnerability or risk, but does not necessarily result in mental disorders, strategies to mitigate risk or to prevent poor outcomes are important considerations in intervention with trauma-exposed children. In their article, "Universal Preventive Interventions for Children in the Context of Disasters and Terrorism," Betty Pfefferbaum and colleagues describe universal intervention strategies that have been used in support of disaster- or terrorism-exposed children, both pre-event and postevent, reviewing existing empirical outcome studies. In addition, they offer useful tools for clinical practice and suggest future directions for disaster-related prevention with children. Meghan Marsac, Katharine Donlon, and Steven Berkowitz review "Indicated and Selective Preventive Interventions," reminding us that the field of preventive interventions, particularly in at-risk trauma-exposed children, is relatively new, but promising, and requires additional study to recommend definitive strategies. The authors discuss research supported, as well as promising approaches to mitigating poor outcomes in at-risk children. Last, Brooks Keeshin and Jeffrey Strawn's article, "Psychological and Pharmacological Treatment of Youth with Posttraumatic Stress Disorder: An Evidence-based Review," provides a critical review of the current evidence for treatment of children with PTSD. The authors conclude that trauma-focused psychotherapies remain the primary evidence-based treatment for PTSD and that pharmacotherapy can be a useful adjunct when prolonged or severe symptoms are present.

In summary, exposure to potentially traumatic experiences is common among children in the United States. Childhood trauma can result from a variety of different adverse experiences taking place in many different environments. Trauma exposure can have a range of complex outcomes, often negatively impacting the biological, psychological, and interpersonal development of children. Clinicians who work with children must be knowledgeable about the epidemiology of childhood trauma, how to screen for exposure and assess outcomes, as well as where to refer for appropriate evidence-based preventive and clinical interventions. This issue provides a concise but comprehensive review of these important areas.

Stephen J. Cozza, MD
Professor of Psychiatry
Associate Director
Center for the Study of Traumatic Stress
Uniformed Services University of the Health Sciences
Bethesda, MD 20814, USA

Judith A. Cohen, MD
Medical Director
Center for Traumatic Stress in Children and Adolescents
Allegheny General Hospital
Professor of Psychiatry
Drexel University College of Medicine
4 Allegheny Center, 8th Floor
Pittsburgh, PA 15212, USA

Joseph G. Dougherty, MD
Program Director
National Capital Consortium
Child and Adolescent Psychiatry Fellowship
Walter Reed National Military Medical Center
Bethesda, MD 20889, USA

E-mail addresses:
stephen.cozza@usuhs.edu (S.J. Cozza)
jcohen1@wpahs.org (J.A. Cohen)
joseph.g.dougherty@health.mil (J.G. Dougherty)

Epidemiology of Traumatic Experiences in Childhood

Benjamin E. Saunders, PhD*, Zachary W. Adams, PhD

KEYWORDS

- Traumatic events • Epidemiology • Child maltreatment • Polyvictimization

KEY POINTS

- Understanding the epidemiology of traumatic experiences in childhood is critical to conducting meaningful trauma research, developing effective trauma services and service delivery systems with the greatest reach, and efficiently allocating resources.
- There are many serious challenges to understanding the epidemiology of childhood traumatic events, including the nature of many forms of traumatic experiences, inadequate national surveillance efforts, and conceptual and methodological differences between studies.
- Studies directly interviewing nationally representative samples of older youth are the most useful in understanding the epidemiology of childhood traumatic events.
- Depending on how various traumatic experiences are defined, 8–12% of American youth have experienced at least one sexual assault; 9–19% have experienced physical abuse by a caregiver or physical assault; 38–70% have witnessed serious community violence; 1 in 10 has witnessed serious violence between caregivers; 1 in 5 has lost a family member or friend to homicide; 9% have experienced Internet-assisted victimization; and 20–25% have been exposed to a natural or man-made disaster.
- Exposure to multiple types of victimization and trauma is very common among youth, characterizing 20% to 48% of all youth depending on the number of victimization types measured.
- Clinicians are encouraged to incorporate effective victimization and other traumatic event screening into their everyday practice.

INTRODUCTION

Understanding the epidemiology of traumatic experiences in childhood is critical to conducting meaningful trauma research, developing effective trauma services and service delivery systems, and efficiently allocating resources for both activities. Without an understanding of the basic topography of these events in the lives of youth,

---

The authors have nothing to disclose.
Department of Psychiatry and Behavioral Sciences, National Crime Victims Research and Treatment Center, Medical University of South Carolina, 67 President Street, MSC 861, Charleston, SC 29425, USA
* Corresponding author.
E-mail address: saunders@musc.edu

Child Adolesc Psychiatric Clin N Am 23 (2014) 167–184
http://dx.doi.org/10.1016/j.chc.2013.12.003
1056-4993/14/$ – see front matter © 2014 Elsevier Inc. All rights reserved.

childpsych.theclinics.com

Acronyms	
DAFSA	Drug or alcohol facilitated sexual assault
MVA	Motor vehicle accident
NatSCEV	National Survey of Children's Exposure to Violence
NCANDS	National Child Abuse and Neglect Data System
NCS-A	National Comorbidity Study-Adolescent supplement
NCVS	National Crime Victimization Survey
NEISS-AIP	National Electronic Injury Surveillance System All Injury Program
NIBRS	National Incident-Based Reporting System
NSA	National Survey of Adolescents
NSA-R	National Survey of Adolescents-Replication
TESI	Traumatic Events Screening Inventory for Children
UCR	Uniform Crime Reports

there is a danger of overfocusing on extraordinary, emotionally gripping, or highly visible types of events and overlooking less obvious or dramatic, but perhaps highly significant forms of trauma. From a public health viewpoint, knowing the prevalence and incidence of trauma types can help increase the reach of interventions, programs, and services. Obtaining even a relatively modest effect with either prevention or intervention services can result in a large public health impact when applied to a highly prevalent form of trauma. Such information can help guide policy-makers as they direct resources, and program and intervention developers as they consider new approaches. Epidemiologic information allows the field to better understand the most critical and most common trauma types, and the most affected populations, thus to achieve the greatest impact with limited resources. Accurate epidemiologic information also can help with the attributive process of explaining associations between traumatic events and outcomes. Without an epidemiologic background on which to place these associations, faulty conclusions may be drawn. As the saying goes, "when you hear hoof beats in Wyoming, think horses not zebras." Epidemiologic data provide the proper background for research, practice, and policy.

Prevalence and incidence of traumatic experiences among specified groups are the most basic pieces of epidemiologic information. Prevalence denotes the number of individual children experiencing a particular type of traumatic event within a certain time period, such as from birth to age 18 or within the past year. Incidence refers to the number of incidents or cases of a trauma type that occurs within a specified time period, such as within the past year, regardless of the number of affected people. Because children and youth may experience more than 1 incident over a time period, incidence rates usually exceed prevalence rates. For example, in a victimization survey of a nationally representative sample of 4008 adult women, 339 of the women indicated they had experienced at least 1 completed rape before the age of 18 years, a childhood rape prevalence rate of 85 per 1000 women.[1] However, because many had experienced more than 1 assault, the 339 victims described 438 incidents of completed rape in childhood, a childhood rape incidence rate of 109 per 1000 women. Therefore, distinguishing whether epidemiologic reports are describing prevalence or incidence rates occurring in which time periods is important to understanding and comparing results across studies.

Unfortunately, despite the importance of epidemiologic information, obtaining precise estimates of the prevalence and incidence of different types of potentially traumatic events that can occur in childhood is actually problematic. This difficulty is due to several factors, including the inherent nature of some of the types of traumatic events that children experience, the assets available to the field for detecting and counting events, and confounding methodological issues between studies. Understanding these problems is necessary to interpreting the available information and drawing proper conclusions. Some of the reasons for the difficulty in understanding the epidemiology of child trauma are discussed herein.

TRAUMATIC EVENT CHARACTERISTICS

Many forms of childhood trauma, particularly interpersonal violence, occur in private circumstances and rarely are observed by others. Frequently only perpetrators and children have knowledge of the events, and neither may want to reveal them. Offenders are fearful of the legal and social consequences if their behavior is discovered. Children often do not tell about incidents for many reasons, including being afraid of getting into trouble; a sense of stigmatization, shame, guilt, or self-blame about the events; fear of the offender; or fear of getting the offender into trouble. Some children (and some offenders) may not understand that what happened to them was wrong, or personally label the incidents as abuse or victimization. For example, a child may think that receiving a severe physical beating from a parent for misbehavior is appropriate, even though they were terrified during the experience.

For these and other reasons, interpersonal violence incidents involving children have very low rates of being officially reported to authorities such as law enforcement or child protective services.[2,3] Studies dealing only with cases reported to authorities such as law enforcement or child welfare agencies will severely underestimate the frequency of these events. Moreover, it is likely that reported cases differ from unreported ones on key characteristics including demographics of the offender and victim, and the nature and severity of the abusive behaviors.[4-7] Detecting interpersonal violence events in victimization surveys of community samples requires respondents to acknowledge them. Unfortunately, the same factors often inhibit disclosure of sensitive incidents even when careful and sophisticated screening approaches are used, also resulting in somewhat of an undercount of these types of events. Therefore, the secretive and stigmatizing nature of some types of traumatic events makes measuring their prevalence and incidence difficult.

These characteristics also may differentially affect responses by members of subpopulations. For example, males may be more concerned than females about revealing incidents of sexual assault, particularly assaults by male offenders, because of concerns about even greater perceived stigmatization. Girls from certain cultural or ethnic groups that value virginity more than others may be less likely to disclose sexual abuse. Children from geographic regions where severe physical punishment is the norm may be less likely to report physical abuse because they do not view it as out of the ordinary. Therefore, some of these challenges to obtaining accurate prevalence and incident rates may interact with factors such as gender, ethnicity, and regional cultures, resulting in differential undercounts for some subgroups. Further research is needed to better understand these relationships.

INADEQUATE SURVEILLANCE EFFORTS

For many forms of childhood trauma, there are few or inadequate ongoing national community surveillance efforts that can reveal basic prevalence, incidence, or case-characteristic trends. For example, in the United States the National Crime Victimization Survey (NCVS) is a very large (N = >90,000 households) nationally representative household victimization survey conducted annually by the US Department of Justice[8] that collects information about the incidence of certain crimes among participants.

Some of these crimes, such as sexual assault, intimate partner violence, and forms of community violence, are likely to be traumatic events for children if they are victims or are present when they occur. However, the presence of children who are not direct victims is not identified with these crimes. Most importantly, information about crimes against children younger than 12 years is not collected at all. In addition, the methods used for collecting information about sensitive types of crime such as rape and sexual assault have been criticized as inadequate, resulting in severe underestimates of the true incidence.[9] This problem with the NCVS has been acknowledged by the Department of Justice and is receiving considerable study.[10] Therefore some parts of the NCVS can be useful in estimating the incidence of some crimes against youth, but it misses a large portion of the types of victimizations of children that are frequently the most traumatic.

Other annual sources of national victimization information, such as the National Child Abuse and Neglect Data System (NCANDS),[11] and the Federal Bureau of Investigation Uniform Crime Reports (UCR) and National Incident-Based Reporting System (NIBRS),[12] collect information only about incidents reported to child protection agencies and law enforcement agencies, respectively. These data do not account for the large numbers of unreported cases of child victimization, and have significant overlap in the cases they detect because of cross-reporting requirements. Therefore, the 3 main federally sponsored surveillance systems for crime and abuse, the NCVS, NCANDS, and UCR/NIBRS, while offering some useful information, fail to give a complete picture of the prevalence and incidence of the victimization of children and youth in the United States.

CONCEPTUAL AND METHODOLOGICAL DIFFERENCES

Because of the lack of systematic, effective, and complete surveillance systems for the victimization of children and youth in the United States, most knowledge about the epidemiology of childhood violence and other traumatic events must be garnered from an essentially serendipitous collection of studies conducted for many different purposes. Because of the ad hoc nature of these studies, there is considerable variation among them regarding vital conceptual and methodological characteristics.[13] These differences result in sometimes widely varying findings that are problematic to meld and interpret.[2] Accordingly, even simple questions, such as what is the annual incidence or childhood prevalence of sexual assault, physical abuse, or other important traumatic events among children, are amazingly difficult to answer. Advocates, service providers, policy-makers, and even some researchers frequently ask why prevalence and incidence estimates of childhood events vary so widely between studies. Most often, conceptual and methodological differences are the sources of most variation. Thus, to understand the epidemiology of childhood trauma properly, one must understand the challenges involved in gaining this information and the underlying reasons for differing results between studies. Several of the most important and common methodological issues that arise between studies are discussed in this section.

Definitions

There are many gray definitional areas in deciding exactly what situations and behaviors constitute potentially traumatic events for children. There is great consensus concerning some types of events, such as violent rape by a stranger, witnessing severe violence in the home or community, or being involved in a serious natural disaster. However, there is debate as to whether some difficult childhood events such as divorce, natural death of a loved one, Internet harassment, or placement in foster care should be considered "traumatic" or should be more properly considered as stressful or distressing. Within event types generally agreed to be traumatic, there are discrepancies about the boundaries of the definitions. When does physical discipline cross the line and become physical abuse? When are parental arguments severe enough to constitute emotional abuse for a child? Exactly what behaviors and situations constitute a sexual assault? When do aggressive interactions between peers become bullying? Different conceptual and operational definitions between studies that supposedly are studying the same phenomenon lead to markedly different results. In general, studies that have broader conceptual and operational definitions of particular incident types will report larger prevalence and incidence rates than those with more conservative and restricted definitions, because more events will be captured by screening.[14]

Sampling Approach

The nature of the sample that participates in a study will affect the prevalence and incidence rates of childhood traumatic events found. Five sampling approaches are commonly used in studies of childhood trauma. Studies involving clinical or service-involved samples often report very high rates of childhood trauma, often 80% to 90%.[15–19] Of course, these are participants who are having significant problems that may be the result of trauma experiences, which accounts for the high rates of reported trauma typically found in these studies. Results from clinical samples can help characterize treatment seekers, but are of little value in determining population estimates.

Similarly, studies of known or reported cases (eg, children in foster care), by definition, have high rates of exposure to trauma events.[20] Although they can provide information about cases detected by authorities, they are not helpful in understanding unreported cases or in making population estimates. Community convenience samples have unknown biases attributable to how they are constructed, which prevent the making of broader population estimates.[15,21] More useful are limited community samples that are representative of a known sampling frame.[22,23] For example, classrooms may be selected at random within a school district and students assessed. These results can be generalized to the population from which the sample was selected (eg, the school system), and the results can be useful when the population sampled is believed to be similar to other populations of interest (eg, children in similar school districts). However, making generalizations beyond the sampled populations can be misleading.

Most useful are studies that use nationally representative community samples.[24–28] Depending on the specific population sampled and sample size, results from these studies frequently can be used to develop national estimates of the prevalence and incidence of traumatic events among children and youth and within important subgroups, such as by gender, race/ethnicity, or rural/urban. Results from these studies offer the broadest picture of the epidemiology of childhood trauma and serve as the best benchmarks for advocates, practitioners and policy-makers.

Respondent

Estimates of the prevalence of childhood trauma can vary significantly by the source of information. Some studies extract information from archival, administrative, or clinical records of service agencies.[29] This information can be useful in understanding service-involved populations if the agencies regularly use effective comprehensive screening methods for many types of child trauma of interest, and accurately record and maintain that information in the record system. Unfortunately, many times these procedures are rarely in place. In addition, there usually is a confound between sampling approach and using agency records as the source of information, in that these cases most likely have been or will be reported to authorities if a service agency knows about it. Thus the results from these samples cannot be generalized to the broader population of youth.

The 4 National Incidence Studies of Child Abuse and Neglect have used "sentinels" as respondents.[30] These studies systematically sampled a set of counties nationwide, and professionals within those counties that would be likely to know about cases of child abuse. Researchers then surveyed the sentinels about abuse cases they knew about within the study period, whether or not they had been reported to authorities. This approach has yielded much higher estimates of abuse than known, reported samples. However, it still requires that someone other than the child or perpetrator knows about the abuse.

Parents or caregivers are a common source of trauma history information, and may know of many of the incidents of trauma a child may have experienced.[26,28] For very young children, caregivers may be the only feasible source of information. For incidents that occurred when an older child was very young, parents also may be the only source of information. However, as children get older they likely will experience many events that are unknown by the parent, resulting in an undercount.

Individuals likely are best able to give the most complete report of the traumatic events they have experienced, at least past a certain age. Victimizations studies have been conducted successfully using children as young as 10 years as respondents.[26,28,31] However, personal trauma history information gathered from individuals also contains error. Beyond the already discussed reluctance to disclose sensitive events, individuals simply may not remember or may misremember events that occurred years ago. Research on the impact of trauma on memory has yielded mixed results, with some studies finding an enhanced memory for traumatic events and others finding memory problems associated with the use of defensive avoidance as a coping mechanism.[32] However, it is clear that memory issues can affect individuals' ability to describe past events in general. Concerns about memory raise questions about studies that ask adults to recall incidents of trauma in childhood. Although adults are likely to remember the serious events that occurred in childhood, the details of the events may be less accurate, and they may not recall less serious incidents. In addition to potentially biased estimates associated with impaired long-term recall of childhood events, retrospective studies of adults actually describe the prevalence of childhood trauma decades in the past. For example, the average age of participants in the National Women's Study[1] and the National Violence Against Women Survey[33] was approximately 40 years, meaning that the incidents of childhood victimization reported occurred 20 to 30 years previously. These studies are useful in understanding more about adult populations and past prevalence rates of childhood victimization, but have little relevance to current epidemiology.

Therefore, studies asking about events that occurred in more time-proximate periods will be more accurate, suggesting that direct surveys of children, youth, and young adults are preferable when trying to determine incidence and prevalence rates of childhood events.

Screening Method

The methods and approaches used to screen for traumatic events in studies can have major effects on results. The impact of factors that inhibit disclosure in victimization surveys can be moderated by the use of more sophisticated screening methods. Self-report questionnaires usually produce lower prevalence estimates in comparison with personal interviews, either in person or by telephone. Techniques such as proper placement of sensitive questions within an interview schedule, use of clarifying introductions to challenge stereotypes and cue the respondent's recall, avoiding single-item "gate" questions, using a larger number of screening questions, using behaviorally specific screening questions, avoiding undefined summary terms such as "abuse," and delaying follow-up questions until after screening questions are completed all contribute to greater disclosure rates.[34–36] However, these techniques must be balanced with the time and resources available for assessment and respondent fatigue. Unfortunately, many studies do not use these techniques, reducing their accuracy.

REVIEW OF IMPORTANT LITERATURE

For the reasons already described, this review focuses on findings from methodologically rigorous studies using national samples of youth in the United States that assess the most serious forms of childhood trauma. These studies give the most generalizable estimates for the prevalence of childhood traumatic events. Findings from studies of more restricted populations carry known and unknown biases that can be misleading when applied to unrelated situations. Studies reporting prevalence estimates from limited populations such as particular service organizations, cities, states, or regions are not included, such as the ACE Study,[37] the Teen Dating Violence Study,[38] the Great Smokey Mountains Study,[23] the Adolescent Alcohol Related Sexual Assault Study,[39] and the Minnesota Student Survey.[40] Likewise, studies from other countries such as the Canadian Incidence Study of Reported Child Abuse and Neglect,[41] the UK Victimization Study,[42] and the Netherlands Prevalence Study on Maltreatment[43] are excluded. Furthermore, retrospective studies of adults[1,33] are not included for the reasons described earlier.

Included studies for estimates of the prevalence of victimization and exposure to interpersonal violence in childhood are limited to those that used large, nationally representative samples of youth reporting on their own histories of trauma and victimization and parents of younger children, and that used methodologically sound screening methods. These studies included: (1) the National Survey of Children's Exposure to Violence[26] (NatSCEV: N = 4549, ages 0–17 years); (2) the National Survey of Children's Exposure to Violence II[28] (NatSCEV II: N = 4503, ages 0–17 years); (3) the National Survey of Adolescents[24,44] (NSA: N = 4023, ages 12–17 years); (4) the National Survey of Adolescents—Replication[45–47] (NSA-R: N = 3614, ages 12–17 years); and (5) the National Comorbidity Study—Adolescent supplement[25,48] (NCS-A: N = 6483, ages 13–17 years). Where lifetime prevalence estimates are reported for age groups, data from adolescents rather than from younger children are used, because information from older youth give the best estimates of prevalence across all of childhood. For other types of potentially traumatic events for which national representative samples and self-report data are not available, data from rigorously designed national clinical samples are reported with appropriate caveats.

Sexual Victimization

The NatSCEV[26] study found that 6% of American youth aged 0 to 17 years had experienced at least 1 episode of sexual victimization (sexual assault, rape, sexual exposure by an adult, sexual harassment, statutory sexual offenses) within the past year, with girls being about 1.5 times more likely to have such a history. Adolescents aged 14 to 17 had much higher past-year (16%) and lifetime (28%) prevalence rates of any kind of sexual victimization than the full sample of children. More specifically, 11% of adolescents in that age cohort (19% of girls) reported experiencing at least 1 sexual assault involving physical contact, and 8% endorsed a history of at least 1 attempted or completed rape (14% of girls) during their lifetimes. Results from the NatSCEV II[28] essentially replicated these rates. Girls aged 14 to 17 had a past-year prevalence of 23% for any type of sexual victimization, 11% for a sexual assault, and 8% for attempted or completed rape. Lifetime prevalence rates for the 14- to 17-year-old age group by gender for any sexual victimization was 20% for males and 35% for females; for any sexual assault, 4% for males and 17% for females; and for any attempted or completed rape, 3% for males and 13% for females.

Both the NSA[24,44] and NSA-R[45–47] studies used sample selection and interview methods similar to those of the 2 NatSCEV studies. However, the NSA and NSA-R had more limited definitions of sexual assault and a broader age range for the adolescents included (12–17 years). Accounting for these differences, the results were remarkably similar between the 2 NatSCEV and 2 NSA studies. The NSA found that an estimated 8% of adolescents, 13% of girls and 3% of boys, endorsed experiencing at least 1 lifetime sexual assault. Among adolescents who endorsed a history of sexual assault in the NSA study, nearly half (46%) reported that they were younger than 13 at the time of their first assault. Figures were similar in the NSA-R study, where 8% of all adolescents endorsed a history of sexual assault.

New analyses of the NSA-R data were performed for the 17-year-olds in the sample (N = 599). This age cohort would have nearly completed childhood, meaning their results provide a more comprehensive estimate of total childhood prevalence of sexual assault. The sample size is somewhat small, but is nationally representative. Within this age cohort, 12% (n = 74) of youth reported a lifetime history of sexual assault, which is similar to the rate found with the somewhat younger cohort of NatSCEV adolescents (11%). The 17-year-old girls reported a sexual assault lifetime prevalence rate of 20%, and the boys a 5% rate. These 74 victims described 113 lifetime sexual assaults, the characteristics of which are presented in **Table 1**. Teens were the offenders in 3 of 5 assaults, adults were the offenders in 2 of 5, and males perpetrated more than 4 of 5 assaults. Strangers committed only about 1 of 6 assaults. Similar-age friends, acquaintances, and dating partners were the most common offenders, committing nearly 3 of every 5 childhood sexual assaults. Relatives were the offenders in 13% of the assaults, and other adults committed 12%. Most sexual assaults (69%) occurred when the victim was an adolescent, and relatively few (7%) occurred in early childhood (age 0–5 years).

A type of sexual assault experienced by youth that is sometimes overlooked is drug- or alcohol-facilitated sexual assault (DAFSA). In these situations girls are sexually assaulted while intoxicated and incapacitated, either voluntarily or involuntarily, by drugs or alcohol. Using the NSA-R data, McCauley and colleagues[49] found that 2% of American adolescent girls had experienced a DAFSA. These types of assault accounted for 18% of all sexual assaults reported by girls in the NSA-R.

Considered together, conservative estimates would be that approximately 8% to 10% of American youth have experienced at least 1 sexual assault, with higher rates of sexual victimization among girls (13%–17%) relative to boys (3%–5%). Put more colloquially, at any point in time approximately 1 out of 6 American girls and 1 out of 25 boys have experienced a sexual assault involving some sort of physical contact. The rates increase to 1 out of 5 girls and 1 out of 20 boys when using data from a 17-year-old age cohort, the best estimate of the full risk during childhood. By far, the highest risk group is teenage girls being assaulted by peers and dating partners, with DAFSA being an important situational factor.

Table 1
National survey of adolescents—replication: sexual assault incident characteristics for 17-year-old respondents

Characteristic	Number	Percentage
Offender Age		
Adult	40	35.4
Teen	67	59.3
Child	5	4.4
Don't know	1	0.9
Offender Gender		
Male	93	82.3
Female	17	15.0
Don't know	3	2.7
Offender Relationship to Victim		
Stranger	18	15.9
Friend/acquaintance	54	47.8
Dating partner	11	9.7
Father	1	0.9
Brother	9	8.0
Other relative	5	4.4
Babysitter	2	1.8
Other adult	12	10.6
Refused	1	0.9
Assault Location		
Home	28	24.8
School	14	12.4
Neighborhood	15	13.3
Community	20	17.7
Elsewhere	35	31.0
Not sure	1	0.9
Age of Victim (y)		
0–5	7	6.5
6–11	26	24.3
12–17	74	69.2
Don't know	6	5.6
Mean (SD); median	12.9 (4.3); 14.0	

Data from Refs.[45–47]

Physical Abuse and Assault

Findings for lifetime prevalence of physical abuse among adolescents were higher in NatSCEV (19%)[26] and NatSCEV II (18%)[28] than in NSA (9%)[44] and NCS-A (4%).[48] This discrepancy is primarily due to differences in how abuse was defined. In NatSCEV, any incidents whereby an adult hit, beat, kicked, or physically hurt a child in any way, aside from spanking on the bottom, were classified as physical abuse. In NSA, however, abuse was defined more conservatively as incidents that required youth to see a doctor, spanking that resulted in noticeable marks, bruises, or welts, or punishments that included burning, cutting, or tying up a youth.[24] Thus, the lower lifetime prevalence estimates in NSA reflect only severe forms of physical punishment and abuse, a more stringent threshold than was used in NatSCEV and NatSCEV II. In addition, the inclusion of younger adolescents in the NSA sample may have suppressed the overall lifetime estimates of childhood physical abuse because younger children would have lower prevalence rates. Indeed, among youth aged 10 to 13 in the NatSCEV sample, lifetime prevalence was lower, at 10%, than among the older children.[26] These trends underscore the importance of considering how victimization definitions and the ages of respondents affect results when comparing prevalence findings across studies.

With regard to physical assault, estimates varied across studies, ranging from 17% lifetime prevalence in NSA[24] to 71% lifetime prevalence among adolescents in NatSCEV.[26] NatSCEV II found a similar rate of 69%.[28] Again, these disparate estimates between studies stem from differences in the criteria used to define physical assault. For instance, in NSA, physical assault was defined by incidents whereby adolescents were attacked either with or without a weapon when intent to kill or injure was still present, threatened with a gun or knife, or beaten to the point of serious injury.[24] In NatSCEV, on the other hand, physical assaults included incidents with and without weapons, with and without injuries, and without perceived life or injury threat.[26] These estimates did not include other forms of threats or harassment, such as teasing or emotional bullying, which was endorsed by 29% of youth in the NatSCEV sample.[26]

Witnessed Violence

In addition to violence directly experienced by youth, witnessing violence perpetrated against others has also been linked to a range of deleterious outcomes.[50] Thus, epidemiologic studies of child victimization have assessed the prevalence of witnessed violence in the home and community. In the NSA-R, approximately 2 of 5 adolescents (38%) reported ever witnessing 1 or more serious incidents of community violence, and 1 in 10 (9%) had witnessed serious violence between parents or caregivers.[51] Boys were more likely than girls to endorse witnessing most forms of violence, including seeing someone shot with a gun, stabbed or cut with a knife, mugged or robbed, or threatened with a weapon. However, 4% of girls, compared with 2% of boys, reported witnessing someone being sexually assaulted. In the NatSCEV sample, 70% of adolescents aged 14 to 17 endorsed a history of any witnessed violence, and approximately one-third reported witnessing family violence.[26] Rates were very similar in NatSCEV II.[28] Again, differences in the types of violence included in these categorizations likely account for these differences in findings. As with several other forms of victimization, rates of past-year witnessed violence were highest among older adolescents, supporting the notion that teens are particularly vulnerable to trauma exposure.

Traumatic Death of a Loved One

Violent death of a loved one can also be a serious trauma for children. Using the NSA-R data, Rheingold and colleagues[52] found that nearly 1 in 5 (18%) of American adolescents had lost a family member or friend to some type of homicide. Of the adolescents, 9% were the survivors of criminal homicide and 7% of vehicular homicide, and 2% reported surviving both types of loss. Of the survivors, 53% had lost a close friend, 42% a nonimmediate family member, and 5% a close family member.

Internet-Assisted Victimization

Another form of interpersonal victimization that has emerged over the past several years is Internet-assisted victimization. According to data from the NatSCEV study,

6% of youth experienced some form of online victimization in the past year, with 9% endorsing a lifetime history of online victimization.[53] These estimates span a range of incidents, including online sexual harassment (6% lifetime prevalence) and online sexual solicitation (5% lifetime prevalence). Given the ubiquity of the Internet and mobile devices today, there is a great need to continue to monitor and build our understanding of this form of victimization and its impact on young people.

Other Potentially Traumatic Events

Disaster

On average, a disaster (natural or man-made) occurs somewhere in the world every day.[54] Although several studies have estimated the prevalence of mental health problems following disasters, few have considered the prevalence of disaster exposure. Responses from the NSA sample, however, indicated that approximately one-quarter of adolescents had been involved in a natural disaster in their lifetimes, among whom approximately 1 in 3 feared that they would be seriously injured or killed in the event.[55] These data generally align with those from a large (N = 935), national sample of adults, which yielded a lifetime prevalence estimate of 22% for exposure to at least 1 disaster.[56]

Motor vehicle accidents

Motor vehicle accidents (MVAs) represent another common form of potentially traumatic event encountered by youth. Unfortunately, the prevalence of these events typically has not been assessed as rigorously as interpersonal victimization. In the NSA sample, 21% of adolescents endorsed lifetime involvement in a serious accident, which could have occurred in a motor vehicle or in another setting.[55] In NSA-R, approximately 10% of adolescents reported a lifetime history of any MVA involvement (Williams JL, Rheingold AA, Knowlton AW, et al, unpublished manuscript, 2013). Other estimates of MVA and other injury incidence and prevalence are available from the National Electronic Injury Surveillance System All Injury Program (NEISS-AIP), operated by the US Consumer Product Safety Commission.[57] This source provides national estimates of various types of fatal and nonfatal incidents that lead to treatment in hospital emergency departments. Data for the NEISS-AIP are gathered from a subsample of a stratified national probability sample of United States hospitals that have at least 6 beds and provide 24-hour emergency department service, and are weighted to produce national estimates. Although figures are likely to underestimate the total number of children and teens who experience MVAs, including those that do not require youth to seek medical attention but may have been psychologically traumatic, the severity of incidents measured increases the likelihood of capturing accidents that may have been perceived as traumatic. According to the NEISS-AIP, in 2011 there were an estimated 310,568 episodes of treatment in United States emergency departments for children younger than 18 years whose injuries occurred while they were occupants during MVAs. This figure corresponds to a rate of 420 incidents per 100,000 children in this age cohort. When other forms of transportation-related injuries were included (eg, bicycle injuries, pedestrian injuries), the estimate rose to 808,721 (approximately 1100 per 100,000 youth).

Other accidents and animal attacks

According to the NEISS-AIP,[57] in 2011 the most common type of injuries treated in emergency departments for children younger than 15 was unintentional falls (2,411,097 estimated falls), followed by unintentionally being struck by or against another person or object (1,461,985 incidents). Among adolescents aged 15 to 24 the ranking was reversed, with an estimated 1,039,781 unintentional struck by/against incidents and 921,958 unintentional falls. Animal bites and stings, which also may be traumatic for children, accounted for an estimated 460,233 episodes of treatment in United States emergency departments for young people (<14 years).

Polyvictimization

There is substantial research demonstrating that exposure to multiple forms of trauma in childhood is very common. In the NSA, 20% of all youth and 41% of the victims of any of the 4 types of victimization measured had experienced more than 1 type.[58] In NatSCEV II, 48% of youth had experienced 2 or more of the 50 types of victimization measured, 15% endorsed 6 or more, and 5% reported exposure to 10 or more different types of victimization.[28] In NatSCEV, 10% of adolescents aged 15 to 18 years had experienced 15 or more types of victimization.[59]

Ford and colleagues[60] applied latent class analysis to the NSA sample and identified 6 distinct victimization classes. Four of these classes, comprising approximately one-third of the total sample, were characterized by polyvictimization. Higher degrees of polyvictimization have been linked to more severe and impairing forms of distress in adolescents.[59–61] Furthermore, different polyvictimization profiles appear to be associated with different patterns of behavioral and emotional outcomes,[60] highlighting the importance of assessing multiple forms of trauma in assessment protocols and considering the impact of cumulative forms of victimization and adversity on youth's functioning.

APPLICATION IN CLINICAL PRACTICE

As noted earlier, clinicians should be aware of the basic epidemiology of childhood trauma because it serves as a background for assessment, intervention selection, and service-program development. Several points from the foregoing review can be applied to clinical practice.

Knowing High-Risk Populations

Clinicians should be aware of populations of youth at particularly high risk. Different forms of trauma are more or less prevalent among certain populations. Some are obvious, such as that children living in high-crime areas are more likely to be exposed to community violence. However, 2 characteristics seem to cut across many types of trauma, age, and gender. First, as children get older the cumulative burden of trauma increases. Because they have lived longer, older children are more likely to have experienced more trauma types, and exposure to a greater number of trauma types is associated with more serious problems.[20,59] Second, adolescence is a particularly dangerous period for many new traumatic events, often rapidly adding to the trauma burden. In addition, girls bear a substantial additional risk primarily because of their high rates of sexual assault, anywhere from 3 to 4 times greater than boys. From the epidemiologic data, it could be argued that teenage girls represent the highest risk group for trauma.

Need for Screening

The significant prevalence and mental health impact of different forms of childhood traumatic events strongly suggest that clinicians should be screening child and youth patients for their lifetime histories of traumatic events as part of everyday practice. Without an understanding of the full scope of trauma experienced, clinicians risk having an incomplete history, misdiagnosing, and ultimately inadequately treating their child and youth patients. Trauma screening should be part of every assessment.

Screening Techniques

Clinicians should be aware of the threats to validity of trauma screening described earlier, and should use screening approaches and techniques that are likely to produce the most accurate data. Principles such as using explanatory introductions, behaviorally specific questions, and multiple screening items apply to both clinical assessment and research. Although busy clinicians must account for time demands when making assessment choices, good screening can be done in a time-efficient manner. Many of the tools used in the research described in this article are available and can be adapted for clinical use.

Case Formulation

As noted by the prevalence rates described, many children seen in clinical service settings will have histories of serious traumatic events, and a large proportion of them are likely to have experienced multiple types.[20] However, they are often referred for services because of an emergent report of one type of trauma and are identified by that moniker (eg, "sexual abuse victim"). There is an understandable tendency to attribute nearly all the problems and difficulties experienced by a child to their exposure to trauma, particularly the events leading to referral. However, clinicians should remember that many children are resilient and that not every episode of violence or other trauma causes serious problems.[62] Clinicians should not assume a child has serious problems based solely on the trauma history. Moreover, clinicians should not assume that the incident leading the child to be referred to services is the most critical one on their trauma history. Building a timeline of traumatic events and difficulties and placing a child's history in an epidemiologic context can help with case formulation, narrow down which events may be the most important to a child with a complicated history of multiple types of victimization, help focus treatment on the most important incidents, and help prevent misattribution of causality.[63]

TOOLS FOR PRACTICE

Two tools used in some of the research described here may be useful to clinicians. Versions of the Juvenile Victimization Questionnaire[64] were used in the NatSCEV and NatSCEV II studies. Versions of the Event History Interview for Children & Adolescents[65] were used in the NSA and the NSA-R surveys. Each can be used to conduct an assessment of the victimization history of youth. Although both are fairly long (30–40 minutes) and somewhat complicated to administer, each produces comprehensive and detailed information about a youth's history and incident characteristics that are directly related to mental health problems. When time is a serious concern, briefer screening tools can be used, such as the Traumatic Events Screening Inventory for Children (TESI)[66] and the UCLA Posttraumatic Stress Disorder Reaction Index.[67]

FUTURE DIRECTIONS

Understanding the true epidemiology of childhood traumatic experiences is challenging for many reasons, including conceptual, definitional, and methodological problems encountered. Fortunately, some of these problems are being moderated as new work incorporates the ideas and techniques of studies such as the NSA and NatSCEV series of studies. In the future, greater methodological consistency will aid in cross-study comparisons. However, new complications are emerging.

A serious methodological challenge is the increase of exclusive usage of cell phones. Many of the best studies to date have used random-digit dialing selection and telephone interviewing methods. Indeed the NCVS now has incorporated this technology as well. However, using this approach when a large and growing proportion of households in the United States do not have landline phones is more challenging and more expensive. In addition, response rates have decreased over time owing to societal concern about telephone fraud, identity theft, and other technology issues, which further affects the external validity of findings. Therefore, some of the most cost-effective methods are becoming more difficult and expensive to use. New technologies, such as online surveys and the use of standing national panels, hold some promise but also present their own challenges to accuracy and generalizability.

A second major issue is the amount of available information about the importance of the many forms of trauma children many experience. A single survey can only assess a limited amount of trauma types, leaving others unassessed. Only a restricted number of incident characteristics can be evaluated, even though many may be known to be significant predictors of outcomes. Each unassessed item is a potential confound to any conclusions. However, developing a survey that adequately assesses and is able to control for the entire spectrum of important trauma types is simply not feasible at this juncture. Therefore, future work will have to make critical judgments about what to include in individual studies, and accounting for previous data will be even more critical to building a useful epidemiologic literature of child trauma.

Finally, the field would benefit from an improved national surveillance system for childhood traumatic events. Current efforts are simply inadequate given the need. The field needs access to consistent incidence data about important forms of traumatic experiences to detect trends and the overall range of child trauma.

SUMMARY

Over the past 2 decades, the importance of psychological trauma in response to exposure to violence and other events has emerged as a vitally important area of research and practice. Research has found that trauma exposure is a key element in child development, psychopathology, and functioning. Consequently, policy-makers, service systems, and individual professionals concerned with children are seeking to become "trauma-informed" and to implement evidence-based programs and interventions for trauma-related problems. Knowing the epidemiology of traumatic experiences in childhood is a fundamental requirement for accomplishing this change effectively. It is fair to say that our current knowledge is based on the handful of rigorous, nationally representative studies completed to date. It is now known that a large proportion of children have had traumatic experiences, many of whom experience multiple types and incidents of traumatic events, and that adolescence is a particularly risky developmental period for trauma. However, considerably more research is needed to answer other important and fundamental questions with precision and authority.

REFERENCES

1. Saunders BE, Kilpatrick DG, Hanson RF, et al. Prevalence, case characteristics, and long-term psychological correlates of child rape among women: a national survey. Child Maltreat 1999;4(3):187–200.
2. Gilbert R, Widom CS, Browne K, et al. Burden and consequences of child maltreatment in high-income countries. Lancet 2009;373:68–81.

3. MacMillan HL, Jamieson E, Walsh CA. Reported contact with child protection services among those reporting child physical and sexual abuse: results from a community survey. Child Abuse Negl 2003;27:1397–408.
4. Drake B, Lee SM, Jonson-Reid M. Race and child maltreatment reporting: are blacks overrepresented? Child Youth Serv Rev 2009;31(3):309–16.
5. Hanson RF, Resnick HS, Saunders BE, et al. Factors related to the reporting of childhood rape. Child Abuse Negl 1999;23(6):559–69.
6. Hanson RF, Kievit LW, Saunders BE, et al. Correlates of adolescent reports of sexual assault: findings from the National Survey of Adolescents. Child Maltreat 2003;8(4):261–72.
7. Ruggiero KJ, Smith DW, Hanson RF, et al. Is disclosure of childhood rape associated with mental health outcome? Results from the National Women's Study. Child Maltreat 2004;9(1):62–77.
8. Truman J, Langton L, Planty M. Criminal victimization, 2012 (NCJ 243389). Washington, DC: U.S. Department of Justice, Office of Justice Programs, Bureau of Justice Statistics; 2013.
9. Kilpatrick DG, McCauley J. Understanding national rape statistics. Harrisburg (PA): VAWnet, a project of the National Resource Center on Domestic Violence; 2009. Available at: http://www.vawnet.org. Accessed November 11, 2013.
10. Kruittschnitt C, Kalsbeek WD, House CC. Estimating the incidence of rape and sexual assault: panel on measuring rape and sexual assault in Bureau of Justice Statistics household surveys. Washington, DC: The National Academes Press; 2013. Available at: http://www.nap.edu/catalog.php?record_id=18605. Accessed November 19, 2013.
11. U.S. Department of Health and Human Services, Administration for Children and Families, Administration on Children, Youth and Families, Children's Bureau. Child maltreatment 2011. 2012. Available at: http://www.acf.hhs.gov/programs/cb/research-data-technology/statistics-research/child-maltreatment. Accessed November 15, 2013.
12. U.S. Department of Justice, Federal Bureau of Investigation. Summary of the Uniform Crime Reporting (UCR) program. Washington, DC: Author; 2013. Available at: http://www.fbi.gov/about-us/cjis/ucr/crime-in-the-u.s/2012/crime-in-the-u.s.-2012/resource-pages/about-ucr/aboutucrmain.pdf/view. Accessed October 4, 2013.
13. Fallon B, Trocme N, Fluke J, et al. Methodological challenges in measuring child maltreatment. Child Abuse Negl 2010;34(1):70–9.
14. Finkelhor D. Childhood victimization: violence, crime, and abuse in the lives of young people. New York: Oxford University Press; 2008.
15. Ford JD, Gagnon K, Connor DF, et al. History of interpersonal violence, abuse, and nonvictimization trauma and severity of psychiatric symptoms among children in outpatient psychiatric treatment. J Interpers Violence 2011;26:3316–37.
16. Jaycox LH, Ebener P, Damesek L, et al. Trauma exposure and retention in adolescent substance abuse treatment. J Trauma Stress 2004;17:113–21.
17. King DC, Abram KM, Romero EG, et al. Childhood maltreatment and psychiatric disorders among detained youths. Psychiatr Serv 2011;62:1430–8.
18. Louwers EC, Korfage IJ, Affourtit MJ, et al. Effects of systematic screening and detection of child abuse in emergency departments. Pediatrics 2012;130:457–64.
19. Muesser KT, Taub J. Trauma and PTSD among adolescents with severe emotional disorders involved in multiple service systems. Psychiatr Serv 2008;59:627–34.

20. Grasso DJ, Saunders BE, Williams LM, et al. Patterns of multiple victimization among maltreated children in Navy families. J Trauma Stress 2013;26(5):597–604.
21. Khoury L, Tang YL, Bradley B, et al. Substance use, childhood trauma experience, and posttraumatic stress disorder in an urban civilian population. Depress Anxiety 2010;27:1077–86.
22. Centers for Disease Control and Prevention. Web-based injury statistics query and reporting system (WISQARS) [online]. Atlanta, GA: National Center for Injury Prevention and Control, Centers for Disease Control and Prevention (producer); 2003. Available at: www.cdc.gov/ncipc/wisqars.
23. Copeland WE, Keeler G, Angold A, et al. Traumatic events and posttraumatic stress in childhood. Arch Gen Psychiatry 2007;64:577–84.
24. Kilpatrick DG, Saunders BE, Smith DW. Research in brief: youth victimization: prevalence and implications (NCJ 194972). Washington, DC: National Institute of Justice, U.S. Department of Justice; 2003.
25. Kessler RC, Avenevoll S, Costello EJ, et al. Design and field procedures in the U.S. National Comorbidity Survey Replication Adolescent Supplement (NCS-A). Int J Methods Psychiatr Res 2009;18(2):69–83.
26. Finkelhor D, Turner HA, Ormrod R, et al. Violence, abuse, and crime exposure in a national sample of children and youth. Pediatrics 2009;124:1411–23.
27. Walsh K, Danielson CK, McCauley JL, et al. National prevalence of posttraumatic stress disorder among sexually revictimized adolescent, college, and adult household-residing women. Arch Gen Psychiatry 2012;69(9):935–42.
28. Finkelhor D, Turner HA, Shattuck A, et al. Violence, crime, and abuse exposure, in a national sample of children and youth: an update. JAMA Pediatr 2013; 167(7):614–21.
29. McIntyre JK, Widom CS. Childhood victimization and crime victimization. J Interpers Violence 2011;26(4):640–63.
30. Sedlak AJ, Mettenburg J, Basena M, et al. Fourth national incidence study of child abuse and neglect (NIS-4): report to Congress. Washington, DC: U.S. Department of Health and Human Services, Administration for Children and Families; 2010.
31. Bony-McCoy S, Finkelhor D. Psychosocial sequelae of violent victimization in a national youth sample. J Consult Clin Psychol 1995;63:726–36.
32. Goodman GS, Quas JA, Ogle CM. Child maltreatment and memory. Annu Rev Psychol 2010;61:325–51.
33. Tjaden P, Thoennes N. Full report of the prevalence, incidence, and consequences of violence against women: findings from the National Violence Against Women Survey. Washington, DC: U.S. Department of Justice, National Institute of Justice; 2000.
34. Testa M, Livingston JA, VanZile-Tamsen C. The impact of questionnaire administration mode on response rate and reporting of consensual and nonconsensual sexual behavior. Psychol Women Q 2005;29(4):345–52.
35. Fisher BS. The effects of survey question wording on rape estimates: evidence from a quasi-experimental design. Violence Against Women 2009; 15(2):133–47.
36. Hamby SL, Koss MP. Shades of gray: a qualitative study of terms used in the measurement of sexual victimization. Psychol Women Q 2003;27(3):243–55.
37. Felitti VJ, Anda RF, Nordenberg D, et al. Relationship of childhood abuse and household dysfunction to many of the leading causes of death in Adults: the Adverse Childhood Experiences (ACE) Study. Am J Prev Med 1998;14(4): 245–58.

38. Banyard VL, Cross C. Consequences of teen dating violence: understanding intervening variables in ecological context. Violence Against Women 2008;14: 998–1013.

39. Young A, Grey M, Abbey A, et al. Alcohol related sexual assault victimization among adolescents: prevalence, characteristics, and correlates. J Stud Alcohol Drugs 2008;69(1):39–48.

40. Eisenberg ME, Ackard DM, Resnick MD. Protective factors and suicide risk in adolescents with a history of sexual abuse. J Pediatr 2007;151:482–7.

41. Trocmé NM, Tourigny M, MacLaurin B, et al. Major findings from the Canadian incidence study of reported child abuse and neglect. Child Abuse Negl 2003; 27(12):1427–39.

42. Radford L, Corral S, Bradley C, et al. The prevalence and impact of child maltreatment and other types of victimization in the UK: findings from a population survey of caregivers, children and young people and young adults. Child Abuse Negl 2013;37:801–13.

43. Euser S, Alink LR, Pannebakker F, et al. The prevalence of child maltreatment in the Netherlands across a 5-year period. Child Abuse Negl 2013;37:841–51.

44. Kilpatrick DG, Saunders BE. Prevalence and consequences of child victimization: results from the national survey of adolescents, final report. Washington, DC: US Department of Justice, Office of Justice Programs; 1997.

45. Kilpatrick DG. Complex patterns of exposure to interpersonal violence and comorbid mental disorders among adolescents and young adults. Presented at the 17th Annual Kent State Psychology Forum. Kent, April 22–25, 2007.

46. Wolitzky-Taylor KB, Ruggiero KJ, McCart MR, et al. Has adolescent suicidality decreased in the United States? Data from two national samples of adolescents interviewed in 1995 and 2005. J Clin Child Adolesc Psychol 2010;39:64–76.

47. McCart MR, Zajac K, Danielson CK, et al. Interpersonal victimization, posttraumatic stress disorder, and change in adolescent substance use prevalence over a ten-year period. J Clin Child Adolesc Psychol 2011;40:136–43.

48. McLaughlin KA, Green JG, Gruber MJ, et al. Childhood adversities and first onset of psychiatric disorders in a national sample of US adolescents. Arch Gen Psychiatry 2012;69(11):1151–60.

49. McCauley J, Conoscenti L, Ruggiero KJ, et al. Prevalence and correlates of drug/alcohol-facilitated and incapacitated sexual assault in a nationally representative sample of adolescent girls. J Clin Child Adolesc Psychol 2009;38(2): 295–300.

50. Jaffee SR, Moffitt TE, Caspi A, et al. Influence of adult domestic violence on children's internalizing and externalizing problems: an environmentally informative twin study. J Am Acad Child Adolesc Psychiatry 2002;41(9):1095–103.

51. Zinzow H, Ruggiero K, Resnick H, et al. Prevalence and mental health correlates of witnessed parental and community violence in a national sample of adolescents. J Child Psychol Psychiatry 2009;50(4):441–50.

52. Rheingold AA, Zinzow H, Hawkins A, et al. Prevalence and mental health outcomes of homicide survivors in a representative sample of adolescents: data from the 2005 National Survey of Adolescents. J Child Psychol Psychiatry 2012;53(6):687–94.

53. Mitchell KJ, Finkelhor D, Wolak J, et al. Youth internet victimization in a broader victimization context. J Adolesc Health 2011;48:128–34.

54. Norris F, Friedman M, Watson P, et al. 60,000 disaster victims speak: part I. An empirical review of the empirical literature, 1981-2001. Psychiatry 2002;65: 207–39.

55. Kilpatrick DG, Saunders BE. National survey of adolescents in the United States, 1995 [Data file]. 1995. Available at: http://www.icpsr.umich.edu/icpsrweb/ICPSR/studies/2833#dev. Accessed November 8, 2013.

56. Briere J, Elliott D. Prevalence, characteristics, and long-term sequelae of natural disaster exposure in the general population. J Trauma Stress 2000;13(4):661–79.

57. U.S Consumer Product Safety Commission. National Electronic injury Surveillance System. 2013. Available at: http://www.cpsc.gov/en/Research-Statistics/NEISS-Injury-Data. Accessed November 11, 2013.

58. Saunders BE. Understanding children exposed to violence: toward an integration of overlapping fields. J Interpers Violence 2003;18(4):356–76.

59. Finkelhor D, Ormrod RK, Turner HA. Lifetime assessment of poly-victimization in a national sample of children and youth. Child Abuse Negl 2009;33:403–11.

60. Ford JD, Elhai JD, Connor DF, et al. Poly-victimization and risk of posttraumatic, depressive, and substance use disorders and involvement in delinquency in a National Survey of Adolescents. J Adolesc Health 2010;46:545–52.

61. Finkelhor D, Ormrod RK, Turner HA. Poly-victimization: a neglected component in child victimization. Child Abuse Negl 2007;31:7–26.

62. Masten AS. Resilience in children threatened by extreme adversity: frameworks for research, practice and translational synergy. Dev Psychopathol 2011;23(2):493–506.

63. Saunders BE. Determining the best practice for treating sexually victimized children. In: Goodyear-Brown P, editor. Handbook of child sexual abuse. Hoboken (NJ): John Wiley & Sons; 2012. p. 173–97.

64. Hamby S, Finkelhor D, Turner H, et al. The Juvenile victimization questionnaire toolkit. 2011. Available at: http://colahtts://cola.unh.edu/ccrc/juvenile-victimization-questionnaire.unh.edu/ccrc/juvenile-victimization-questionnaire. Accessed November 22, 2013.

65. National Crime Victims Research and Treatment Center, Medical University of South Carolina. Event history interview for children & adolescents Ver. 1.02. Charleston (SC): Author; 2007.

66. Ribbe D. Psychometric review of traumatic event screening instrument for children (TESI-C). In: Stamm BH, editor. Measurement of stress, trauma, and adaptation. Lutherville (MD): Sidran Press; 1996. p. 386–7.

67. Steinberg A, Brymer M. The UCLA PTSD reaction index. In: Reyes G, Elhai J, Ford J, editors. Encyclopedia of psychological trauma. New York: John Wiley & Sons, Ltd; 2008. p. 673–4.

The Biological Effects of Childhood Trauma

Michael D. De Bellis, MD, MPH*, Abigail Zisk, AB

KEYWORDS

- Childhood trauma • Developmental traumatology • Developmental psychopathology
- Posttraumatic stress symptoms • Stress • Biological stress systems
- Brain development • Genes

KEY POINTS

- Trauma in childhood is a grave psychosocial, medical, and public policy problem that has serious consequences for its victims and for society.
- Chronic interpersonal violence in children is common worldwide.
- Developmental traumatology, the systemic investigation of the psychiatric and psychobiological effects of chronic overwhelming stress on the developing child, provides a framework and principles when empirically examining the neurobiological effects of pediatric trauma.
- Despite the widespread prevalence of childhood trauma, less is known about trauma's biological effects in children than in adults with child trauma histories and even less is known about how these pediatric mechanisms underlie trauma's short-term and long-term medical and mental health consequences.

INTRODUCTION

Trauma in childhood has serious consequences for its victims and for society. For the purposes of this critical review, childhood trauma is defined according to the *Diagnostic and Statistical Manual of Mental Disorders* (Fourth Edition) (*DSM-IV*) and the *Diagnostic and Statistical Manual of Mental Disorders* (Fifth Edition) (*DSM-V*) as exposure to actual or threatened death, serious injury, or sexual violence.[1,2] This includes experiences of direct trauma exposure, witnessing trauma, or learning about trauma that happened to a close friend or relative. In children, motor vehicle accidents, bullying, terrorism, exposure to war, child maltreatment (physical, sexual, and emotional abuse; neglect) and exposure to domestic and community violence are common types of childhood traumas that result in

Healthy Childhood Brain Development and Developmental Traumatology Research Program, Department of Psychiatry and Behavioral Sciences, Duke University Medical Center, Box 104360, Durham, NC 27710, USA
* Corresponding author.
E-mail address: michael.debellis@duke.edu

Child Adolesc Psychiatric Clin N Am 23 (2014) 185–222
http://dx.doi.org/10.1016/j.chc.2014.01.002
1056-4993/14/$ – see front matter © 2014 Elsevier Inc. All rights reserved.

Abbreviations	
ACTH	Adrenocorticotrophic hormone (also called "corticotropin")
AVP	Arginine vasopressin
BDNF	Brain-derived neurotrophic factor
CRF	Corticotropin-releasing factor
CRH	Corticotropin-releasing hormone
CSF	Cerebrospinal fluid
HPA	Hypothalamic-pituitary axis
LC	Locus coeruleus
LHPA	Limbic-hypothalamic-pituitary-adrenal
PFC	Prefrontal cortex
PTSD	Posttraumatic stress disorder
PTSS	Posttraumatic stress symptoms
SNPs	Single nucleotide polymorphisms
SNS	Sympathetic nervous system

distress, posttraumatic stress disorder (PTSD), and posttraumatic stress symptoms (PTSS). Childhood traumas, in particular those that are interpersonal, intentional, and chronic, are associated with greater rates of PTSD,[3] PTSS,[4,5] depression[6] and anxiety,[7] and antisocial behaviors[8] and greater risk for alcohol and substance use disorders.[9–12]

The traditional categorical clusters of symptoms that form the diagnosis of PTSD are each associated with differences in biological stress symptoms and brain structure and function and are thought to individually contribute to delays in or deficits of multisystem developmental achievements in behavioral, cognitive, and emotional regulation in traumatized children and lead to PTSS and comorbidity.[13] Thus, this article examines PTSD as a dimensional diagnosis encompassing a range of pathologic reactions to severe stress rather than as a dichotomous variable.

Developmental traumatology, the systemic investigation of the psychiatric and psychobiological effects of chronic overwhelming stress on the developing child, provides the framework used in this critical review of the biological effects of pediatric trauma.[13] This field builds on foundations of developmental psychopathology, developmental neuroscience, and stress and trauma research. The *DSM-IV* (Text Revision) diagnosis of PTSD is made when criterion A, a type A trauma, is experienced and when 3 clusters of categorical symptoms are present for more than 1 month after traumatic event(s). These 3 clusters are criterion B: intrusive re-experiencing of the trauma(s); criterion C: persistent avoidance of stimuli associated with the trauma(s); and criterion D: persistent symptoms of increased physiologic arousal.[1] These criteria are complex and each criterion is thought to be associated with dysregulation of at least 1 major biological stress system as well as several different brain circuits. This makes both the psychotherapeutic and the psychopharmacologic treatment of individuals with early trauma complex and challenging.

Criterion symptoms have an experimental basis in classical and operant conditioning theory, where animals learn to generalized behaviors based on previous experiences, or reinforcements,[14] and in animal models of learned helplessness, where animals under conditions of uncontrollable shock do not learn escape behaviors and have exaggerated fear responses as well as social isolation and poor health.[15] For example, cluster B re-experiencing and intrusive symptoms can best be conceptualized as a classically conditioned response that is mediated by the serotonin system and is similar in some ways to the recurrent intrusive thoughts experienced in obsessive-compulsive disorder, where serotonin and norepinephrine transmitter deficits play an important role.[16] An external or internal conditioned stimulus (eg, the traumatic trigger) activates unwanted and distressing recurrent and intrusive memories of the traumatic experience(s) (eg, the unconditioned stimulus). Other criterion B symptoms, however, such as nightmares or night terrors, may involve the dysregulation of multiple neurotransmitter systems (serotonin, norepinephrine, dopamine, choline, and γ-aminobutyric acid[17]). Criterion C symptoms represent both avoidant behaviors and negative alterations in cognitions. In the *DSM-V*, criterion C was divided into avoidant behaviors and criterion D negative alterations in cognitions.[2] Avoidant behaviors can be thought of as ways to control painful and distressing re-experiencing of symptoms. These symptoms are likely associated with the dopamine system and overactivation of the opioid system and with anhedonia and numbing of responses.[18] In the *DSM-IV*, the former criterion D persistent symptoms of increased physiologic arousal and reactivity is now criterion E and likely involves dysregulation of several biological stress systems,[13,19] as discussed later in further detail.

This article reviews the known differences in pediatric victims' stress biology compared with those children who have not experienced trauma. These differences are likely the causes of the greater rates of psychopathology (PTSD, depression, disruptive behaviors, suicidality, and substance use disorders) and of the common medical disorders (cardiovascular disease, obesity, chronic pain syndromes, gastrointestinal disorders, and immune dysregulation) seen in child victims.[20] Throughout, the relationship to biological stress systems and common stress symptoms is associated. On many levels, childhood trauma can be regarded as "an environmentally induced complex developmental disorder."[13]

Exposure to a traumatic event or series of chronic traumatic events (eg, child maltreatment) activates the body's biological stress response systems.[21–23] Stress activation has behavioral and emotional effects that are similar to individual PTSS symptoms.[24] Furthermore, an individual's biological stress response system is made up of different, interacting systems that work together to direct the body's attention toward protecting the individual against environmental life threats and to shift metabolic resources away from homeostasis and toward a fight-or-flight (and/or freezing) reaction.[19,25] The stressors associated with the traumatic event are processed by the body's sensory systems through the brain's thalamus, which then activates the amygdala, a central component of the brain's fear detection and anxiety circuits. Cortisol levels become elevated through transmission of fear signals to neurons in the prefrontal cortex (PFC), hypothalamus, and hippocampus and activity increases in the locus coeruleus (LC) and sympathetic nervous system (SNS). Subsequent changes in catecholamine levels contribute to changes in heart rate, metabolic rate, blood pressure, and alertness.[19] This process also leads to the activation of other biological stress systems.

In the review of the pertinent literature section, we will examine the main biological stress response systems, with a focus on the limbic-hypothalamic-pituitary-adrenal (LHPA) axis and the LC-norepinephrine/SNS or catecholamine system. The serotonin system, oxytocin and the oxytocin system, the immune system, and new data in genetic and epigenetic factors and gene-environment interactions that influence these systems and contribute to an individual's experience of vulnerability and resilience to childhood trauma are also reviewed. For each of these systems, an explanation is provided of the mechanisms that drive them, followed by an examination of how these systems compare in children and adults who have been exposed to childhood trauma, thereby highlighting how early life adversity can disrupt the body's ability to regulate its response to stress.

Experiencing trauma during development along with dysregulation of biological stress systems can have an adverse impact on childhood brain development[13] and brain imaging studies in children who experienced trauma and adults with trauma histories are discussed. Recently, the field of neuroscience has become increasingly aware of gender as an important moderator of experience, so peer-reviewed publications are reviewed that highlight gender differences, if available. Little is known about trauma's neurobiological, genetic, and epigenetic effects in children compared with those adults with trauma histories. Because longitudinal psychobiological research in pediatric trauma is a severely understudied area, most of this review is based on cross-sectional studies. Although studies are highlighted where longitudinal research is available, more longitudinal research in trauma-exposed children is needed to understand the pediatric mechanisms underlying trauma's short-term and long-term adverse effects in adolescence and adulthood. The clinical applications of this knowledge are reviewed and how stress related biomarkers may provide important tools for clinicians and researchers to objectively examine predictors of PTSS and to monitor treatment response is discussed. Suggestions for future directions are then offered.

A literature search of PubMed and PsychINFO articles published to 2013 using keywords and MeSH terms, "childhood," "trauma," "stress," and/or "posttraumatic stress," which overlapped individually with "hypothalamic-pituitary axis (HPA)," "corticotropin-releasing hormone," "corticotropin-releasing factor," "immune," "serotonin," "dopamine," "oxytocin," "brain," "brain imaging," "brain structure," "brain function," "cognitive," "genes," "polymorphisms," and "epigenetics" that were limited to the English language, were reviewed and selected for this critical review. Trauma studies involving physical head trauma or medical illnesses were not included. The criteria were that the articles be peer reviewed and methodologically sound, with emphasis placed on the paucity of longitudinal studies in this field. When reviews were needed to describe the foundations of biological stress systems and brain development, meta-analyses or peer-reviewed critical reviews published by known stress researchers were cited.

REVIEW OF THE PERTINENT LITERATURE: THE NEUROBIOLOGY OF BIOLOGICAL STRESS SYSTEMS
Limbic-Hypothalamic-Pituitary-Adrenal Axis

The LHPA axis plays a central role in regulating the body's response to stress and is the most studied biological stress system in animals and humans. Activation of the LHPA axis triggers the hypothalamus to secrete corticotropin-releasing hormone (CRH). This neuropeptide, also called corticotropin-releasing factor (CRF), is a key mediator of the stress response.[26] The term CRH is used when describing its function in the neuroendocrine system and the term CRF is commonly used when describing its function as a neurotransmitter. The term CRH is the older term, however, and authors are not always consistent in using these rules.

CRH stimulates the release of adrenocorticotrophic hormone (ACTH) by binding to CRH receptors in the anterior pituitary. ACTH in turn binds to G protein–coupled receptors in the adrenal cortex, especially in the zona fasciculata of the adrenal glands. ACTH also stimulates the secretion of cortisol, a glucocorticoid hormone that plays an important role throughout the central nervous system. Cortisol activates glucocorticoid and mineralocorticoid receptors, which are located and expressed throughout the brain. Glucocorticoid receptors act as transcription factors and regulate gene expression for metabolism and immune function as well as for cognitive and brain development.[27] Increased levels of cortisol suppress the immune system, stimulates gluconeogenesis, and inhibit its own secretion via negative feedback to glucocorticoid receptors in the hippocampus.[19]

CRF is widely distributed throughout the brain and is involved in the stress response and in learning and memory.[28] Cortisol regulates the stress response system both in the hippocampus and medial PFC, where it works to attenuate the stress response, and in the medial and central nuclei of the amygdala, where it works to promote the stress response via CRF-1 receptors.[29] Through negative feedback, cortisol controls its own secretion, inhibiting the hypothalamus' release of CRH and the pituitary's release of ACTH, thereby bringing the body back to a state of homeostasis rather than arousal.[19] Cortisol levels have a consistent diurnal pattern, where levels are typically close to their peak during morning awakening, rise further in the 20-minute period after awakening, and then progressively fall, reaching the nadir in the afternoon in children,[30] adolescents,[31] and adults.[32] Furthermore, cortisol levels and pituitary volumes increase with age.[33]

The LHPA Axis and Childhood Trauma

Exposure to severe stress and trauma in youth can disrupt the regulatory processes of the LHPA axis across the life span in both animals and humans.[26,27,34–36] In animals, injections of CRF in early life produce a delayed effect in later life that is associated with reduced cognitive function, reduced number of CA3 hippocampal neurons, and decreased branching of hippocampal pyramidal neurons.[37,38] Although the pediatric trauma literature suggests that the LHPA system is dysregulated in youth exposed to trauma, the cortisol regulation data seem contradictory, where baseline morning and 24-hour cortisol concentrations showed no differences,[39,40] were higher,[41–47] or, in a few studies, lower[47–49] compared with youth without trauma. Additionally, no cortisol response differences,[39,50,51] blunted cortisol responses,[52] and increased cortisol concentration responses[53,54] have been reported in maltreated children and adults with histories of childhood maltreatment under psychological and pharmacologic challenges. Other measures of the LHPA axis, such as ACTH, also show these contradictory findings, where both blunted[39,55] and increased[50,53,54,56] ACTH levels have been reported in maltreated depressed children and adults with histories of childhood maltreatment under psychological and pharmacologic challenges. Furthermore, in a meta-analysis, lower morning but higher afternoon/evening cortisol levels, a flatter diurnal rhythm, and greater daily cortisol output were seen in adults retrospectively reporting trauma,[47] whereas another meta-analysis demonstrated that individuals with adulthood trauma exposure and adults with PTSD showed no differences in cortisol levels,[57] indicating that the developing LHPA axis is vulnerable to dysregulation as a result of childhood trauma.

As outlined by De Bellis and colleagues,[13,39,42] the discrepant findings described previously may be related to several mediator and moderator mechanisms. A detailed examination of the factors associated with these mechanisms is important in studies endophenotyping an individual's response to the effects of early trauma on the development of biological stress systems. Endophenotyping is a term used to describe emotional and behavioral symptoms into stable phenotypes or observable traits with genetic associations. Identifying endophenotypes in traumatized children will be an important new tool for novel approaches to treatments, such as personalized medicine.[58] Several of these mediation and moderation mechanisms for the biological effects of trauma on the developing child can be found in a previously published critical review by De Bellis,[13] and 12 updated mechanisms are discussed later for the LHPA system because this system is the most studied, providing the most data to synthesize into mechanisms (**Fig. 1**). Other biological stress systems are reviewed and these mechanisms discussed only if there are published data available.

Permanent changes occur as a result of childhood trauma onset

Elevated central CRH and CRF occur with the onset of trauma. Although this CRF elevation persists into adulthood, initial elevations of ACTH and cortisol levels become attenuated with chronic exposure to elevated CRH (also known as CRF). High CRH in turn causes adaptive down-regulation of pituitary CRH and neural CRF receptors after trauma onset. These ideas agree with McEwen's[26] theory of allostatic load, which hypothesizes that organisms adapt to re-regulate psychobiological responses to chronic stress to prevent physical harm to the organism. Increasing allostatic load over the life-span, however, increases vulnerability to stress disorders in response to new stressors. Thus, this down-regulation of CRF receptors may be an adaptive mechanism that regulates pituitary hypertrophy (a finding seen in maltreated children with PTSD[59]), whereas a down-regulation of CRF receptors makes neurons less responsive to CRF-induced neuronal damage and seizures.[60,61] The opposite of chronic stress (ie, environmental enrichment) delays seizures and neuronal damage in seizure prone animals through a CRF mechanism.[62] In support of this idea, higher levels of cerebrospinal fluid (CSF) CRF are seen in juvenile primates raised under unpredictable and adverse early rearing conditions,[63] which longitudinally persist into young adult-hood.[64] CSF CRF levels are higher in adults with childhood trauma histories.[20] In combat-related PTSD, elevated levels of central CRH were found[65,66]; childhood trauma is also a risk factor for a diagnosis of PTSD after combat experiences.[67] Chronically elevated CRF causes generalized arousal, anxiety, aggression, hypervigilance, and stimulation of the SNS, all core symptoms of the PTSD hyperarousal cluster.[24] It also causes inhibition of feeding and sexual behavior, core symptoms of major depression, another common outcome of traumatic experiences in childhood.[68]

Childhood trauma re-regulates biological stress systems

The long-term consequence of early trauma experiences and elevated CRF resets the regulation of the LHPA axis so that ACTH and cortisol secretions are set at lower 24-hour levels during baseline and nonstressful conditions. Adult studies of victims of childhood trauma consistently show lower cortisol levels.[47,69] In a meta-analysis, one of the most robust findings was that the longer the time since the trauma, the lower the morning cortisol, daily cortical volume, ACTH, and postdexamethasone cortisol levels.[47] Because the adult PTSD studies focus on past trauma, the latter hypothesis may best explain the main differences in the data in childhood PTSD studies, where higher baseline cortisol levels were reported in most pediatric studies,[41–47] whereas lower 24-hour cortisol levels were seen in adults maltreated in youth.[69] This attenuation hypothesis is supported by data from the only longitudinal psychobiological study published to date, where nonstress cortisol levels were assessed at 6 time points from childhood through young adulthood in sexually abused and nonabused girls. In this study, nonstress cortisol activity was initially significantly higher in sexually abused girls (post abuse disclosure) compared with nonabused girls, but cortisol activity was significantly attenuated starting in adolescence and significantly lower during young adult follow-up compared with those who were nonabused.[70]

Priming also called sensitization occurs as a result of childhood trauma

Priming occurs as a reflection of chronic compensatory adaptation of the LHPA axis long after trauma exposure, and it may be more likely to occur after pubertal maturation. Thus, studies that show greater cortisol or ACTH response after childhood trauma exposure may be the result of priming. LHPA axis regulation is affected by

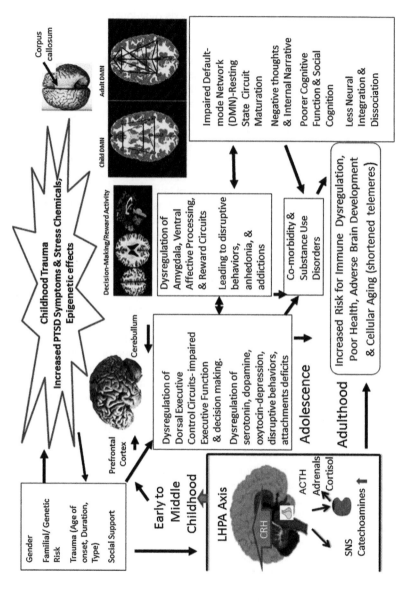

Fig. 1. Developmental traumatology model of the biological effects of trauma.

other hormones that are stress mediated, such as arginine vasopressin (AVP) and the catecholamines, both of which act synergistically with CRH.[19] A primed system hyper-responds during acute stress or during the occurrence of traumatic reminders because of the interactive neuroendocrine and neurotransmitter effects activated by current life stressors on the dysregulated LHPA axis. Another term used to describe priming is *sensitization*, defined as enhanced neuroendocrine, autonomic, and behavioral responsiveness to stress as well as LHPA axis dysregulation.[20,71] Thus, when a new emotional stressor or traumatic reminder is experienced, the LHPA axis response is enhanced (higher ACTH and higher cortisol levels). This has been seen in findings of increased ACTH secretion in depressed, abused youth who were continuing to experience chronic adversity[50] and in depressed women with a history of abuse who reported more recent chronic mild stress than abused women without major depressive disorder, who had blunted ACTH responses to CRF.[56] In a study of post-institutionalized children that examined the effect of interactions between children and their caregivers, basal cortisol levels increased in response to parental interactions only in children who had previously been exposed to severe neglect from institutional rearing.[72] In addition, a prolonged elevation in cortisol levels occurred only when the previously neglected children were interacting with their caregivers, because interactions with unfamiliar adults led to similar cortisol levels in previously neglected and non-neglected children. These results, therefore, illustrate that previously neglected children generalized caregiver interactions as traumatic reminders and stressful experiences and thus demonstrated a disruption in the regulatory processes of the LHPA axis in response to these social interactions. Moreover, in adults with a history of child abuse, higher cortisol levels occur after exposure to traumatic reminders compared with neutral memories.[73] These results are the effects of priming or sensitization.

Trauma timing and duration influence biological stress systems

Timing of trauma, such as duration (single episode or chronic), age of trauma onset, and stage of development, influence cortisol levels posttrauma. Cross-sectional studies show that trauma in infant primates[74] and very young or prepubertal children living in orphanages show low morning and daytime cortisol production,[75] suggesting that prepubertal children may be more sensitive to negative feedback control mechanisms for cortisol output than older school-age children who show higher cortisol levels.[41–47] Sexually abused prepubertal children with major depression exhibited significantly lower mean baseline ACTH concentrations over the first 4 hours after sleep onset compared with control children.[76] Results of these cross-sectional studies suggest tight down-regulation of ACTH and cortisol due to elevated central CRF in very young children. Pituitary volumes increased with age[59] along with increasing cortisol levels, which are also associated with increasing body fat.[77] Significantly larger pituitary volumes are seen in pubertal and postpubertal maltreated children and adolescents with PTSD compared with nonmaltreated controls.[59] Thus, elevated central CRH levels may lead to pituitary hypertrophy in traumatized children, which may be most pronounced during very early childhood and puberty, due to trophic factors. An adaptive response to elevated CRH levels, particularly during the sensitive periods of very early childhood and adolescence to elevated CRH levels, must be down-regulation of CRH receptors, or the resultant high cortisol levels would result in medical illness and brain structure damage. Tight control of cortisol secretion in infancy and attenuation of cortisol secretion after trauma onset and in response to increasing levels of cortisol that occur with increasing age and puberty are in accord with the theory of allostatic load,[26] which hypothesizes that organisms adapt to chronic stress to prevent physical harm.

Individual differences in response to childhood trauma are associated with different types of biological stress system regulation

Individual differences in behavioral and emotional responses are associated with different types of LHPA axis dysregulation. Most studies show LHPA axis dysregulation consistent with elevated central CRF in youth who experience childhood trauma and depressive and anxiety symptoms[39,41–47,50,78–80] or comorbid internalizing and externalizing behaviors,[42,79] whereas traumatized children with marked disruptive behavioral disorders or antisocial behaviors show lower cortisol levels.[81] In addition, in a study of adults with moderate to severe child maltreatment histories and no diagnosable psychopathology, lower concentrations of cortisol and ACTH were seen in response to the Trier Social Stress Test compared with healthy adults without maltreatment histories,[82] further suggesting that elevated central CRF is likely seen as a result of maltreatment even in resilient outcomes.

Early trauma type and trauma severity influence biological stress systems

Certain trauma types and increased overall trauma severity are more likely to result in LHPA dysregulation. For example, children who suffered from physical and sexual abuse occurring in the first 5 years of life were more likely to experience internalizing symptoms and LHPA axis dysregulation than those who suffered from abuse, neglect, or emotional abuse occurring after age 5.[40] Increasing severity of childhood trauma is associated with dysregulation of the LHPA axis. Children who experienced multiple maltreatment types or those who experienced severe sexual abuse were more likely to have elevated cortisol levels.[44] Furthermore, in maltreated children with PTSD, 24-hour urinary cortisol concentrations correlated positively with increased trauma duration, and with PTSD intrusive and hyperarousal symptoms.[42]

Genetic factors influence biological stress system responses to childhood trauma

LHPA-related genetic factors influence the effect of childhood trauma on the LHPA axis and its associated outcomes. Gene × environment interplay is important for the expression of both negative and resilience outcomes after childhood trauma. Gene × environment investigations are a relatively new area of study, so these data should be considered preliminary because this part of the field is still in its infancy.

Polymorphisms are normal variations in genes that code for important proteins that build the body and its functions. Single nucleotide polymorphisms (SNPs) are the most common type of genetic variation. Specific polymorphisms that are needed to form LHPA axis–related structures (CRH and glucocorticoid receptors) seem to moderate the effect of child abuse on the risk for childhood neuroticism and adult depressive symptoms. The brain's CRH type 1 receptors (CRHR1s) are located throughout the brain[27] and, when activated, produce symptoms of anxiety and depression.[24,83]

There are few studies of gene × environment interplay in children. In one study, physically abused, emotionally abused, and neglected children who carried 2 copies of the TAT haplotype of the CRHR1 had significantly higher levels of neuroticism, a prelude to anxiety and depression, than nonmaltreated children who had 2 copies of the TAT haplotype.[84] In this study, however, sexually abused children and children who had experienced 3 or 4 types of abuse and who had 2 copies of the TAT haplotype seemed to be protected from neuroticism compared with children who experienced other types of maltreatment.[84] In a follow-up study of these children, only maltreated children who carried 2 copies of the TAT haplotype exhibited a blunted slope of diurnal cortisol change, a sign of increasing allostatic load and dysregulation of the LHPA axis. The CRHR1 haplotype groups (0 or 1 copy vs 2 copies), however, were not related to internalizing symptoms.[85]

In contrast, a study of adult carriers of both the TCA (ie, T alleles formed of SNP rs7209436 and C allele formed by SNP rs4792887) and TAT haplotypes (ie, A allele formed of SNP rs110402) as well as the 2 SNPs (rs7209436 and rs242924) located in intron 1 of the CRHR1 gene were significantly protected from having major depression despite histories of child abuse.[86] This finding was replicated in a large study of women with child maltreatment[87] and in African American men and women[88] but not replicated in a study of European men and women who experienced childhood maltreatment.[87] Alternatively, adults with moderate to severe child maltreatment histories and the GG polymorphisms of the CRHR1 gene (rs110402) showed a significant interaction with maltreatment for increased cortisol responses to dexamethasone/CRH pharmacologic challenge compared with those adults with maltreatment and the A allele.[88] Higher cortisol is a well-replicated finding in adults with major depression.[19,89] Furthermore, sex effects may be important in gene × environment interplay. In another study of adults with child abuse histories, the protective effect of the CRHR1 polymorphisms (rs110402 A allele) against developing adult depression and with decreased cortisol response in the dexamethasone/CRH pharmacologic challenge were observed only in men, not in women,[90] a finding opposite to the one described previously.[87]

Gene × environment interplay was seen in a prospective study of the FKBP5 gene, a gene that inhibits glucocorticoid receptor–mediated glucocorticoid activity.[91] In this study, 884 Caucasians with no history of depression were enrolled at age 12 to 14 years and followed for 10 years.[92] Those who were homozygous for the minor alleles and had traumatic (but not separation [i.e., loss of parent through death or divorce]) events (in particular, severe child maltreatment) prior to age 24 years showed an increased incidence of depression on follow-up, suggesting that the minor allele of the FKBP5 polymorphism and childhood trauma interacted to predict adult depression. Three variants in the FKBP5 gene (rs4713916, rs1360780, and rs3800373) were associated with a failure of cortisol responses to return to baseline in healthy adults after psychosocial stress, suggesting a genotype-dependent risk of chronically elevated plasma cortisol levels in the context of acute stress as a possible mechanism for the increased risk of stress-related mental disorders, such as depression and PTSD in adults with these alleles.[93] Cross-sectional studies have also found interaction for adults who carry the minor FKBP5 allele and have child maltreatment histories because they have increased rates of depression,[94] PTSD,[95,96] and suicide risk.[97] In a cross-sectional study, the less common FKBP5 haplotype (H2) was associated with an increased risk of overt aggressive behavior in adult male prisoners who had a history of physical abuse.[98] In an imaging study, healthy young adults were genotyped for 6 FKBP5 polymorphisms (rs7748266, rs1360780, rs9296158, rs3800373, rs9470080, and rs9394309) previously associated with psychopathology and/or LHPA axis function.[99] Interactions between each SNP and increased levels of emotional neglect were associated with heightened reactivity to angry and fear faces in the dorsal amygdala, which suggests a neurobiological mechanism linking PTSS and depressives symptoms of hyperarousal and hypervigilience to negative affect and to psychopathology.[99] Hence, investigations of gene × environment interplay suggest that risk genes may interact with childhood trauma to produce different adult emotional, behavioral, and neurobiological outcomes.

Epigenetic factors influence biological stress system responses to childhood trauma
LHPA-related epigenetic factors influence the effect of childhood trauma on the LHPA axis and its associated negative behavioral and emotional outcomes. Epigenetics is also a relatively new area of study, so the limited data to date are described. The epigenome consists of chromatin, the protein-based structure around DNA, and

a covalent modification of the DNA itself by the methylation of cytosine rings found at CG dinucleotides.[100] The epigenome determines the accessibility of the DNA to convert genetic information into the messenger RNA necessary for gene function. Early traumatic experiences are associated with hyper- and demethylation of specific regulatory sites in key biological stress system genes, including the gene encoding of the glucocorticoid receptor[101] and the neuropeptide AVP, which is co-localized with CRH and released with CRH from the paraventricular nucleus of the hypothalamus during stress.[102] Increased methylation of key biological stress system genes can silence a gene's activity by making the gene inaccessible for transcription, whereas demethylation may make a gene accessible for transcription. Thus, childhood trauma can have a long-term impact on gene activity without changing an individual's DNA sequence (ie, genes).[103,104] Epigenetic effects may account for the inconsistent main gene and gene × environment results in the studies previously reported.

Animal studies have provided the first evidence of epigenetic effects caused by early trauma. Rats developing in optimal environments show less stress reactivity.[105] Because lactating female Long-Evans rats exhibit individual variation in the frequency of pup licking/grooming, high or low levels of pup licking/grooming are considered a maternal phenotype.[106] As adults, the offspring of high licking/grooming mothers show lower plasma ACTH and cortisol responses to acute stress in comparison with animals reared by low licking/grooming mothers.[106,107] The offspring of high licking/grooming mothers also show significantly increased hippocampal glucocorticoid receptor mRNA and protein expression, enhanced glucocorticoid negative feedback sensitivity, and decreased hypothalamic CRF mRNA levels, which all indicate decreased stress reactivity as a result of optimal quality of care.[105] Furthermore, DNA methylation patterns differ in high licking/grooming versus low licking/grooming offspring. The glucocorticoid receptor promoter sequence in the hippocampus of adult offspring of low licking/grooming mothers is hypermethylated and functionally less sensitive to cortisol feedback. Maternal behaviors also affect other biological systems that are associated with the LHPA axis. Prolonged periods of maternal separation alter the methylation state of the promoter for the AVP gene in the pup, increasing hypothalamic vasopressin AVP synthesis and LHPA responses to stress, along with memory deficits and learned helplessness behaviors.[108]

In a rodent model of infant maltreatment, abuse and neglect during infancy decreases brain-derived neurotrophic factor (BDNF) gene expression in the adult PFC.[109] In addition, these investigators found that chronic treatment with a DNA methylation inhibitor lowered levels of methylation in male and female rats exposed to early maltreatment. They also showed not only that infant trauma was associated with poor mothering in the next generation but also that these epigenetic changes in DNA methylation were passed from one generation to the next generation, even if the offspring of an abusive dam (mother rat) was cross-fostered with a nonmaltreating dam, thereby indicating heritability of these epigenetic changes.[109]

Increased methylation in a neuron-specific glucocorticoid receptor (NR3C1) promoter was seen in human postmortem hippocampus obtained from suicide victims with a history of childhood abuse compared with suicide victims without child abuse histories and controls who died of non–suicide-related causes, demonstrating an association between early trauma and epigenetic alterations.[101] Decreased hippocampal glucocorticoid receptor expression due to epigenetic changes likely increased LHPA activity and enhanced the risk of both depression and suicide in adults who were child abuse victims.[101] These findings link the previously described data from rats to humans and suggest a common effect of quality of parental care on the epigenetic regulation of hippocampal glucocorticoid receptor expression that can lead to health or the LPHA axis dysregulation seen in childhood PTSD and PTSS and adult depression.

In addition, a preliminary investigation showed that experiencing foster care during childhood is associated with changes in methylation of genes related to both the HPA axis and the immune system.[110] This study, therefore, supports the idea that childhood trauma may be linked to changes in genetic expression and resulting mental and medical health problems.

Gender differences influence the effects of childhood trauma on biological stress systems

Gender differences influence the effect of childhood trauma on the HPA axis. Research involving men and women who were exposed to early trauma but who did not have any psychopathologic diagnoses has shown stronger associations between trauma and increased CRF levels in men than in women.[111] In children, girls with histories of physical abuse had higher levels of urinary oxytocin, a neuroendocrine peptide that down-regulates cortisol and is associated with complex social behaviors, and lower levels of salivary cortisol after an experimental stressor compared with nonabused girls, whereas abused and nonabused boys did not differ in their hormonal responses.[112] Early trauma and gender differences are an area of research that warrants further investigations, because a prospective investigation showed that maltreated males may be more likely to be arrested for violent offenses as adults,[113] thus becoming prisoners and less likely to be involved in retrospective research studies. This fact can lead to a selection bias in retrospective studies and a possibly mistaken idea that females are more vulnerable to early trauma. Early trauma experiences may lead to greater down-regulation of cortisol due to high levels of CRF and other stress markers in males compared with females, findings that are commonly seen in individuals with antisocial behaviors.[81]

Social support buffers biological stress system dysregulation and its associated negative behavioral and emotional outcomes

As adults, the offspring of high licking/grooming mothers show decreased stress and cortisol reactivity as a result of optimal quality of care.[105] In preschool children, quality of childcare is associated with a buffering of hypothalamic-pituitary-adrenal axis to stress.[114] In adult studies, social support was associated with a decrease in the cortisol response to the Trier Social Stress Test in men.[115] Furthermore, decreased cortisol response and activity in the dorsal anterior cingulate, a brain region involved in distress separation, were seen in response to an exclusion neuroimaging task when daily social support was part of the research paradigm.[116] Further research is needed on the impact of social support in traumatized children.

Individual biological stress systems dysregulation in response to childhood trauma and the genes associated with the function of these systems influence other biological systems during development to contribute to psychopathology

The LHPA modulates the LC-norepinephrine/SNS system and the immune system.[19] When the hypothalamus releases CRH in response to stress, the LC becomes activated indirectly through the central amygdala.[19] Serotonin modulates LHPA activity.[117] Furthermore, having more than 1 type of a depression risk allele in 2 different biological stress systems (ie, the risk CRHR1 polymorphisms in the LHPA axis and the short allele of serotonin transporter gene promoter polymorphism [5-HTTLPR] in the serotonin system) is associated with current depressive symptoms in adults with less severe levels of child abuse and neglect as measured on the Childhood Trauma Questionnaire.[118]

Childhood trauma adversely influences development

Biological stress systems dysregulation in response to childhood trauma adversely influences cellular, cognitive, and brain development.[42,119,120] Human brain maturation is marked by the acquisition of progressive skills in physical, behavioral, cognitive, and emotional domains. Myelin, a fatty white substance produced by glial cells, is a vital component of the brain. Myelin encases the axons of neurons, forming an insulator, the myelin sheath, and is responsible for the color of white matter. Myelination of newly formed neuronal networks increases neural connectivity and parallels these developmental changes. Brain development occurs with an overproduction of neurons in utero; increases in neuron size, synapses, and neural connections during childhood and adolescence; selective elimination of some neurons (apoptosis) with corresponding decreases in some connections and strengthening of others; and corresponding increases in myelination to hasten these connections. Synapses, dendrites, cell bodies, and unmyelinated axons, which form the brain's gray matter, decrease during development.[121] Glucocorticoids are important for normal brain maturation, including initiation of terminal maturation, remodeling axons and dendrites, and affecting cell survival.[26,122] Both suppressed and elevated glucocorticoid levels can impair brain development and function.[26,122] During brain maturation, stress, and elevated levels of stress hormones and neurotransmitters may lead to adverse brain development through apoptosis,[123–125] delays in myelination,[126] abnormalities in developmentally appropriate pruning,[127,128] the inhibition of neurogenesis,[129–131] or stress-induced decreases in brain growth factors.[132] Maternal deprivation increases the death of infant rat brain cells.[133] Consequently, dysregulation of a maltreated child's major stress systems likely contributes to adverse brain development and leads to psychopathology.[13]

Telomeres are the repetitive TTAGGG sequence at the end of linear chromosomes and with each division, telomeres get shorter and are considered a molecular clock for cellular aging.[134] In a cross-sectional study of children who were previously institutionalized, telomere length was shorter than children without such histories.[135] In a prospective longitudinal study of children, from ages 5 to 10 years, children who experienced 2 or more types of violence (measured as bullying, witnessing domestic violence, and physical abuse), have increased telomere erosion, a marker of premature cellular aging, compared with children who did not experience violence.[120] This landmark study suggests that children who experience trauma have decreased telomere maintenance, a potential mechanism (premature aging) for adverse brain development, mental health problems, and chronic health problems in adults with a childhood history of trauma.[13,136]

The Locus Coeruleus–Norepinephrine/Sympathetic Nervous System/Catecholamine System and Childhood Trauma

When the hypothalamus releases CRH in response to a stressor, the LC-norepinephrine/SNS system becomes activated indirectly through the central amygdala. Activation of the LC causes an increase in the release of norepinephrine throughout the brain and results in symptoms of PTSD and anxiety.[13] The LC is an ancient brain structure that increases activation of the SNS, a part of the autonomic nervous system that controls the fight-or-flight or freeze response.[13] The catecholamines (epinephrine, dopamine, and norepinephrine) and corresponding increased activity in the SNS work to generally prepare an individual for action by redistributing blood away from the skin, intestines, and kidneys and to the brain, heart, and skeletal muscles[137] and by diverting energy through a central dopamine mechanism that inhibits the PFC, from a thinking and planning mode to a survival and alertness mode.[138,139]

Sexually abused girls with dysthymia demonstrated greater 24-hour levels of total urinary catecholamines than nonabused girls.[140] Maltreated boys and girls with PTSD showed greater levels of urinary catecholamines at baseline than nonmaltreated healthy children and nonmaltreated children with generalized anxiety disorder.[42] Urinary catecholamines positively correlated with duration of PTSD trauma and number of PTSD internalizing and child dissociative symptoms.[42] In a study of children who experienced motor vehicle accidents, significantly elevated plasma noradrenaline concentrations were seen prospectively, at both months 1 and 6, after the accident, compared with the non-PTSD and control groups, further suggesting that higher catecholamines occur as a result of trauma and PTSD.[141] In a study of police academy recruits, those with early trauma exposure demonstrated heightened 3-methoxy-4-hydroxyphenylglycol (the major metabolite of norepinephrine) response after watching critical incident videos.[142] An adult positron emission tomography imaging study demonstrated significantly reduced norepinephrine transporter availability in the LC in PTSD, which would lead to chronic stimulation of the LC as a result of increased levels of norepinephrine. This finding positively correlated with PTSD hypervigilance symptoms. Furthermore, in a gene × environment analysis, adult carriers of the Val allele of the catechol O-methyltransferase polymorphism (a gene involved in dopamine degradation) with a history of sexual abuse showed a higher disposition toward anger, symptoms commonly seen in PTSD patients, compared with adults homozygous for the Met allele. The Val allele is associated with increased dopamine neurotransmission in the PFC, which is associated with deficits in executive function[138,139] and increased risk for impulsive anger. On the other hand, adults with early trauma and the Val/Val genotype showed increasing levels of dissociation corresponding to increased exposure to higher levels of childhood trauma.[143] Dissociation is a failure to integrate sense of self with current and past memories and emotions and is a pathologic defense to ward off anxiety that is also associated with nonintentional antisocial behaviors. Dissociation is a different construct from depression and anxiety. Thus, studies in both children and adults have consistently demonstrated higher LC-norepinephrine/SNS system activity associated with childhood trauma and PTSD, whereas down-regulation of this system due to trauma may be associated with antisocial behavior and dissociation.

The Serotonin System and Childhood Trauma

Serotonin is a critical element of the stress response system.[13] Serotonergic neurons project diffusely from the central serotonin raphe nuclei in midbrain to important cortical and subcortical brain regions (eg, PFC, amygdala, and hippocampus) that play known roles in regulating emotions (eg, mood), behaviors (eg, aggression and impulsivity),[144,145] cognitive function, motor function, appetite, and the regulation of many physiologic processes (eg, cardiovascular, circadian, neuroendocrine respiratory, and sleep functions[144,146]). Serotonin is an important regulator of morphogenetic activities during early brain development, influencing cell proliferation, migration, and differentiation, thus influencing child brain development.[147] In preclinical animal studies, decreased levels of serotonin activity are associated with increased levels of aggressive behaviors in rodents and primates exposed to early adversity.[148] Mice genetically engineered to lack the serotonin transport gene show increased LHPA axis activation to stress, suggesting that serotonin modulates LHPA activity.[117] Disruptions in serotonin's regulatory functioning are linked with several psychopathologic disorders that are commonly seen in children and adults with childhood trauma. For example, decreased levels of serotonin activity have been associated with mental health problems, such as depression and anxiety,[149] as well as with aggressive behaviors in individuals with personality disorders, such as borderline personality disorder.[150]

Early trauma dysregulates serotonin in humans. The serotonin transporter protein is involved in the reuptake of serotonin from the synapse and is critical to serotonin regulation in the brain. The short allele of 5-HTTLPR interacts with maltreatment in the development of childhood depression. The short allele is associated with reduced transcriptional activity of serotonin, so that there is less central serotonin available in the brain, whereas the long allele has at least twice the basal level of transcriptional activity of the short variant.[151] Most studies regarding the effects of 5-HTTLPR are in adults maltreated as children. A large epidemiologic study demonstrated that there were no main genetic effects, but carriers of the S allele had a higher risk of developing depressive and suicidal symptoms when exposed to stressful life events and childhood maltreatment.[152] Children who were homozygous for the short allele of 5-HTTPR demonstrated a significantly elevated vulnerability to depression but only in the presence of maltreatment, but the presence of positive supports reduced this risk.[153] Having 2 short-short alleles of the 5-HTTLPR gene moderated the association between bully victimization and emotional problems, such that frequently bullied children were at an increased risk as adolescents for depression or anxiety; the short-long and long-long genotypes did not confer an increased risk.[154] Other studies, however, have not shown an increased vulnerability to depression as a function of interactions between the short allele and maltreatment. Instead, they have shown increased risk with the long-long allele.[85,155] One study of 595 youth suggests that genetic variation has a negligible effect on promoting resilience among maltreated children.[156] Nonmaltreated children with the short-short genotype were more likely to have higher resilient functioning, whereas maltreated children with the short-short genotype were more likely to have lower resilience.[156] This study agrees with controversial meta-analyses that have found that adverse childhood events had a main effect on depressive outcomes regardless of 5-HTTLPR polymorphisms.[157,158] The discrepant findings in adults may be caused by failure to include trauma versus a stressful life event, trauma age of onset, trauma duration, and trauma type in the gene × environment interaction analyses. An interaction showing that adults with histories of child maltreatment, who were also carriers of the short 5-HTTLPR allele were found in another meta-analysis to be at increased risk for depression.[159] On the other hand, in a forensic sample of 237 men with elevated levels of child abuse and neglect (as measured by the Childhood Trauma Questionnaire), measures of psychopathy were highest among carriers of the 5-HTTPR long allele and carriers of the low-activity monoamine oxidase A (MAOA) gene.[160] Thus, resilience is a complex issue, because psychopathy as an outcome may be more harmful to society than depressive symptoms.

Genes associated with the serotonin system have been linked to other adverse outcomes in the presence of childhood trauma. The MAOA gene codes for an enzyme that selectively degrades the biogenic amines dopamine, serotonin, and norepinephrine after reuptake from the synaptic cleft and influences behavioral regulation.[161] Meta-analyses revealed that the association between early family adversity (particularly between neglect or physical abuse) and the short version of the MAOA gene was significantly associated with a general index of mental health problems, antisocial behavior, attentional problems, and hyperactivity in boys.[162] Adolescent boys with the short MAOA allele who were exposed to maltreatment or poor-quality family relations had more alcohol-related problems than maltreated boys with the longer MAOA allele.[163] Early use of alcohol in youth was predicted by an interaction of the short alleles of 5-HTTLPR and maltreatment.[164] Furthermore, women with a history of sexual abuse and the short MAOA allele were more likely to demonstrate alcoholism and antisocial personality disorder than were women with a history of sexual abuse and the long allele.[165]

Furthermore, genetic polymorphisms can have additive genetic effects. Children who were homozygous for the short allele of 5-HTTLPR, had the Val66Met variant of the BDNF gene, and had been maltreated were at increased risk of depression.

In summary, the serotonin system and the genes regulating the serotonin system are influenced by early trauma. The field has not yet advanced, however, to the point where treatment can be tailored to an individual child. More work needs to be done on gene-gene interactions, possible epigenetic effects, trauma variables, and other factors, such as social supports, to achieve this aim.

The Oxytocin System and Childhood Trauma

Oxytocin plays an important role in interpersonal relationships. Involved in the regulation of an individual's sexual response and milk production, this hormone is also responsible for the regulation of a wider range of social interactions, including social memory and cognition, emotion recognition, empathy, and attachment.[166] In addition, the oxytocin system is involved in the regulation of the body's response to stress. Research in rats demonstrated a relationship between oxytocin and the mother's relationship with her offspring, because those mothers who engaged in more licking/grooming behaviors exhibited higher levels of oxytocin receptor binding in the amygdala.[167] Similarly, rat mothers who demonstrated high levels of licking/grooming had increased levels of oxytocin gene expression and a subsequent increase in dopamine reward production. Mothers who demonstrated lower levels of licking/grooming behaviors had lower levels of oxytocin gene expression, highlighting the important role that oxytocin plays in the attachment bond.[168]

Research involving humans has similarly demonstrated that negative life events can disrupt the body's regulation of oxytocin. Decreased levels of oxytocin have been found in women exposed to early maltreatment—a relationship that was shown especially strong when the form of maltreatment was emotional abuse.[20] Gender differences have also been found in the relationship between childhood trauma and oxytocin regulation. Focusing on oxytocin response to an experimental stressor in abused girls and abused boys, girls exposed to physical abuse exhibited higher levels of oxytocin as well as decreased levels of cortisol in response to the experimental stress, whereas there was no difference in hormone response to the stress in the abused boys.[112] In the Adverse Childhood Experiences Study, a relationship was found between exposure to early trauma and increased promiscuity.[136] To explain this relationship, the researchers pointed out that disruptions in oxytocin regulation of social attachments during childhood can lead to high oxytocin and thus adult relationship problems because women abused as children were more likely to form fast and less discriminate personal attachments during adulthood that can lead to re-victimization.[136]

A strong moderating effect of a positive social environment, however, has also been found in adults with a specific allele of the oxytocin receptor gene OXTR who had been exposed to early stress, because increased resilience in adulthood was found only in those individuals who had been surrounded by a positive family environment during childhood.[169] Further research is needed on the impact of oxytocin on emotional and behavioral outcomes in traumatized children.

The Immune System and Childhood Trauma

Activation of the immune system involves the production of cytokines, which promote an inflammatory reaction to infection or pathogens in the body. Although one of the main effects of this reaction is to produce the physical symptoms of sickness (eg, fever, nausea, and fatigue), activation of cytokines that promote inflammation are implicated in depression, a common outcome of early trauma.[170] A recent systematic review provided evidence that supports the relationship between proinflammatory cytokines and increased levels of depression and anxiety in adolescents.[171] Higher levels of plasma antinuclear antibody titers have been found in girls who have been sexually abused, suggesting that exposure to this form of stress may inhibit the body's means of suppressing the B lymphocytes or the lymphocytes that produce antibodies, thereby leading to the increased levels of the antibody titers found in the abused girls.[172] Increased levels of inflammatory cytokines as well as decreased levels of anti-inflammatory cytokines have been associated with adult PTSD and exposure to chronic stress.[173,174] In women who had experienced early maltreatment, those who had been diagnosed with PTSD had higher activation levels of T cells than those who did not have PTSD. More specifically, investigators found a positive correlation between T-cell activation levels and intrusive symptoms of PTSD.[175] Similar results were found in a study of women with PTSD secondary to physical or sexual abuse during childhood, where these women demonstrated increased inflammatory and immune activity.[176] Other investigators demonstrated that greater concentrations of interleukin-6, a proinflammatory cytokine, were seen during the Trier Social Stress Test in adults with child maltreatment histories compared with adults without such histories.[177] Furthermore a longitudinal study of a New Zealand birth cohort (n = 1037) demonstrated that adults with histories of poverty, social isolation, or maltreatment had elevated rates of depression and age-related metabolic disease risks in adulthood, including higher body mass index, total cholesterol, and glycated hemoglobin; low levels of high-density lipoprotein; low maximum oxygen consumption; and higher levels of C-reactive protein, a measure of inflammation.[178] Furthermore, children exposed to a greater number of these adverse childhood risk factors had greater age-related disease risk in adult life.[178] The increased activation of cytokines and dysregulation of the immune system, along with the other biological stress response systems, such as the HPA axis and the LC/SNS systems, that occurs in response to early adversity, can lead to hypertension, accelerated atherosclerosis, metabolic syndrome, impaired growth, immune system suppression, and poorer medical health in adults with child trauma histories.[179]

The Effect of Childhood Trauma on Neuropsychological Functioning and Cognitive Development

Cross-sectional studies examining maltreatment trauma in childhood have shown lower IQs and deficits in language and academic achievement in maltreated children compared with children who have not been exposed to maltreatment.[180–185] The link between early trauma and IQ has been demonstrated through a twin study, where after controlling for the effect of shared heritability, domestic violence was associated with lower IQ (eg, mean of 8 points) in exposed versus nonexposed children.[186] Exposure to trauma in childhood has also been associated with executive deficits.[187–189]

Fewer studies have examined the effect of child maltreatment on a broader, more comprehensive range of neuropsychological functioning. A study comparing previously institutionalized children exposed to long periods of neglect with those exposed to brief periods of institutionalization as well as children raised in their biological families found that the children who experienced prolonged neglect performed more poorly in the domains of visual attention, memory, learning, and inhibitory control but that these previously institutionalized children did not demonstrate deficits when the tasks involved auditory or executive processing.[190] These results, therefore, highlight that specific domains of cognitive functioning may be more sensitive to early neglect than others. Lower performance in IQ, complex visual attention, visual memory, language, verbal memory and learning, planning, problem solving, speeded naming, and reading and mathematics achievement were seen in neglected children with and without PTSD compared with socioeconomically similar controls.[191] Furthermore, PTSD symptom number and the failure to supervise, witnessing violence, and emotional abuse variables were each associated with lower scores in IQ, academic achievement, and neurocognitive domains.[191] Neglected children with PTSD due to witnessing interpersonal violence, however, had lower performance levels on the NEPSY Memory for Faces Delayed than both neglected children who witnessed domestic violence and did not have PTSD and children not exposed to maltreatment or violence, indicting that PTSD was associated with impaired consultation of memory.[191] Childhood PTSD subsequent to witnessing interpersonal violence has also been associated with lower levels of performance on the California Verbal Learning Test–Children's Version compared with those without PTSD, whereas both PTSD and non-PTSD groups of youth exposed to domestic violence demonstrated deficits in executive functioning, attention, and IQ standardized scores.[192]

In a study comparing the performance of abused youth with PTSD, abused youth without PTSD, and nonmaltreated youth on comprehensive neuropsychological testing, both groups of maltreated youth performed worse than the control youth, with deficits in IQ, academic achievement, and all neurocognitive domains except for fine motor functioning.[193] The maltreated youth with PTSD showed greater deficits in visuospatial abilities than the maltreated youth without PTSD, and sexual abuse was found negatively associated with language and memory scores. A negative relationship was found between the number of maltreatment types experienced and academic achievement, demonstrating that cumulative trauma leads to neuropsychological problems that are unrelated to PTSD symptoms.[193] Data from the National Survey of Child and Adolescent Well-Being study demonstrated that maltreated children who experienced maltreatment during multiple developmental periods had more externalizing and internalizing problems and lower IQ scores than children maltreated in only 1 developmental period, suggesting that trauma duration has negative and cumulative cognitive effects.[194]

Longitudinal prospective studies involving adolescents and adults exposed to maltreatment in childhood agree with the cross-sectional studies and have demonstrated lower IQ scores and deficits in reading ability.[195–200] The research on the effects of early trauma on cognitive function indicates that early trauma is associated with adverse cognitive development and that this is likely reflected in adverse brain development.

The Effect of Childhood Trauma on Brain Development

An early, unexpected, trauma, maternal deprivation, increases the death of both neurons and glia cells in cerebral and cerebellar cortexes in infant rats.[133] Increased exposure to cumulative life stress (eg, exposure to severe marital conflict or severe chronic illness of a close family member or friend) was associated with poorer spatial working memory performance and decreased volumes of white and gray matter in the PFC of nonmaltreated youth.[201] Pediatric imaging studies demonstrated that both cerebral and cerebellar volumes are smaller in abused and neglected youth compared with nonmaltreated youth.[202–206] In a research study, maltreated subjects with PTSD had 7.0% smaller intracranial and 8.0% smaller cerebral volumes than nonmaltreated children.[119] The total midsagittal area of corpus callosum, the major interconnection between the 2 hemispheres that facilitates intercortical communication, was smaller in maltreated children.[119] Smaller cerebral volumes were significantly associated with earlier onset of PTSD trauma and negatively associated with duration of abuse.[119] PTSD symptoms of intrusive thoughts, avoidance, hyperarousal, and dissociation correlated negatively with intracranial volume and total corpus callosum measures.[119] Another study showed smaller brain and cerebral volumes and attenuation of frontal lobe asymmetry in children with maltreatment-related PTSD or subthreshold PTSD compared with archival nonmaltreated controls.[203]

These 2 studies did not, however, control for low socioeconomic status, which influences brain maturation through ecological variables.[119,207] In another study that controlled for socioeconomic status, children with maltreatment-related PTSD had smaller intracranial, cerebral cortex and PFC, PFC white matter, and right temporal lobe volumes and areas of the corpus callosum and its subregions and larger frontal lobe CSF volumes than controls.[205] The total midsagittal area of corpus callosum and middle and posterior regions remained smaller, whereas right, left, and total lateral ventricles and frontal lobe CSF were proportionally larger than controls, after adjustment for cerebral volume.[205] Brain volumes also positively correlated with age of onset of PTSD trauma and negatively correlated with duration of abuse.[205] The larger lateral ventricles were only seen in maltreated males, suggesting that males are more vulnerable to the neurotoxic effects of childhood maltreatment. Smaller cerebellar volumes were seen in male and female maltreated children with PTSD.[204] Younger age of onset and longer trauma duration were significantly correlated with smaller cerebellum volumes.[204] Smaller cerebellum volumes were also seen in previously institutionalized youth.[202] The cerebellum is a complex posterior brain structure that is involved in cognitive functions,[208] decision-making, reward circuits,[209,210] and the default mode network that is associated with understanding social intentions.[211] Child maltreatment is also associated with adverse effects in individual brain structures that are involved in reward and default network processing. In a large study of 61 medically healthy youth (31 male and 30 female) with chronic PTSD secondary to abuse, who had similar trauma and mental health histories, and 122 healthy nonmaltreated controls (62 male and 60 female), the midsagittal area of the corpus callosum subregion 7 (splenium) was smaller in both boys and girls with maltreatment-related PTSD compared with their gender-matched comparison subjects.[212] Youth with PTSD did not show the normal age-related increases in the area of the total corpus callosum and its region 7 (splenium) compared with nonmaltreated children.[212] This was an important finding for several reasons. The maltreated and control children were not prenatally exposed to substances and had no pregnancy or birth trauma, were psychotropically naïve, and had no history of substance abuse or dependence, thus excluding confounds commonly seen in maltreated children[213,214] and not addressed in exclusion criteria in most neurobiological studies published to date. The axons in the splenium of the corpus callosum myelinate during adolescence and are important to the posterior reward circuits and the posterior default networks.[215] Additionally, clinical symptoms of PTSD intrusive, avoidant, and hyperarousal symptoms; symptoms of childhood dissociation; and child behavioral checklist internalizing T score significantly and negatively correlated with corpus callosum measures.[212] Children with maltreatment-related PTSD had reduced fractional anisotropy values on diffusion tensor imaging brain scans of white matter, indicating less myelin integrity in the medial and posterior corpus, a region that contains interhemispheric projections from brain structures involved in circuits that mediate emotional and memory processing, core disturbances associated with trauma history.[216] Smaller corpus callosum area measures were seen in another anatomic MRI brain study of neglected children with psychiatric disorders compared with nonmaltreated children with psychiatric disorders, suggesting that smaller corpus callosum measures may be a consequence of maltreatment.[217]

Furthermore, areas of executive function show evidence of adverse brain development in children with maltreatment-related PTSD. Decreased N-acetylaspartate (NAA) concentrations are associated with increased metabolism and loss of neurons.[218] For example, brain NAA levels decrease when someone has neuronal loss, such as a stroke. A preliminary investigation suggested that maltreated children and adolescents with PTSD demonstrated lower NAA/creatine ratios in the medial PFC compared with sociodemographically matched controls.[219] These findings suggest neuronal loss in the medial PFC, an executive brain region, in pediatric maltreatment-related PTSD. Another group found that decreased left ventral and left inferior prefrontal gray matter volumes in maltreated children with PTSD symptoms negatively correlated with bedtime salivary cortisol levels, further suggesting that early trauma damages executive regions.[220] One functional imaging study of maltreated children and adolescents with PTSD symptoms showed significant decreases in inhibitory processes compared with nonmal treated controls,[221] and another showed impaired cognitive control in adopted children with histories of maltreatment who were formerly raised in foster care.[222] These investigations strongly suggest that childhood maltreatment interferes with executive or control circuits, whose dysregulation is an important contributor to adolescent and adult mental health and substance use disorders. Thus, childhood trauma can have detrimental effects on the brain networks that establish an individual's ability to think, and regulate their sense of self, motivations, and behaviors.

Another important contributor to memory and the default mode network is the hippocampus. Unlike findings in adult PTSD, where several studies reported hippocampal atrophy,[223] maltreated children and adolescents with PTSD or subthreshold PTSD showed no anatomic differences in limbic (hippocampal or amygdala) structures cross-sectionally[119,203,205] or longitudinally.[224] Investigators have demonstrated, however, functional brain differences in the amygdala and hippocampus of maltreated youth compared with nonmal treated children.[222,225] One study suggests that hippocampal atrophy may be a latent developmental effect of childhood maltreatment.[226]

Child maltreatment is also associated with adverse development of brain reward regions involved in recognizing emotions and social cognition, such as the superior temporal gyrus[206] and the orbital frontal cortex.[227] In carefully screened young adult subjects, those with a history of verbal abuse and no other forms of maltreatment had reduced fractional anisotropy on diffusion tensor imaging brain scans of white matter in the arcuate fasciculus in left superior temporal gyrus, the cingulum bundle by the posterior tail of the left hippocampus, and the left body of the fornix, indicating decreased integrity in these language neural pathways.[228] Furthermore, fractional anisotropy values negatively correlated with verbal abuse experiences.[228] In healthy adult women, a history of sexual abuse was specifically associated with hippocampal, corpus callosum, or frontal cortex reductions if it occurred during specific developmental age periods, indicating vulnerable windows for the brain effects of child trauma.[217]

Functional neuroimaging studies of adults with PTSD related to childhood maltreatment have shown decreased levels of executive and attentional function as reflected by decreased activation in the dorsal control networks with corresponding increased activation of the amygdala and hippocampus and other structures of the affective emotional networks during emotional challenge tasks, suggesting dorsal control network deficits in adult PTSD secondary to childhood trauma.[229–231] Research using functional neuroimaging of children and adolescents exposed to maltreatment has shown similar executive, attentional, and affective emotional dysregulation.[221,222,232–234] Furthermore, previously institutionalized children demonstrated decreased prefrontal white matter microstructural organization on measures of diffusion tensor imaging that was associated with neurocognitive deficits in spatial planning and a visual learning and memory task compared with non-neglected controls.[235]

In another study of healthy adult women with a history of childhood sexual abuse, investigators found higher T2 relaxation time (an indirect index of resting blood volume) in the cerebellar vermis than in nonmaltreated women, which correlated strongly with Limbic System Checklist ratings of temporal lobe epilepsy and their frequency of substance use.[236] In studies of carefully characterized healthy adults who only experienced corporal punishment without other forms of maltreatment, T2 relaxation times were increased in dopamine-rich brain decision-making and reward regions (caudate and putamen, dorsolateral PFC, substantia nigra, thalamus, and accumbens).[237] In the latter study, regional T2 relaxation times were significantly associated with increased use of drugs and alcohol.[237] These studies provide further evidence that specific types of abuse and neglect contribute to the intergenerational cycle of emotional and behavioral problems as well as addiction by their detrimental impact on the brain.

Genetic factors interact with childhood trauma to influence brain structure and function. For example, adults with the Val66Met polymorphism of BDNF who had a history of child maltreatment had a greater likelihood of depressive disorders and a smaller hippocampus, highlighting a child trauma × polymorphism interaction for hippocampal volume reductions.[238] Epigenetic factors also play a role in brain function. In a genome-wide study of promoter methylation in individuals with severe abuse during childhood trauma, decreased promoter transcriptional activity associated with decreased hippocampal expression of the Alsin variants were seen.[239] Adults who were maltreated as children and committed suicide showed similar hypermethylation in the nerve growth factor–induced protein A binding site within a glucocorticoid receptor variant that was associated with decreased glucocorticoid receptor expression in the hippocampus.[101] Mice without the expression of the Alsin gene exhibited more anxiety compared with wild-type mice.[240]

Furthermore, there are gender × maltreatment effects on brain development. Gender differences were demonstrated using anatomic MRI. Maltreated boys with PTSD had smaller cerebral volumes and larger lateral ventricular volumes than maltreated girls with PTSD, even though the 2 groups had similar trauma, mental health histories, and IQ.[212] In addition, research has shown a relationship between the type of trauma and gender, because neglect has been shown to have a strong association with smaller corpus callosum size in boys, whereas sexual abuse was strongly linked to decreased corpus callosum size in girls.[217] In a functional MRI study comparing maltreated youth with PTSD symptoms to nonmaltreated youth during performance on an emotional oddball task, left precuneus/posterior middle cingulate hypoactivation to fear versus calm or scrambled face targets were seen in maltreated versus control male youth and may represent dysfunction and less resilience in attentional networks in maltreated male youth.[241] These findings were not seen in maltreated female youth with PTSD symptoms and gender by maltreatment effects were not attributable to demographic, clinical, or maltreatment parameters, suggesting that maltreated male youth may be dedicating significant functional neural resources to processing affective stimuli in lieu of cognitive processes, which may lead to impulsive decision making during states of fear emotion and thus less resilience in maltreated male youth.[241]

Thus, the data to date strongly suggest that childhood trauma is associated with adverse brain development in multiple brain regions that have a negative impact on emotional and behavioral regulation, motivation, and cognitive function. Molecular aging may contribute to these mechanisms and lead to a premature aging but less than optimal brain maturation process in traumatized children as they become adults.

CLINICAL PRACTICE APPLICATION

Understanding the biological effects of maltreatment provides important information that can be used in practice. The first approach is to ensure a safe environment for child and adolescent patients. It is unlikely that any treatment or buffering of the biological stress systems will occur if a child continues to live in an extremely adverse environment. As outlined in this issue, evidence-based interventions show promise in treating traumatized children. Similar interventions have shown not only promise in treating traumatized adults but also that the treatment "heals" some of the dysregulations reviewed in neurobiological stress systems. Many of victims of trauma have sleep problems.[242,243] In a longitudinal investigation of sexually abused girls, self-reported sleep disturbances were seen approximately 10 years post abuse disclosure compared with control girls and were related to current depression, PTSD, and revictimization.[244] It was recently demonstrated that sleep has a restorative function; during sleep, potentially neurotoxic waste products (eg, β amyloid) are cleared from the brain.[245] Furthermore, inhibition of catecholamines enhance this waste removal.[245] Therefore, a first step in helping patients with trauma symptoms is to address any sleep hygiene issues they may have, with behavioral methods and/or medications if needed.

A review of recent functional MRI studies demonstrated that cognitive-behavioral therapy can alleviate dysregulation of the fear response and negative emotions associated with anxiety disorders and predict treatment outcomes.[246] Furthermore, greater left amygdala activity on functional MRI in pediatric patients with non–trauma-related anxiety was associated with greater improvement in anxiety symptoms post treatment.[247] Evidenced-based trauma therapies likely work by changing brain responses. Studies of brain function and trauma in pediatric patients, however, are in their infancy. Psychopharmacologic treatments that target biological stress systems are beyond the scope of this article.[248,249] Cognitive-behavioral therapy is the treatment of choice with the most evidenced-based studies suggesting its effects in children. Most child psychiatrists start with sleep hygiene, then a selective serotonin reuptake inhibitor for symptoms of anxiety and depression or an adrenergic agent, such as clonidine, propranolol, and guanfacine, to down-regulate biological stress systems, if trauma-focus cognitive behavioral therapy and improved sleep have less than optimal results. Other medications are used to treat comorbid disorders, such as attention-deficit/hyperactivity disorder. Because some childhood traumas (child maltreatment) are associated with family histories of mood and anxiety disorders, clinicians should be careful with antipsychotic drugs because they may be more likely to cause tardive dyskinesia in these child victims.[248] Although medications are useful for treating certain symptoms, double-blind studies are needed. It is likely that with further imaging and genetic studies, specific treatments and medication regimens may be tailored for specific PTSD symptoms and individuals in the future. The biological effects of PTSD and its treatment continue, however, to be understudied.

IMPORTANT TOOLS FOR PRACTICE

Understanding the biological effects of maltreatment provides important tools that can be useful in practice. Besides self-report instruments to study changes in moods, emotions, and behaviors during psychotherapeutic and/or pharmacologic treatments, sleep can be objectively measured using biomarkers, such as actographs, which are noninvasive digital monitoring devices that can be worn on the wrist and measure daily activity, sleep awakenings, and sleep efficiency. Other biomarkers that can be used to monitor and tailor treatment and help prevent the negative biological effects of trauma are monitoring measures of heart rate, body mass index, and posttrauma and follow-up salivary cortisol and amylase concentrations because these measures predict PTSD,[250] and decreasing these levels during treatment may predict remission.

FUTURE DIRECTIONS

The largest contributor to childhood trauma in the United States is family dysfunction; almost half of child-onset mental disorders and approximately a third of adult-onset mental disorders are preceded by child abuse and neglect and family dysfunction.[251] Although the mental disorders found in maltreating parents and child victims are serious, they are amenable to prevention and treatment.

Given how detrimental childhood trauma is to an individual's development, more efforts and social resources are needed for prevention. Studies show that child maltreatment is amenable to primary prevention. Child maltreatment prevention programs, such as home visiting[252] during an expectant mother's first pregnancy, aimed at addressing mental health and parenting concerns of high-risk new mothers, show great promise in preventing child abuse and neglect. For example, home visiting of an expectant mother by nurses for low-income, at-risk families has been a well-replicated strategy for preventing child abuse and neglect.[253,254] Several studies of this Nurse-Family Partnership program have demonstrated improved grade-point averages and achievement test scores in math and reading in grades 1 through 3 in children during their age 9 follow-up assessment[255]; decreased internalizing symptoms and decreased rates of tobacco, alcohol, and marijuana use along with improved reading and math scores at age 12 follow-up assessment[256]; and decreased antisocial behaviors at age 19 follow-up assessment.[257] When a parent becomes maltreating, however, even an intensive program of home visitation by nurses in addition to standard treatment is not enough to prevent recidivism of physical abuse and neglect.[258] Maltreated children in foster care showed less self-destructive behavior, substance use, and total risk behavior problem standardized scores and higher grades than maltreated children who were reunified with their biological families when interviewed during their 6-year follow-up.[259] These studies indicate that there are 2 opportunities to break the cycle of maltreatment. The first opportunity is during an expectant parent's first pregnancy, to aid in fostering a loving and caring environment for the parent/child dyad and to avoid the neurobiological consequences of childhood maltreatment. These types of early prevention programs are cost effective.[260] If this cannot be done, however, the second opportunity is to treat victims of maltreatment after the fact.

There are important evidence-based interventions (eg, trauma-focused cognitive behavior therapy) for the treatment of PTSD and depression[261] and for antisocial behaviors in youth with early trauma (eg, multisystemic therapy[262]). Many of these interventions are discussed in the Prevention and Intervention Section elsewhere in this issue. The long-term effectiveness of these programs are not known, however. There are not enough professionals trained in evidence-based practices to treat all child victims, and some youth and their families are simply noncomplaint with these treatments. Therefore, understanding the neurobiological consequences of chronic stress on a child's developing brain and body is still needed so that the adverse medical and mental health outcomes of early life stress can be treated.[263] A society that places its focus on an infrastructure of primary prevention would be choosing the less costly option for victims and for itself.

SUMMARY

This article outlines how childhood trauma has detrimental consequences on the biological stress systems and cognitive and brain development. Trauma in childhood is costly for its victims and for society. Resilience is not a common outcome of childhood trauma. In a longitudinal study of individuals who had experienced abuse and neglect during childhood, only 22% of those who had been abused or neglected achieved resiliency based on a comprehensive assessment of healthy adult functioning by the time they reached young adulthood.[264] Girls who grew up in poverty and were not maltreated were more likely to show resilience.[264] Although there are some important evidenced-based treatments for child victims, it is in the national interest to put in place an infrastructure of primary child trauma prevention as the less costly option for future victims and for society. Understanding the neurobiological consequences of child trauma will assist in treating child and adult victims, who tend to be more treatment refractory and may have a different endophenotype from individuals with medical (including mental health) disorders who do not have such histories. Nevertheless, more work is needed to understand the neurobiological consequences of chronic stress on a child's developing brain and body so that the adverse medical and mental health outcomes of early life stress can be treated in those cases (eg, warfare, natural disasters, and child maltreatment) where prevention and effective early intervention may not occur. Such understanding of the neurobiology and genetic influences of child trauma on child development will lead to novel and effective approaches to treatments (eg, personalized medicine).

REFERENCES

1. American Psychiatric Association. Diagnostic and statistical manual of mental disorders. Text Revision. 4th edition. Washington, DC: American Psychiatric Press; 2000.
2. American Psychiatric Association. Trauma- and stressor-related disorders, in diagnostic and statistical manual of mental disorders. 5th edition. Arlington (VA): American Psychiatric Publishing; 2013.
3. Widom CS. Posttraumatic stress disorder in abused and neglected children grown up. Am J Psychiatry 1999;156:1223–9.
4. Ford JD, Stockton P, Kaltman S, et al. Disorders of extreme stress (DESNOS) symptoms are associated with type and severity of interpersonal trauma exposure in a sample of healthy young women. J Interpers Violence 2006;21(11): 1399–416.
5. Carrion VG, Weems CF, Ray RD, et al. Toward an empirical definition of pediatric PTSD: the phenomenology of PTSD symptoms in youth. J Am Acad Child Adolesc Psychiatry 2001;41:166–73.
6. Widom CS, DuMont K, Czaja SJ. A prospective investigation of major depressive disorder and comorbidity in abused and neglected children grown up. Arch Gen Psychiatry 2007;64:49–56.
7. Copeland W, Keeler G, Angold A, et al. Traumatic events and posttraumatic stress in childhood. Arch Gen Psychiatry 2007;64:577–84.
8. Luntz BK, Widom CS. Antisocial personality disorder in abused and neglected children grown up. Am J Psychiatry 1994;151:670–4.
9. Clark DB, Lesnick L, Hegedus A. Trauma and other stressors in adolescent alcohol dependence and abuse. J Am Acad Child Adolesc Psychiatry 1997; 36:1744–51.

10. De Bellis MD. Developmental traumatology: a contributory mechanism for alcohol and substance use disorders. Psychoneuroendocrinology 2001;27: 155–70.

11. Dube SR, Miller JW, Brown DW, et al. Adverse childhood experiences and the association with ever using alcohol and initiating alcohol use during adolescence. J Adolesc Health 2006;38(4):444.e1–10.

12. Dube SR, Felitti VJ, Dong M, et al. Childhood abuse, neglect, household dysfunction and the risk of illicit drug use: the adverse childhood experiences Study. Pediatrics 2003;111(3):564–72.

13. De Bellis MD. Developmental traumatology: the psychobiological development of maltreated children and its implications for research, treatment, and policy. Dev Psychopathol 2001;13(3):539–64.

14. Kirsch I, Lynn SJ, Vigorito M. The role of cognition in classical and operant conditioning. J Clin Psychol 2004;60(4):369–92.

15. Maier SF, Watkins LR. Stressor controllability and learned helplessness: the roles of the dorsal raphe nucleus, serotonin, and corticotropin-releasing factor. Neurosci Biobehav Rev 2005;29:829–41.

16. Dell'Osso B, Nestadt G, Allen A, et al. Serotonin-Norepinephrine reuptake inhibitors in the treatment of obsessive-compulsive disorder: a critical review. J Clin Psychiatry 2006;67:600–10.

17. Pagel JF. The neuropharmacology of nightmares. In: Lader M, Cardinali DP, Pandi-Perumal SR, editors. Sleep and sleep disorders: a neuropsychopharmacological approach. New York: Springer Science; 2006. p. 243–50.

18. Argyropoulos SV, Nutt DJ. Anhedonia revisited: is there a role for dopamine-targeting drugs for depression? J Psychopharmacol 2013;27:869–77.

19. Chrousos GP, Gold PW. The concepts of stress and stress system disorders: overview of physical and behavioral homeostasis. J Am Med Assoc 1992; 267(9):1244–52.

20. Heim C, Newport DJ, Mletzko T, et al. The link between childhood trauma and depression: insights from HPA axis studies in humans. Psychoneuroendocrinology 2008;33(6):693–710.

21. McEwen BS. The neurobiology of stress: from serendipity to clinical relevance. Brain Res 2000;886:172–89.

22. Tsigos C, Chrousos GP. Hypothalamic-pituitary-adrenal axis, neuroendocrine factors and stress. J Psychosom Res 2002;53(4):865–71.

23. LeDoux J. Fear and the brain: where have we been, and where are we going? Biol Psychiatry 1998;44:1229–38.

24. Charney DS, Deutch AY, Krystal JH, et al. Psychobiologic mechanisms of post-traumatic-stress-disorder. Arch Gen Psychiatry 1993;50(4):294–306.

25. Cannon WB. The wisdom of the body. Physiol Rev 1929;9:399–431.

26. McEwen BS. Physiology and neurobiology of stress and adaptation: central role of the brain. Physiol Rev 2007;87:873–904.

27. Lupien SJ, McEwen BS, Gunnar MR, et al. Effects of stress throughout the lifespan on the brain, behaviour and cognition. Nat Rev Neurosci 2009;10: 434–45.

28. De Souza EB. Corticotropin-releasing factor receptors: physiology, pharmacology, biochemistry and role in central nervous system and immune disorders. Psychoneuroendocrinology 1995;20:789–819.

29. Herman JP, Ostrander MM, Mueller NK, et al. Limbic system mechanisms of stress regulation: hypothalamo-pituitary-adrenocortical axis. Prog Neuropsychopharmacol Biol Psychiatry 2005;29(8):1201–13.

30. Rosmalen JG, Oldehinkel AJ, Ormel J, et al. Determinants of salivary cortisol levels in 10–12 year old children: a population-based study of individual differences. Psychoneuroendocrinology 2005;30:483–95.
31. Susman EJ, Dockray S, Schiefelbein VL, et al. Morningness/eveningness, morning-to-afternoon cortisol ratio, and antisocial behavior problems during puberty. Dev Psychol 2007;43(4):811–22.
32. Schmidt-Reinwald A, Pruessner JC, Hellhammer DH, et al. The cortisol response to awakening in relation to different challenge tests and a 12-hour cortisol rhythm. Life Sci 1999;64:1653–60.
33. Hayakawa K, Konishi Y, Matsuda T, et al. Development and aging of brain midline structures: assessment with MR imaging. Radiology 1989;172:171–7.
34. Plotsky PM, Meaney MJ. Early, postnatal experience alters hypothalamic corticotropin-releasing factor (CRF) mRNA, median eminence CRF content and stress-induced release in adult rats. Brain Res Mol Brain Res 1993;18: 195–200.
35. Meaney MJ. Maternal care, gene expression, and the transmission of individual differences in stress reactivity across generations. Annu Rev Neurosci 2001;24: 1161–92.
36. Sanchez MM, Ladd CO, Plotsky PM. Early adverse experience as a developmental risk factor for later psychopathology: evidence from rodent and primate models. Dev Psychopathol 2001;13(3):419–49.
37. Brunson KL, Kramar E, Lin B, et al. Mechanisms of late-onset cognitive decline after early-life stress. J Neurosci 2005;25:9328–38.
38. Brunson KL, Eghbal-Ahmadi M, Bender R, et al. Long-term, progressive hippocampal cell loss and dysfunction induced by early-life administration of corticotropin-releasing hormone reproduce the effects of early-life stress. Proc Natl Acad Sci U S A 2001;98:8856–61.
39. De Bellis MD, Chrousos GP, Dorn LD, et al. Hypothalamic-pituitary-adrenal axis dysregulation in sexually abused girls. J Clin Endocrinol Metab 1994; 78:249–55.
40. Cicchetti D, Rogosch FA, Gunnar MR, et al. The differential impacts of early physical and sexual abuse and internalizing problems on daytime cortisol rhythm in school-aged children. Child Dev 2010;81(1):252–69.
41. Carrion VG, Weems CF, Ray RD, et al. Diurnal salivary cortisol in pediatric post-traumatic stress disorder. Biol Psychiatry 2002;51:575–82.
42. De Bellis MD, Baum A, Birmaher B, et al. A.E. Bennett research Award. Developmental traumatology: part I: biological stress systems. Biol Psychiatry 1999; 45:1259–70.
43. Gunnar MR, Morison SJ, Chisholm K, et al. Salivary cortisol levels in children adopted from Romanian orphanages. Dev Psychopathol 2001;13:611–28.
44. Cicchetti D, Rogosch FA. Diverse patterns of neuroendocrine activity in maltreated children. Dev Psychopathol 2001;13:677–93.
45. Delahanty DL, Nugent NR, Christopher NC, et al. Initial urinary epinephrine and cortisol levels predict acute PTSD symptoms in child trauma victims. Psychoneuroendocrinology 2005;30:121–8.
46. Pfeffer CR, Altemus M, Heo M, et al. Salivary cortisol and psychopathology in children bereaved by the September 11, 2001, terror attacks. Biol Psychiatry 2007;61:957–65.
47. Miller GE, Chen E, Zhou ES. If it goes up, must it come down? Chronic stress and the hypothalamic–pituitary–adrenocortical axis in humans. Psychol Bull 2007;133:25–45.

48. Goenjian AK, Yehuda R, Pynoos RS, et al. Basal cortisol, dexamethasone suppression of cortisol, and MHPG in adolescents after the 1988 earthquake in Armenia. Am J Psychiatry 1996;153:929–34.
49. King JA, Mandansky D, King S, et al. Early sexual abuse and low cortisol. Psychiatry Clin Neurosci 2001;55:71–4.
50. Kaufman J, Birmaher B, Perel J, et al. The corticotropin-releasing hormone challenge in depressed abused, depressed nonabused, and normal control children. Biol Psychiatry 1997;42:669–79.
51. Murali R, Chen E. Exposure to violence and cardiovascular and neuroendocrine measures in adolescents. Ann Behav Med 2005;30(2):155–63.
52. MacMillan HL, Georgiades K, Duku EK, et al. Cortisol response to stress in female adolescents exposed to childhood maltreatment: results of the youth mood project. Biol Psychiatry 2009;66(1):62–8.
53. Heim C, Mletzko T, Purselle D, et al. The Dexamethasone/Corticotropin-releasing factor test in men with major depression: role of childhood trauma. Biol Psychiatry 2008;63:398–405.
54. Heim C, Newport DJ, Heit S, et al. Pituitary-adrenal and autonomic responses to stress in women after sexual and physical abuse in childhood. J Am Med Assoc 2000;284:592–7.
55. Santa Ana EJ, Saladin ME, Back SE, et al. PTSD and the HPA axis: differences in response to the cold pressor task among individuals with child vs. adult trauma. Psychoneuroendocrinology 2006;31(4):501–9.
56. Heim C, Newport DJ, Bonsall R, et al. Altered pituitary-adrenal axis responses to provocative challenge tests in adult survivors of childhood abuse. Am J Psychiatry 2001;158:575–81.
57. Klaassens ER, Giltay EJ, Cuijpers P, et al. Adulthood trauma and HPA-axis functioning in healthy subjects and PTSD patients: a meta-analysis. Psychoneuroendocrinology 2012;37(3):317–31.
58. Simon GE, Perlis RH. Personalized medicine for depression: can we match patients with treatments? Am J Psychiatry 2010;167:1445–55.
59. Thomas LA, De Bellis MD. Pituitary volumes in pediatric maltreatment related PTSD. Biol Psychiatry 2004;55:752–8.
60. Ehlers CL, Henriksen SJ, Wang M, et al. Corticotropin releasing factor produces increases in brain excitability and convulsive seizures in rats. Brain Res 1983;278:332–6.
61. Weiss SB, Post RM, Gold PW, et al. CRF-induced seizures and behavior: interaction with arnygdala kindling. Brain Res 1986;372:345–51.
62. Korbey SM, Heinrichs SC, Leussis MP. Seizure susceptibility and locus ceruleus activation are reduced following environmental enrichment in an animal model of epilepsy. Epilepsy Behav 2008;12:30–8.
63. Coplan JD, Andrews MW, Rosenblum LA, et al. Persistent elevations of cerebrospinal fluid concentrations of corticotropin-releasing factor in adult nonhuman primates exposed to early-life stressors: implications for the pathophysiology of mood and anxiety disorders. Proc Natl Acad Sci U S A 1996;93:1619–23.
64. Coplan JD, Smith EL, Altemus M, et al. Elevations in cisternal cerebrospinal fluid corticotropin-releasing factor concentrations in adult primates. Biol Psychiatry 2001;50:200–4.
65. Baker DG, West SA, Nicholson WE, et al. CSF corticotropin-releasing hormone levels and adrenocortical activity in combat veterans with posttraumatic stress disorder. Am J Psychiatry 1999;156:585–8.

66. Bremner JD, Licinio J, Darnell A, et al. Elevated CSF corticotropin-releasing factor concentrations in posttraumatic stress disorder. Am J Psychiatry 1997;154: 624–9.
67. Bremner JD, Southwick SM, Johnson DR, et al. Childhood physical abuse and combat-related posttraumatic stress disorder in Vietnam Veterans. Am J Psychiatry 1993;150:235–9.
68. Kaufman J, Plotsky PM, Nemeroff CB, et al. Effects of early adverse experiences on brain structure and function: clinical implications. Biol Psychiatry 2000;48: 778–90.
69. Yehuda R, Kahana B, Binder-Brynes K, et al. Low urinary cortisol excretion in Holocaust survivors with posttraumatic stress disorder. Am J Psychiatry 1995; 152:982–6.
70. Trickett PK, Noll JG, Susman EJ, et al. Attenuation of cortisol across development for victims of sexual abuse. Dev Psychopathol 2010;22(1):165–75.
71. Yehuda R. Advances in understanding neuroendocrine alterations in PTSD and their therapeutic implications. Ann N Y Acad Sci 2006;1071:137–66.
72. Fries AB, Shirtcliff EA, Pollak SD. Neuroendocrine dysregulation following early social deprivation in children. Dev Psychobiol 2008;50(6):588–99.
73. Elzinga BM, Schmahl C, Vermetten E, et al. Higher cortisol levels following exposure to traumatic reminders in abuse-related PTSD. Neuropsychopharmacology 2003;28:1656–65.
74. Boyce WT, Champoux M, Suomi SJ, et al. Salivary cortisol in nursery-reared rhesus monkeys: reactivity to peer interactions and altered circadian activity. Dev Psychobiol 1995;28:257–67.
75. Gunnar MR, Vazquez DM. Low cortisol and a flattening of expected daytime rhythm: potential indices of risk in human development. Dev Psychopathol 2001;13:515–38.
76. De Bellis MD, Dahl RE, Perel J, et al. Nocturnal ACTH, cortisol, growth hormone, and prolactin secretion in prepubertal depression. J Am Acad Child Adolesc Psychiatry 1996;35:1130–8.
77. Dimitriou T, Maser-Gluth C, Remer T. Adrenocortical activity in healthy children is associated with fat mass. Am J Clin Nutr 2003;77:731–6.
78. Hart J, Gunnar M, Cicchetti D. Altered neuroendocrine activity in maltreated children related to symptoms of depression. Dev Psychopathol 1996;8: 201–14.
79. Cicchetti D, Rogosch FA. The impact of child maltreatment and psychopathology on neuroendocrine functioning. Dev Psychopathol 2001;13:783–804.
80. Kaufman J. Depressive disorders in maltreated children. J Am Acad Child Adolesc Psychiatry 1991;30:257–65.
81. Susman EJ. Psychobiology of persistent antisocial behavior: stress, early vulnerabilities and the attenuation hypothesis. Neurosci Biobehav Rev 2006;30: 376–89.
82. Carpenter LL, Carvalho JP, Tyrka AR, et al. Decreased adrenocorticotropic hormone and cortisol responses to stress in healthy adults reporting significant childhood maltreatment. Biol Psychiatry 2007;62:1080–7.
83. Stenzel-Poore MP, Heinrichs SC, Rivest S, et al. Overproduction of corticotropin-releasing factor in transgenic mice: a genetic model of anxiogenic behavior. J Neurosci 1994;14(5):2579–84.
84. DeYoung C, Cicchetti D, Rogosch FA. Moderation of the association between childhood maltreatment and neuroticism by the corticotropin-releasing hormone receptor 1 gene. J Child Psychol Psychiatry 2011;52:898–906.

85. Cicchetti D, Rogosch FA, Oshri A. Interactive effects of corticotropin releasing hormone receptor 1, serotonin transporter linked polymorphic region, and child maltreatment on diurnal cortisol regulation and internalizing symptomatology. Dev Psychopathol 2011;23:1125–38.

86. Bradley RG, Binder EB, Epstein MP, et al. Influence of child abuse on adult depression: moderation by the corticotropin-releasing hormone receptor gene. Arch Gen Psychiatry 2008;65(2):190–200.

87. Polanczyk G, Caspi A, Williams B, et al. Protective effect of CRHR1 gene variants on the development of adult depression following childhood maltreatment: replication and extension. Arch Gen Psychiatry 2009;66: 978–85.

88. Tyrka AR, Price LH, Gelernter J, et al. Interaction of childhood maltreatment with the corticotropin-releasing hormone receptor gene: effects on hypothalamic-pituitary-adrenal axis reactivity. Biol Psychiatry 2009;66:681–5.

89. Spijker AT, van Rossum EF. Glucocorticoid sensitivity in mood disorders. Neuroendocrinology 2012;95:179–86.

90. Heim CM, Bradley RG, Deveau TC, et al. Effect of childhood trauma on adult depression and neuroendocrine function: sex-specific moderation by CRH receptor 1 gene. Front Behav Neurosci 2009;3:1–10.

91. Wochnik GM, Ruegg J, Abel GA, et al. FK506-binding proteins 51 and 52 differentially regulate dynein interaction and nuclear translocation of the glucocorticoid receptor in mammalian cells. J Biol Chem 2005;280:4609–16.

92. Zimmermann P, Brückl T, Nocon A, et al. Interaction of FKBP 5 gene variants and adverse life events in predicting depression onset: results from a 10-year prospective community study. Am J Psychiatry 2011;168:1107–16.

93. Ising M, Depping AM, Siebertz A, et al. Polymorphisms in the FKBP5 gene region modulate recovery from psychosocial stress in healthy controls. Eur J Neurosci 2008;28:389–98.

94. Appel K, Schwahn C, Mahler J, et al. Moderation of adult depression by a polymorphism in the FKBP5 gene and childhood physical abuse in the general population. Neuropsychopharmacology 2011;36:1982–91.

95. Binder EB, Bradley RG, Liu W, et al. Association of FKBP5 polymorphisms and childhood abuse with risk of posttraumatic stress disorder symptoms in adults. J Am Med Assoc 2008;299:1291–305.

96. Xie P, Kranzler HR, Poling J, et al. Interaction of FKBP5 with childhood adversity on risk for post-traumatic stress disorder. Neuropsychopharmacology 2010;35: 1684–92.

97. Roy A, Gorodetsky E, Yuan Q, et al. Interaction of FKBP5, a stress-related gene, with childhood trauma increases the risk for attempting suicide. Neuropsychopharmacology 2010;35:1674–83.

98. Bevilacqua L, Carli V, Sarchiapone M, et al. Interaction between FKBP5 and childhood trauma and risk of aggressive behavior. Arch Gen Psychiatry 2012; 69:62–70.

99. White MG, Bogdan R, Fisher PM, et al. FKBP5 and emotional neglect interact to predict individual differences in amygdala reactivity. Genes Brain Behav 2012; 11(7):869–78.

100. Razin A. CpG methylation, chromatin structure and gene silencing-a three-way connection. EMBO J 1998;17:4905–8.

101. McGowan PO, Sasaki A, D'Alessio AC, et al. Epigenetic regulation of the glucocorticoid receptor in human brain associates with childhood abuse. Nat Neurosci 2009;12(3):342–8.

102. Murgatroyd C, Spengler D. Epigenetics of early child development. Front Psychiatr 2011;2(16):1–15.
103. McGowan PO. Epigenomic mechanisms of early adversity and HPA dysfunction: considerations for PTSD research. Front Psychiatr 2013;4(110):1–6.
104. McGowan PO, Szyf M. The epigenetics of social adversity in early life: implications for mental health outcomes. Neurobiol Dis 2010;39:66–72.
105. Zhang TY, Labonté B, Wen XL, et al. Epigenetic mechanisms for the early environmental regulation of hippocampal glucocorticoid receptor gene expression in rodents and humans. Neuropsychopharmacology 2013;38(1):111–23.
106. Champagne FA, Francis DD, Mar A, et al. Variations in maternal care in the rat as a mediating influence for the effects of environment on development. Physiol Behav 2003;79:359–71.
107. Kurata A, Morinobu S, Fuchikami M, et al. Maternal postpartum learned helplessness (LH) affects maternal care by dams and responses to the LH test in adolescent offspring. Horm Behav 2009;56:112–20.
108. Murgatroyd C, Patchev AV, Wu Y, et al. Dynamic DNA methylation programs persistent adverse effects of early-life stress. Nat Neurosci 2009;12:1559–66.
109. Roth TL, Lubin FD, Funk AJ, et al. Lasting epigenetic influence of early-life adversity on the BDNF gene. Biol Psychiatry 2009;65(9):760–9.
110. Bick J, Naumova O, Hunter S, et al. Childhood adversity and DNA methylation of genes involved in the hypothalamus-pituitary-adrenal axis and immune system: whole-genome and candidate-gene associations. Dev Psychopathol 2012; 24(4):1417–25.
111. DeSantis SM, Baker NL, Back SE, et al. Gender differences in the effect of early life trauma on hypothalamic-pituitary-adrenal axis functioning. Depress Anxiety 2011;28(5):383–92.
112. Seltzer LJ, Ziegler T, Connolly MJ, et al. Stress-induced elevation of oxytocin in maltreated children: evolution, neurodevelopment, and social behavior. Child Dev 2013. [Epub ahead of print]. http://dx.doi.org/10.1111/cdev.12136.
113. Widom CS. Child abuse, neglect, and violent criminal behavior. Am J Psychiatry 1989;27(2):251–71.
114. Gunnar MR. Quality of early care and buffering of neuroendocrine stress reactions: potential effects on the developing human brain. Prev Med 1998;27:208–11.
115. Heinrichs M, Baumgartner T, Kirschbaum C, et al. Social support and oxytocin interact to suppress cortisol and subjective responses to psychosocial stress. Biol Psychiatry 2003;54:1389–98.
116. Eisenberger NI, Taylor SA, Gable SL, et al. Neural pathways link social support to attenuated neuroendocrine stress responses. Neuroimage 2007;35:1601–12.
117. Li Q, Wichems C, Heils A, et al. Reduction of 5-hydroxytryptamine (5-HT)(1A)-mediated temperature and neuroendocrine responses and 5-HT(1A) binding sites in 5-HT transporter knockout mice. J Pharmacol Exp Ther 1999;291(3): 999–1007.
118. Ressler KJ, Bradley RG, Mercer KB, et al. Polymorphisms in CRHR1 and the Serotonin Transporter Loci: genegeneenvironment interactions on depressive symptoms. Am J Med Genet B Neuropsychiatr Genet 2009;153B:812–24.
119. De Bellis MD, Keshavan M, Clark DB, et al. A.E. Bennett research Award. Developmental traumatology, Part II: brain development. Biol Psychiatry 1999;45: 1271–84.
120. Shalev I, Moffitt TE, Sugden K, et al. Exposure to violence during childhood is associated with telomere erosion from 5 to 10 years of age: a longitudinal study. Mol Psychiatry 2013;18:576–81.

121. Paus T. Mapping brain maturation and cognitive development during adolescence. Trends Cogn Sci 2005;9(2):60–8.
122. McEwen BS. The neurobiology and neuroendocrinology of stress. Implications for post-traumatic stress disorder from a basic science perspective. Psychiatr Clin North Am 2002;25(2):469–94, ix.
123. Edwards E, Harkins K, Wright G, et al. Effects of bilateral adrenalectomy on the induction of learned helplessness. Behavioral Neuropsychopharmacology 1990;3:109–14.
124. Sapolsky RM, Uno H, Rebert CS, et al. Hippocampal damage associated with prolonged glucocorticoid exposure in primates. J Neurosci 1990;10: 2897–902.
125. Simantov R, Blinder E, Ratovitski T, et al. Dopamine induced apoptosis in human neuronal cells: inhibition by nucleic acids antisense to the dopamine transporter. Neuroscience 1996;74:39–50.
126. Dunlop SA, Archer MA, Quinlivan JA, et al. Repeated prenatal corticosteroids delay myelination in the ovine central nervous system. J Matern Fetal Med 1997;6:309–13.
127. Todd RD. Neural development is regulated by classical neuro-transmitters: dopamine D2 receptor stimulation enhances neurite outgrowth. Biol Psychiatry 1992;31:794–807.
128. Lauder JM. Neurotransmitters as morphogens. Prog Brain Res 1988;73:365–88.
129. Gould E, McEwen BS, Tanapat P, et al. Neurogenesis in the dentate gyrus of the adult tree shrew is regulated by psychosocial stress and NMDA receptor activation. J Neurosci 1997;17:2492–8.
130. Gould E, Tanapat P, Cameron HA. Adrenal steroids suppress granule cell death in the developing dentate gyrus through an NMDA receptor-dependent mechanism. Brain Res Dev Brain Res 1997;103:91–3.
131. Gould E, Tanapat P, McEwen BS, et al. Proliferation of granule cell precursors in the dentate gyrus of adult monkeys is diminished by stress. Proc Natl Acad Sci U S A 1998;95:3168–71.
132. Pizarro JM, Lumley LA, Medina W, et al. Acute social defeat reduces neurotrophin expression in brain cortical and subcortical areas in mice. Brain Res 2004; 1025:10–20.
133. Zhang LX, Levine S, Dent G, et al. Maternal deprivation increases cell death in the infant rat brain. Brain Res Dev Brain Res 2002;133:1–11.
134. Harley CB, Futcher AB, Greider CW. Telomeres shorten during ageing of human fibroblasts. Nature 1990;345:458–60.
135. Drury SS, Theall K, Gleason MM, et al. Telomere length and early severe social deprivation: linking early adversity and cellular aging. Mol Psychiatry 2012;17: 719–27.
136. Anda RF, Felitti VJ, Bremner JD, et al. The enduring effects of abuse and related adverse experiences in childhood: a convergence of evidence from neurobiology and epidemiology. Eur Arch Psychiatry Clin Neurosci 2006;256(3):174–86.
137. De Bellis MD, Putnam FW. The psychobiology of childhood maltreatment. Child Adolesc Psychiatr Clin N Am 1994;3(4):663–78.
138. Arnsten AF. Stress impairs prefrontal cortical function in rats and monkeys: role of dopamine D1 and norepinephrine alpha-1 receptor mechanisms. Prog Brain Res 2000;126:183–92.
139. Arnsten AF. The biology of being frazzled. Science 1998;280:1711–2.
140. De Bellis MD, Lefter L, Trickett PK, et al. Urinary catecholamine excretion in sexually abused girls. J Am Acad Child Adolesc Psychiatry 1994;33:320–7.

141. Pervanidou P, Kolaitis G, Charitaki S, et al. The natural history of neuroendocrine changes in pediatric posttraumatic stress disorder after motor vehicle accidents: progressive divergence of noradrenaline and cortisol concentrations over time. Biol Psychiatry 2007;62:1095–102.

142. Otte C, Neylan TC, Pole N, et al. Association between childhood trauma and catecholamine response to psychological stress in police academy recruits. Biol Pyschiatry 2005;57(1):27–32.

143. Savitz JB, van derMerwe L, Newman TK, et al. The relationship between childhood abuse and dissociation. Is it influenced by catechol-O-methyltransferase (COMT) activity? Int J Neuropsychopharmacol 2008;11:149–61.

144. Lesch KP, Mossner R. Genetically driven variation in serotonin update: is there a link to affective spectrum, neurodevelopmental and neurodegenerative disorders? Biol Psychiatry 1998;44(3):179–92.

145. Siever LJ. Neurobiology of aggression and violence. Am J Psychiatry 2008; 165(4):429–42.

146. Lucki I. The spectrum of behaviors influenced by serotonin. Biol Psychiatry 1998;44(3):151–62.

147. Lauder JM. Neurotransmitters as growth regulatory signals: role of receptors and second messengers. Trends Neurosci 1993;16:233–40.

148. Veenema AH. Early life stress, the development of aggression and neuroendocrine and neurobiological correlates: what can we learn from animal models? Front Neuroendocrinol 2009;30(4):497–518.

149. Ressler KJ, Nemeroff CB. Role of serotonergic and noradrenergic systems in the pathophysiology of depression and anxiety disorders. Depress Anxiety 2000; 12(Suppl 1):2–19.

150. Goodman M, New A, Siever L. Trauma, genes, and the neurobiology of personality disorders. Ann N Y Acad Sci 2004;1032:104–16.

151. Lesch KP, Heils A. Serotonergic gene transcriptional control regions: targets for antidepressant drug development? Int J Neuropscyhopharmacol 2000;3:67–79.

152. Caspi A, Sugden K, Moffitt TE, et al. Influence of life stress on depression: moderation by a polymorphism in the 5-HTT gene. Science 2003;301(5631): 386–9.

153. Kaufman J, Yang BZ, Douglas-Palumberi H, et al. Social supports and serotonin transporter gene moderate depression in maltreated children. Proc Natl Acad Sci U S A 2004;101(49):17316–21.

154. Sugden K, Arseneault L, Harrington H, et al. Serotonin transporter gene moderates the development of emotional problems among children following bullying victimization. J Am Acad Child Adolesc Psychiatry 2010;49:830–40.

155. Banny AM, Cicchetti D, Rogosch FA, et al. Vulnerability to depression: a moderated mediation model of the roles of child maltreatment, peer victimization, and serotonin transporter linked polymorphic region genetic variation among children from low socioeconomic status backgrounds. Dev Psychopathol 2013; 25:599–614.

156. Cicchetti D, Rogosch FA. GeneEnvironment interaction and resilience: effects of child maltreatment and serotonin, corticotropin releasing hormone, dopamine, and oxytocin genes. Dev Psychopathol 2012;24:411–27.

157. Munafo MR, Durrant C, Lewis G, et al. Gene Environment interactions at the serotonin transporter locus. Biol Psychiatry 2009;65:211–9.

158. Risch N, Herrell R, Lehner T, et al. Interaction between the serotonin transporter gene (5-HTTLPR), stressful life events, and risk of depression: a meta-analysis. J Am Med Assoc 2009;301:2462–71.

159. Karg K, Burmeister M, Shedden K, et al. The serotonin transporter promoter variant (5-HTTLPR), stress, and depression meta-analysis revisited: evidence of genetic moderation. Arch Gen Psychiatry 2011;68:444–54.
160. Sadeh N, Javdani S, Verona E. Analysis of monoaminergic genes, childhood abuse, and dimensions of psychopathy. J Abnorm Psychol 2013;122(1):167–79.
161. Shih JC, Chen K, Ridd MJ. Monoamine oxidase: from genes to behavior. Annu Rev Neurosci 1999;22:197–217.
162. Kim-Cohen J, Caspi A, Taylor A, et al. MAOA, maltreatment, and gene–environment interaction predicting children's mental health: new evidence and a meta-analysis. Mol Psychiatry 2006;11:903–13.
163. Nilsson KW, Sjoberg RL, Wargelius HL, et al. The monoamine oxidase A (MAO-A) gene, family function and maltreatment as predictors of destructive behaviour during male adolescent alcohol consumption. Addiction 2007;102: 389–98.
164. Kaufman J, Yang BZ, Douglas-Palumberi H, et al. Genetic and environmental predictors of early alcohol use. Biol Psychiatry 2007;61(11):1228–34.
165. Ducci F, Enoch MA, Hodgkinson C, et al. Interaction between a functional MAOA locus and childhood sexual abuse predicts alcoholism and antisocial personality disorder in adult women. Mol Psychiatry 2008;13(3):334–47.
166. Bartz JA, Zaki J, Bolger N, et al. Social effects of oxytocin in humans: context and person matter. Trends Cogn Sci 2011;15(7):301–9.
167. Francis DD, Champagne FC, Meaney MJ. Variations in maternal behaviour are associated with differences in oxytocin receptor levels in the rat. J Neuroendocrinol 2000;12(12):1145–8.
168. Shahrokh DK, Zhang TY, Diorio J, et al. Oxytocin-dopamine interactions mediate variations in maternal behavior in the rat. Endocrinology 2010;151(5):2276–86.
169. Bradley B, Davis TA, Wingo AP, et al. Family environment and adult resilience: contributions of positive parenting and the oxytocin receptor gene. Eur J Psychotraumatol 2013;4.
170. Dantzer R, O'Connor JC, Freund GG, et al. From inflammation to sickness and depression: when the immune system subjugates the brain. Nat Rev Neurosci 2008;9(1):46–56.
171. Mills NT, Scott JG, Wray NR, et al. Research review: the role of cytokines in depression in adolescents: a systematic review. J Child Psychol Psychiatry 2013;54(8):816–35.
172. De Bellis MD, Burke L, Trickett PK, et al. Antinuclear antibodies and thyroid function in sexually abused girls. J Trauma Stress 1996;9(2):369–78.
173. Gill JM, Saligan L, Woods S, et al. PTSD is associated with an excess of inflammatory immune activities. Perspect Psychiatr Care 2009;45(4):262–77.
174. Smith AK, Conneely KN, Kilaru V, et al. Differential immune system DNA methylation and cytokine regulation in post-traumatic stress disorder. Am J Med Genet B Neuropsychiatr Genet 2011;156B(6):700–8.
175. Lemieux A, Coe CL, Carnes M. Symptom severity predicts degree of T cell activation in adult women following childhood maltreatment. Brain Behav Immun 2008;22(6):994–1003.
176. Altemus M, Cloitre M, Dhabhar FS. Enhanced cellular immune response in women with PTSD related to childhood abuse. Am J Psychiatry 2003;160(9): 1705–7.
177. Carpenter LL, Gawuga CE, Tyrka AR, et al. Association between Plasma IL-6 response to acute stress and early-life adversity in healthy adults. Neuropsychopharmacology 2010;35:2617–23.

178. Danese A, Moffitt TE, Harrington H, et al. Adverse childhood experiences and adult risk factors for age-related disease: depression, inflammation, and clustering of metabolic risk markers. Arch Pediatr Adolesc Med 2009;163(12):1135–43.

179. Pervanidou P, Chrousos GP. Metabolic consequences of stress during childhood and adolescence. Metabolism 2012;61(5):611–9.

180. Aber JL, Allen JP, Carlson V, et al. The effects of maltreatment on development during early childhood: recent studies and their theoretical, clinical, and policy implications. In: Carlson V, Cicchetti D, editors. Child maltreatment: theory and research on the causes and consequences of child abuse and neglect. New York: Cambridge University Press; 1989. p. 579–619.

181. Carrey NJ, Butter HJ, Persinger MA, et al. Physiological and cognitive correlates of child abuse. J Am Acad Child Adolesc Psychiatry 1995;34(8):1067–75.

182. Culp RE, Watkins RV, Lawrence H, et al. Maltreated children's language and speech development: abused, neglected, and abused and neglected. First Lang 1991;11:377–89.

183. Eckenrode J, Laird M, Doris J. School performance and disciplinary problems among abused and neglected children. Dev Psychol 1993;29:53–62.

184. McFadyen RG, Kitson WJ. Language comprehension and expression among adolescents who have experienced childhood physical abuse. J Child Psychol Psychiatry 1996;37(5):551–62.

185. Trickett PK, McBride-Chang C. The developmental impact of different forms of child abuse & neglect. Dev Rev 1995;15:311–37.

186. Koenen KC, Moffitt TE, Caspi A, et al. Domestic violence is associated with environmental suppression of IQ in young children. Dev Psychopathol 2003;15(2): 297–311.

187. Beers SR, De Bellis MD. Neuropsychological function in children with maltreatment-related posttraumatic stress disorder. Am J Psychiatry 2002;159:483–6.

188. DePrince AP, Weinzierl KM, Combs MD. Executive function performance and trauma exposure in a community sample of children. Child Abuse Negl 2009; 33(6):353–61.

189. Fishbein D, Warner T, Krebs C, et al. Differential relationships between personal and community stressors and children's neurocognitive functioning. Child Maltreat 2009;14(4):299–315.

190. Pollak SD, Nelson CA, Schlaak MF, et al. Neurodevelopmental effects of early deprivation in postinstitutionalized children. Child Dev 2010;81(1):224–36.

191. De Bellis MD, Hooper S, Spratt EG, et al. Neuropsychological findings in childhood neglect and their relationships to pediatric PTSD. J Int Neuropsychol Soc 2009;15:868–78.

192. Samuelson KW, Krueger CE, Burnett C, et al. Neuropsychological functioning in children with posttraumatic stress disorder. Child Neuropsychol 2010;16(2): 119–33.

193. De Bellis MD, Woolley DP, Hooper SR. Neuropsychological findings in pediatric maltreatment: relationship of PTSD, dissociative symptoms, and abuse/neglect indices to neurocognitive outcomes. Child Maltreat 2013;18(3):171–83.

194. Jaffee SR, Maikovich-Fong AK. Effects of chronic maltreatment and maltreatment timing on children's behavior and cognitive abilities. J Child Psychol Psychiatry 2011;52(2):184–94.

195. Lansford JE, Dodge KE, Pettit GS, et al. A 12-year prospective study of the long-term effects of early child physical maltreatment on psychological, behavioral, and academic problems in adolescence. Arch Pediatr Adolesc Med 2002; 156(8):824–30.

196. Mills R, Alati R, O'Callaghan M, et al. Child abuse and neglect and cognitive function at 14 years of age: findings from a birth cohort. Pediatrics 2011;127(1):4–10.
197. Noll JG, Shenk CE, Yeh MT, et al. Receptive language and educational attainment for sexually abused females. Pediatrics 2010;126(3):e615–22.
198. Perez C, Widom CS. Childhood victimization and long-term intellectual and academic outcomes. Child Abuse Negl 1994;18(8):617–33.
199. Strathearn L, Gray PH, O'Callaghan F, et al. Childhood neglect and cognitive development in extremely low birth weight infants: a prospective study. Pediatrics 2001;108(1):142–51.
200. Trickett PK, McBride-Chang C, Putnam FW. The classroom performance and behavior of sexually abused girls. Dev Psychopathol 1994;6:183–94.
201. Hanson JL, Chung MK, Avants BB, et al. Structural variations in prefrontal cortex mediate the relationship between early childhood stress and spatial working memory. J Neurosci 2012;32(23):7917–25.
202. Bauer PM, Hanson JL, Pierson RK, et al. Cerebellar volume and cognitive functioning in children who experienced early deprivation. Biol Psychiatry 2009;66:1100–6.
203. Carrion VG, Weems CF, Eliez S, et al. Attenuation of frontal asymmetry in pediatric posttraumatic stress disorder. Biol Psychiatry 2001;50:943–51.
204. De Bellis M, Kuchibhatla M. Cerebellar volumes in pediatric maltreatment-related posttraumatic stress disorder. Biol Psychiatry 2006;60(7):697–703.
205. De Bellis MD, Keshavan M, Shifflett H, et al. Brain structures in pediatric maltreatment-related posttraumatic stress disorder: a sociodemographically matched study. Biol Psychiatry 2002;52:1066–78.
206. De Bellis MD, Keshavan MS, Frustaci K, et al. Superior temporal gyrus volumes in maltreated children and adolescents with PTSD. Biol Psychiatry 2002;51:544–52.
207. Hackman D, Farah MJ, Meaney MJ. Socioeconomic status and the brain: mechanistic insights from human and animal research. Nat Rev Neurosci 2010;11:651–9.
208. Riva D, Giorgi C. The cerebellum contributes to higher functions during development. Brain 2000;123:1051–61.
209. Bellebaum C, Daum I. Cerebellar involvement in executive control. Cerebellum 2007;6:184–92.
210. Thoma P, Bellebaum C, Koch B, et al. The cerebellum is involved in reward-based reversal learning. Cerebellum 2008;7:433–43.
211. Fransson P. How default is the default mode of brain function? Further evidence from intrinsic BOLD signal fluctuations. Neuropsychologia 2006;44:2836–45.
212. De Bellis MD, Keshavan MS. Sex differences in brain maturation in maltreatment-related pediatric posttraumatic stress disorder. Neurosci Biobehav Rev 2003;27(1–2):103–17.
213. Conners NA, Bradley RH, Mansell LW, et al. Children of mothers with serious substance abuse problems: an accumulation of risks. Am J Drug Alcohol Abuse 2004;30:85–100.
214. Smith DK, Johnson AB, Pears KC, et al. Child maltreatment and foster care: unpacking the effects of prenatal and postnatal parental substance use. Child Maltreat 2007;12:150.
215. Fair DA, Cohen AL, Dosenbach NU, et al. The maturing architecture of the brain's default network. Proc Natl Acad Sci U S A 2008;105(10):4028–32.
216. Jackowski AP, Douglas-Palumberi H, Jackowski M, et al. Corpus callosum in maltreated children with posttraumatic stress disorder: a diffusion tensor imaging study. Psychiatry Res 2008;162:256–61.

217. Teicher MH, Dumont NL, Ito Y, et al. Childhood neglect is associated with reduced corpus callosum area. Biol Psychiatry 2004;56(2):80–5.
218. Prichard JW. MRS of the brain-prospects for clinical application. In: Young IR, Charles HC, editors. MR spectroscopy: clinical applications and techniques. London: The Livery House; 1996. p. 1–25.
219. De Bellis MD, Keshavan MS, Spencer S, et al. N-acetylaspartate concentration in the anterior cingulate in maltreated children and adolescents with PTSD. Am J Psychiatry 2000;157:1175–7.
220. Carrion VG, Weems CF, Richert K, et al. Decreased prefrontal cortical volume associated with increased bedtime cortisol in traumatized youth. Biol Psychiatry 2010;68(5):491–3.
221. Carrion VG, Garrett A, Menon V, et al. Posttraumatic stress symptoms and brain function during a response-inhibition task: an fMRI study in youth. Depress Anxiety 2008;25(6):514–26.
222. Mueller SC, Maheu FS, Dozier M, et al. Early-life stress is associated with impairment in cognitive control in adolescence: an fMRI study. Neuropsychologia 2010;48(10):3037–44.
223. Smith ME. Bilateral hippocampal volume reduction in adults with post-traumatic stress disorder: a meta-analysis of structural mri studies. Hippocampus 2005; 15:798–807.
224. De Bellis MD, Hall J, Boring AM, et al. A pilot longitudinal study of hippocampal volumes in pediatric maltreatment-related posttraumatic stress disorder. Biol Psychiatry 2001;50:305–9.
225. Carrion VG, Haas BW, Garrett A, et al. Reduced hippocampal activity in youth with posttraumatic stress symptoms: an FMRI study. J Pediatr Psychol 2010; 35(5):559–69.
226. Carrion VG, Weems CF, Reiss AL. Stress predicts brain changes in children: a pilot longitudinal study on youth stress, posttraumatic stress disorder, and the hippocampus. Pediatrics 2007;119(3):509–16.
227. Hanson JL, Chung MK, Avants BB, et al. Early stress is associated with alterations in the orbitofrontal cortex: a tensor based morphometry investigation of brain structure and behavioral risk. J Neurosci 2010;30(22):7466–72.
228. Choi J, Jeong B, Rohan ML, et al. Preliminary evidence for white matter tract abnormalities in young adults exposed to parental verbal abuse. Biol Psychiatry 2009;65:227–34.
229. Bremner JD, Narayan M, Staib L, et al. Neural correlates of memories of childhood sexual abuse in women with and without posttraumatic stress disorder. Am J Psychiatry 1999;156:1787–95.
230. Bremner JD, Vermetten E, Schmahl C, et al. Positron emission tomographic imaging of neural correlates of a fear acquisition and extinction paradigm in women with childhood sexual-abuse-related post-traumatic stress disorder. Psychol Med 2005;35(6):791–806.
231. Shin LM, McNally RJ, Kosslyn SM, et al. Regional cerebral blood flow during script-imagery in childhood sexual abuse-related PTSD: a PET investigation. Am J Psychiatry 1999;156(4):575–84.
232. De Bellis MD, Hooper SR. Neural substrates for processing task-irrelevant emotional distracters in maltreated adolescents with depressive disorders: a pilot study. J Trauma Stress 2012;25(2):198–202.
233. Maheu FS, Dozier M, Guyer AE, et al. A preliminary study of medial temporal lobe function in youths with a history of caregiver deprivation and emotional neglect. Cogn Affect Behav Neurosci 2010;10(1):34–49.

234. Tottenham N, Hare TA, Millner A, et al. Elevated amygdala response to faces following early deprivation. Dev Sci 2011;14(2):190–204.
235. Hanson JL, Adluru N, Chung MK, et al. Early neglect is associated with alterations in white matter integrity and cognitive functioning. Child Dev 2013; 84(5):1566–78.
236. Anderson CM, Teicher MH, Polcari A, et al. Abnormal T2 relaxation time in the cerebellar vermis of adults sexually abused in childhood: potential role of the vermis in stress-enhanced risk for drug abuse. Psychoneuroendocrinology 2002;27:231–44.
237. Sheu YS, Polcari A, Anderson CM, et al. Harsh corporal punishment is associated with increased T2 relaxation time in dopamine-rich regions. Neuroimage 2010;53:412–9.
238. Carballedo A, Morris D, Zill P, et al. Brain-derived neurotrophic factor Val66Met polymorphism and early life adversity affect hippocampal volume. Am J Med Genet B Neuropsychiatr Genetics 2013;162:183–90.
239. Labonté B, Suderman M, Maussion G, et al. Genome-wide epigenetic regulation by early-life trauma. Arch Gen Psychiatry 2012;69(7):722–31.
240. Devon RS, Orban PC, Gerrow K, et al. ALS2-deficient mice exhibit disturbances in endosome trafficking associated with motor behavioral abnormalities. Proc Natl Acad Sci U S A 2006;103(25):9595–600.
241. Crozier JC, Wang L, Huettel SA, et al. Neural correlates of cognitive and affective processing in maltreated youth with posttraumatic stress symptoms: Does gender matter? Dev Psychopathol 2014;26:491–513.
242. Pillar G, Malhotra A, Lavie P. Post-traumatic stress disorder and sleep—what a nightmare! Sleep Med Rev 2000;4(2):183–200.
243. Harvey AG, Jones C, Schmidt DA. Sleep and posttraumatic stress disorder: a review. Clin Psychol Rev 2003;23:377–407.
244. Noll JG, Trickett PK, Susman EJ, et al. Sleep disturbances and childhood sexual abuse. J Pediatr Psychol 2006;31(5):469–80.
245. Xie L, Kang H, Xu Q, et al. Sleep drives metabolite clearance from the adult brain. Science 2013;342:373–7.
246. Porto PR, Oliveira L, Mari J, et al. Change the brain? a systematic review of neuroimaging in anxiety disorders. J Neuropsychiatry Clin Neurosci 2009;21: 114–25.
247. McClure EB, Adler A, Monk CS, et al. fMRI predictors of treatment outcome in pediatric anxiety disorders. Psychopharmacology 2007;191:97–105.
248. DeBellis MD. Medication considerations with maltreated children. In: Talley F, editor. Handbook for the treatment of abused and neglected children. Binghamton (NY): Haworth Press Inc; 2005. p. 423–72.
249. Donnally C. Psychopharmacotherapy for children and adolescents. In: Foa EB, Keane TM, Friedman MJ, et al, editors. Effective treatments for PTSD: practice guidelines from the international society for traumatic stress studies. New York (NY): The Guilford Press; 2009. p. 568.
250. Pervanidou P. Biology of post-traumatic stress disorder in childhood and adolescence. J Neuroendocrinol 2008;20(5):632–8.
251. Green JG, McLaughlin KA, Berglund PA, et al. Childhood adversities and adult psychiatric disorders in the National Comorbidity Survey Replication, I: associations with first onset of DSM-IV disorders. Arch Gen Psychiatry 2010;67: 113–23.
252. Mikton C, Butchart A. Child maltreatment prevention: a systematic review of reviews. Bull World Health Organ 2009;87:353–61.

253. Kitzman H, Olds DL, Henderson CR Jr, et al. Effect of prenatal and infancy home visitation by nurses on pregnancy outcomes, childhood injuries, and repeated childbearing: a randomized controlled trial. J Am Med Assoc 1997;278:644–52.

254. Olds DL, Eckenrode J, Henderson CR Jr, et al. Long-term effects of home visitation on maternal life course and child abuse and neglect: fifteen-year follow- up of a randomized trial. J Am Med Assoc 1997;278(8):637–43.

255. Olds DL, Kitzman H, Hanks C, et al. Effects of nurse home visiting on maternal and child functioning: age-9 follow-up of a randomized trial. Pediatrics 2007; 120:e832.

256. Kitzman H, Olds DL, Cole R, et al. Enduring effects of prenatal and infancy home visiting by nurses on children. Arch Pediatr Adolesc Med 2010;164(5): 412–8.

257. Eckenrode J, Campa M, Luckey DW, et al. Long-term effects of prenatal and in-fancy nurse home visitation on the life course of youths 19-year follow-up of a randomized trial. Arch Pediatr Adolesc Med 2010;164(1):9–15.

258. MacMillan HL, Thomas BH, Jamieson E, et al. Effectiveness of home visitation by public-health nurses in prevention of the recurrence of child physical abuse and neglect: a randomised controlled trial. Lancet 2005;365:1786–93.

259. Taussig HN, Clyman RB, Landsverk J. Children who return home from foster care: a 6-year prospective study of behavioral health outcomes in adolescence. Pediatrics 2001;108(1):1–7.

260. Foster ME, Prinz RJ, Sanders MR, et al. The costs of a public health infrastruc-ture for delivering parenting and family support. Child Youth Serv Rev 2008;30: 493–501.

261. Cohen JA, Mannarino AP, Deblinger E, et al. Cognitive-behavioral therapy for children and adolescents. In: Foa EB, Keane TM, Friedman MJ, et al, editors. Effective treatments for PTSD: practice guidelines from the International Society for Traumatic Stress Studies. New York (NY): The Guilford Press; 2009. p. 223–44.

262. Curtis NM, Ronan KR, Borduin CM. Multisystemic Treatment: a meta-analysis of outcome studies. J Fam Psychol 2004;18(3):411–9.

263. Felitti VJ, Anda RF, Nordenberg D, et al. Relationship of childhood abuse and household dysfunction to many of the leading causes if death in adults. Am J Prev Med 1998;14:245–58.

264. McGloin JM, Widom CS. Resilience among abused and neglected children grown up. Dev Psychopathol 2001;13(4):1021–38.

Assessing the Effects of Trauma in Children and Adolescents in Practice Settings

Cassandra Kisiel, PhD[a],*, Lisa Conradi, PsyD[b],
Tracy Fehrenbach, PhD[a], Elizabeth Torgersen, BA[a],
Ernestine C. Briggs, PhD[c]

KEYWORDS

- Trauma assessment • Measures • Children • Adolescent • Traumatic stress

KEY POINTS

- A comprehensive approach to trauma assessment, including rationale and benefits and key domains to assess, is delineated.
- Trauma-specific assessment measures for use in practice settings, including the use of multiple informants and techniques, are reviewed.
- Factors to consider when selecting and implementing assessment measures in different contexts and settings, including clinics, schools, and disaster response, are discussed.
- Other key considerations in the assessment process, including the role of development, culture, and agency/staff considerations, are described.
- Suggestions for establishing an effective assessment process with youth, caregivers, and families, including strategies for creating a safe environment for assessment and techniques for the translation of trauma assessment information in clinical practice, are provided.

REVIEW OF LITERATURE ON CHILD/ADOLESCENT TRAUMA ASSESSMENT

Assessment is an important part of identifying and effectively addressing the needs of children exposed to trauma. A trauma assessment refers to a comprehensive process conducted by a trained mental health provider/clinician to gain a more thorough understanding of the range of trauma exposures and the areas in which a child or

There are no disclosures to report for any of the authors.

[a] Department of Psychiatry and Behavioral Sciences, Northwestern University Feinberg School of Medicine, 710 North Lake Shore Drive, 12th Floor, Chicago, IL 60611, USA; [b] Chadwick Center for Children and Families, Rady Children's Hospital, San Diego, 3020 Children's Way, MC 5131, San Diego, CA 92123, USA; [c] Department of Psychiatry and the Behavioral Sciences, Center for Child and Family Health, Duke University School of Medicine, 411 West Chapel Hill Street, Suite 200, Durham, NC 27701, USA
* Corresponding author.
E-mail address: c-kisiel@northwestern.edu

Child Adolesc Psychiatric Clin N Am 23 (2014) 223–242
http://dx.doi.org/10.1016/j.chc.2013.12.007

adolescent has been impacted by trauma.[1–5] An assessment is far more comprehensive than a trauma screening. A screening tool refers to a brief measure or tool that is universally administered to children typically by frontline or direct service staff. These tools typically detect exposure to potentially traumatic events and/or endorsement of possible traumatic stress symptoms/reactions. Screening tools are generally used for identification and not for diagnostic purposes; a trauma assessment can determine whether clinical symptoms of traumatic stress are present and characterize the severity of symptoms and their impact on the child's functioning. Although a trauma assessment may use information collected during the trauma screening process (and may include some of the same tools), it typically includes a more in-depth exploration of the nature and severity of the traumatic events, current trauma-related symptoms, and functional impairment. This approach is often used to understand whether a child is on target developmentally (eg, in social/emotional and behavioral domains), to guide treatment planning and monitor progress in treatment or services over time.[6]

Based on recent recommendations, an ideal trauma assessment usually occurs over the course of 2 to 3 sessions and includes a clinical interview; use of objective and psychometrically sound measures; behavioral observations of the child; and collateral contacts with family, other providers (eg, caseworker), and important individuals in the child's life.[6] It also includes many interpersonal goals and processes, such as helping the client feel safe and comfortable in the treatment setting, engaging the client as an active partner in treatment, fostering the therapeutic alliance and relationship, providing psychoeducation on normal responses to trauma, and validating the child's experience through the sharing of assessment data and feedback both initially and over time. Nevertheless, it is understood that there can be practical constraints within clinical settings where an initial assessment needs to be completed after one session (eg, for insurance/billing purposes, to establish a diagnosis, to create a treatment plan). If this is the case, it is suggested that the most essential information is collected initially with additional information gathered over time as a part of an ongoing assessment process (as described below; see **Box 1** on Practical Tips).

Most clinicians generally conduct assessments with their clients as part of routine clinical practice. Research suggests, however, that some clinicians, particularly those in private practice, use informal means of assessment that rely heavily on clinical judgment and client reports. Results from a recent study suggest that only 37% of respondents used formal clinical outcome measures as part of routine clinical practice.[7] Moreover, the study found that clinicians who assessed outcomes in practice were more likely to be younger in age, have a cognitive-behavioral orientation, conduct more hours of therapy per week, provide services for children and adolescents, and work in institutional settings. Additional evidence also suggests that the infrequent use of structured assessment tools in regular clinical practice also represents a historical trend.[7] As the field continues to evolve, however, an even greater emphasis will likely be placed on accountability and use of formal assessment strategies across settings.

Rationale and Benefits of Trauma Assessment

Trauma assessment offers a structured framework for gathering information and identifying and addressing the needs of traumatized children and families (including salient symptoms, risk behaviors, and functional difficulties); identifying the strengths of the child, caregivers, and family that can be used in the treatment process; summarizing assessment information in a meaningful way so that it can be translated and shared with all relevant service providers to inform planning;[8] and engaging children and families in treatment and sharing feedback through this process.[4,6] The many benefits associated with the use of standardized assessments include validation of clinical

---

Box 1
Practical tips for clinical assessment

Sometimes the comprehensive assessment strategies described in this article are not feasible given constraints in either time or resources. Below are 5 tips to help clinicians get the most critical details when these time constraints exist.

- Focus on orienting the client to the assessment process and determining his/her key concerns. This modest investment will not only enhance engagement but will help guide attention to the most pressing issues.

- Think about safety first and address any safety concerns before the end of the session.

- Consider having the client complete some measures before arriving to the appointment. Some options include using technology to make these forms accessible, sending the scales as part of the clinic package, and/or having clients complete some of these forms in the waiting room before or after their appointment.

- Check out your initial impressions and hypotheses with the client to ensure that you are not missing any critical concerns. Many clients will feel validated by this experience and will appreciate the opportunity to actively partner in their care.

- Complete the most essential measures at the outset if time is limited. Set the expectation for ongoing assessment as it will be easier to gather additional information and monitor progress (eg, symptom reduction throughout treatment).

---

judgment,[7] critical feedback for both clinicians and clients on functioning and progress over time,[9] gathering information that may not be disclosed during an interview, and better outcomes for clients. Furthermore, information gathered from a trauma-focused clinical assessment is designed to facilitate selection of appropriate evidence-based interventions and treatment planning. Recent literature suggests the importance of gathering clinically meaningful assessment information that can target specific needs and strengths within the child and family and then be translated directly into treatment and services that are appropriate to these unique needs.[1,5,10] Several trauma-focused tools have been developed for use in clinical and research settings and have been reviewed extensively in recent articles[1,3,6,11,12]; nevertheless, the utility of these tools in treatment planning and clinical practice has been less clear and worthy of further consideration.[10,11]

Some guidelines for implementing a comprehensive trauma assessment approach include the following: (1) assessing for a range of traumatic events, domains of impact, and strengths; (2) gathering information from multiple perspectives and informants; (3) incorporating a variety of assessment techniques; (4) balancing the need for accuracy and consistency with the need for flexibility in approach based on context or setting; (5) assessing child and caregiver responses to trauma over time; (6) creating a safe environment for conducting the assessment; and (7) working with the caregiver/family and across service providers to make sense of the assessment information and translate it for use in practice. These issues are described in detail below.

Key Domains to Assess

Although exposure to trauma and the presence of mental health symptoms following this exposure are the most common reasons a child is referred for a trauma-focused treatment, the assessment and the service/treatment recommendations should never be limited to any single event that led to the referral. Rather, assessing for a wide range of potentially traumatic events, both historical and current, and the impact of these experiences across areas of functioning over time is essential. The following is a listing of key domains and questions to consider when conducting a comprehensive trauma assessment.

Trauma exposure/developmental history

What traumatic events have occurred? Has the child experienced multiple forms of trauma? How chronic and severe were these trauma experiences? Is the child still experiencing the trauma? At what age/developmental stage did the child experience any traumatic events? What are the other relevant trauma circumstances (eg, relationship of perpetrator, reactions of others following disclosure)?

Posttraumatic stress disorder diagnosis/symptoms

What were the effects of the trauma on the child? What symptoms is the child currently experiencing, and how severe are they? Is the child exhibiting intrusive thoughts, avoidance behaviors, negative changes in thoughts and mood, re-experiencing of the event, or changes in his/her baseline level of arousal or reactivity?

Other trauma-related symptoms/complex trauma responses

What other symptoms or responses is the child exhibiting in addition to or separate from posttraumatic stress disorder (PTSD)? How has the trauma impacted the child's developmental processes (eg, regression in any areas of development following the trauma); ability to form attachments and maintain positive relationships; cognitive processes, and learning (eg, difficulties in child's ability to sustain attention, focus on tasks, problem solve, or process information following the trauma); ability to regulate mood (eg, difficulties in the child's ability to modulate his/her emotions, tolerate intense emotions, or label/express feelings following the trauma); behavioral problems (eg, problems with impulse control, oppositional behaviors); dissociative symptoms (eg, problems with blanking or spacing out, persistent forgetfulness, alterations or shifts in consciousness); or physiologic responses (eg, difficulty regulating bodily functions following the trauma, including sleeping, eating, and elimination)?

Emotional/behavioral manifestations (including risk behaviors)

Are there additional manifestations that may not already be captured, including internalizing behaviors (eg, depression, anxiety, withdrawal) or externalizing behaviors (eg, bullying, stealing)? Is there a risk for harm to self or others (self-mutilation, sexual offending)?

Functional difficulties

What is the child's social history? How many close friends does he/she have? Does he/she have experiences with bullying, gangs, or substance abuse? What is the child's education history? Has he/she ever received special education services or an individualized education plan? Are there any other educational-related concerns?

Caregiver and family functioning

Where is the child living? What is the family's history of trauma, substance abuse, and mental health problems? Was there exposure to substances in utero? What is the child's relationship with caregivers/siblings/other family members? How is the family system functioning overall?

Strengths (child, caregiver, community)

What are the child's, caregiver's, and family's strengths and resources within the broader community? How can these strengths be supported, strengthened, and used to improve the child's functioning and resilience?

As noted above, it is important to assess for symptoms of PTSD as well as broader traumatic stress reactions, including mental health symptoms and functional outcomes,[1,3,11] which may be even more common than PTSD symptoms among children particularly following exposure to complex, or chronic, interpersonal trauma.[1,2,5] It is also important to consider mental health needs that may be independent of the child's trauma history. Comparing a child's functioning before and after the traumatic event or events is ideal but may be more straightforward when assessing the impact of a disaster or another single incident trauma; the process of assessment may be more complex if the child has endured years of ongoing or repeated traumas starting at an early age.[1,3] In addition, assessing caregivers' functioning (at least to some degree) is important to understand any potential or ongoing safety concerns and mental health needs that may impact their caregiving, determine their capacity to support their child and his/her recovery from trauma, and any need for services for caregivers.[5,6]

An essential part of trauma assessment sometimes overlooked is the child's and caregiver's strengths or resiliency. Paying attention to strengths during the assessment process—including individual, caregiver, family, and broader environmental strengths—serves many purposes. First, discussing strengths can put the youth and family at ease at the beginning of an assessment and may also help parents/caregivers reframe their perspective; this is especially important when they are overwhelmed by the child's needs. Asking about strengths may also encourage the child and family to begin to make meaning of the traumatic event in a way that considers potential positive outcomes (eg, becoming more connected to community members after a community-based trauma). Assessing strengths can also allow the clinician to recognize if the trauma has negatively impacted areas in which the youth previously excelled, which might otherwise be overshadowed by current needs. Strengths are an important area for more detailed assessment in the context of trauma exposure and responses.[5]

This comprehensive assessment information serves as the foundation for a more accurate and complete understanding of the child, his/her family system, and environment, for identifying primary concerns and presenting problems, and recommending appropriate treatment and services that meet this range of needs. It is important that these recommendations also incorporate the child's and caregiver's existing strengths (eg, hobbies/interests/competencies) and build upon strengths that may emerge as a method for supporting the child in his/her recovery from trauma and to meet his/her highest potential.[5,13]

REVIEW OF ASSESSMENT INSTRUMENTS FOR USE IN PRACTICE SETTINGS

Assessment measures come in a variety of formats including child self-report or caregiver-report (paper and pencil) measures, provider report tools, semi-structured diagnostic tools, and clinical interviews. Many types of assessment tools exist, each offering their own unique benefits and challenges. These tools are available for multiple informants to complete to gather the most comprehensive picture of the child based on a range of perspectives.[6]

Child Report

A child self-report measure may be used if a child has the developmental capacity to read and comprehend a tool (usually ages 8 and above, but will vary across children). Some youth may appreciate the ability to write their answers down in a paper-and-pencil format, whereas others may be more comfortable and also benefit from the opportunity to verbalize their responses (eg, by reading the child report measure aloud with the clinician).

Self-report tools can provide the clinician with various types of information. When feasible and developmentally appropriate, it is important to have the child's report of his/her personal experience of the traumatic event or events, including the aspects considered most difficult. Depending on the child, some of these details may be gathered as a part of a clinical interview (as described below under section on Using a Range of Assessment Approaches and Techniques). This self-report may also be considered primary in the assessment of internalizing symptoms, attributions, or beliefs the child has developed in relation to the trauma (eg, his/her role or responsibility in the trauma and general sense of esteem and safety), which may be less apparent than externalizing symptoms and difficult for caregivers to observe.[3]

Caregiver Report

In addition to a child's self-report of symptoms, it is important to have a caregiver's perspective on how the child is functioning. In particular, for young children (ages 0–8) or children with developmental delays who cannot fully verbalize information themselves, the caregiver report is often the main source of information. For children of all ages, a caregiver report of a child's behaviors and responses also offers an important perspective in terms of how the child is functioning at home with family members and in other important contexts.

Provider Report

Provider report measures can be completed by the clinician or another provider (eg, direct service staff) who has extensive knowledge of the child and reviews and integrates all available information on a child, including interviews with caregivers and teachers, measures, other collateral reports, and behavioral observations. This strategy is particularly helpful in allowing providers to make sense of the wealth of information available and integrating it all into one place. This composite picture allows the provider to have a comprehensive understanding of the child and his/her functioning based on several sources of information.[6]

Table 1 provides an overview of a range of trauma-specific assessment measures including the source, domains assessed, recommended settings, and context, format, number of items, age ranges, cost, and languages available. These reviews have been adapted from information available on the National Child Traumatic Stress Network (NCTSN) Measure Review Database (www.nctsn.org). A targeted list of recommended measures are outlined, including those assessing trauma exposures, PTSD symptoms/diagnoses, complex trauma responses, as well as other symptom patterns. A more detailed discussion of these measures can be found in other recent publications,[3,6,11,12] and guidelines for how to select appropriate measures are outlined below in the section on Considerations for Selecting and Implementing Assessment Measures. Additional reviews of measures assessing broader complex trauma responses, mental health symptoms, and functional difficulties are also reviewed in detail elsewhere, as noted in **Table 1**.

Using a Range of Assessment Approaches and Techniques

Regardless of the age of the child, the clinician will need to make an effort to gather information from a variety of sources including key adults in the youth's life, and multiple reporters who interact with the youth in different settings (eg, all involved caregivers, teachers). In addition to using a range of measures, it is important to gather information using other formats including clinical interviews, collateral interviews, and behavioral observations.

The clinical interview is an important component of the assessment process to support and enhance information collected through standardized measures. As a part of this process, a clinician should take great care in asking highly personal and sensitive questions and be aware that youth may be hesitant sharing information in this manner, especially if doing so for the first time. Therefore, it may be beneficial to gather sensitive information first from primary caregivers and professionals who are familiar with the child's functioning (eg, as part of a collateral interview) and may be aware of his/her trauma exposure history (eg, caseworker) before asking the youth directly about the trauma. This order may allow the clinician to put a child at ease by already "knowing some pieces of information," sharing this knowledge with the child as a means of engagement, and relying on the child for clarification, feedback, and potential disclosure of new information by the child (eg, traumas unknown to adult caregivers). In an ideal scenario, the youth, especially if in grade school or older, will be made aware of the identified needs/concerns as well as the strengths that have been expressed by the various adults during the assessment, so that presenting problems can be discussed openly and with transparency. This information should always be communicated to the child in an accurate but developmentally appropriate and sensitive manner.

Finally, behavioral observations of the child and his/her family are also important to consider. Observing a child's body language, emotional responses, and choices about what he/she shares and does not share provides insight into how the child is coping, how open he/she is to receiving help, and the attributions he/she has concerning the trauma. Observing the child and family members together also provides useful information on family roles, development, attachment, and interpersonal functioning. For instance, family members may reorganize or shift how they relate to the child following the trauma (eg, becoming overprotective, overinvolved, or even dismissive). Observing these dynamics and sharing this feedback with the family may be beneficial for the clinician and the treatment process.

Making Sense of Discrepant Information

Integrating information from the assessment process can be straightforward when the results of assessment measures and clinical observations support one another. At other times, integrating this information may be more challenging due to differences in the way reporters characterize the child's functioning, and the complexity of many children's trauma histories and presentations. It is not uncommon for the caregiver and child report of symptoms and functioning to have some discrepancies. The clinician is still charged with the task of identifying treatment goals even when the caregiver and child disagree about the symptom presentation. Therefore, when inconsistent reports exist, clinicians must draw on other sources of information such as the clinical interview, observation, and collateral sources to determine which report most accurately reflects the child's current functioning. In clinical practice, abused children may be likely to report fewer symptoms than their caregivers. When a caregiver denies problems that a child reports, it may be a signal for the clinician to address family and systemic needs. It is important for clinicians to understand that discrepant reports may have many different meanings, including the following: (1) children may exhibit different observable behaviors in different settings; (2) adults may have different inherent ability or sensitivity to observe and report different types of behaviors (eg, internalized vs externalized) and thus be more reliable reporters of specific types of problems; and/or (3) all observers, including the clinician and other providers, may bring their own biases to

Table 1
Selected and recommended child and adolescent trauma-focused assessment tools[a]

Measure	Source	Domains/ Recommended Setting(s)	Items	Ages	Format	Language(s)	Cost
Child & Adolescent Needs & Strengths (CANS)–Trauma Comprehensive	Kisiel et al, 2010[29]	TE, PTSD, CTR, FI, INT, EXT, STR, ATT CS	110	0–18	Clinician	English	Free
Child PTSD Symptom Scale (CPSS)	Foa et al, 2001[30]	PTSD, FI CS	24	8–18	Youth	English, Armenian[b]	Free
Child's Reaction to Traumatic Events Scale–Revised (CRTES-R)	Jones et al, 2002[31]	PTSD CS	23	6–18	Youth	English, Spanish	Free
Child Sexual Behavior Inventory (CSBI)	Friedrich, 1997[32]	FI, SB CSA	38	2–12	Caregiver	English, Dutch, French, German[c]	$2.20
Child Stress Disorders Checklist (CSDC)	Saxe et al, 2003[33]	PTSD, FI, EXT SS, CS	36	2–18	Observer	English	Free
Children's Impact of Traumatic Events Scale–Revised (CITES-R)	Wolfe et al, 1991[34]	PTSD, SB CSA	78	8–16	Clinician	English	Free
Children's PTSD Inventory (CPTSD-I)	Saigh et al, 2000[35]	TE, PTSD CS	50	6–18	Youth	English, French, Spanish	$161
Clinician-Administered PTSD Scale for Children & Adolescents (CAPS-CA)	Nader et al, 1996[36]	PTSD, FI, STR DIS, CS	32	8–15	Youth	English	$115
Diagnostic Infant & Preschool Assessment (DIPA)	Scheeringa & Haslett, 2010[37]	TE, PTSD, INT, EXT, ATT CS	517	0–6	Caregiver	English	Free
Kauai Recovery Index (KRI)	Hamada et al, 2003[38]	TE, PTSD DIS	24	6–15	Youth	English	Free
Posttraumatic Stress Disorder Semi-Structured Interview & Observational Record (PTSDSSI)	Scheeringa & Zeanah, 1994[39]	TE, PTSD, FI CS	29	0–7	Parent/ caregiver	English, German, Hebrew, Spanish	Free

Measure	Reference	Constructs	Items	Ages	Reporter	Languages	Cost
PTSD in Preschool Aged Children (PTSD-PAC)	Levendosky et al, 2002[40]	PTSD, CS	18	2–5	Caregiver	English	Free
Structured Interview for Disorders of Extreme Stress–Adolescent Version (SIDES-A)	Pelcovitz et al, 2005[41]	CTR, FI, INT, EXT, SB, ATT, CS	50	12–18	Clinician	English, Spanish	Free
Trauma & Attachment Belief Scale (TABS)	Pearlman, 2003[42]	TE, INT, ATT, CS	84	9–99	Youth	English	$47
Trauma Symptom Checklist for Children (TSCC)	Briere, 1996[43]	PTSD, CTR, INT, CSA, DIS, CS	54	8–16	Youth	English, Chinese, Dutch, French[d]	$172
Trauma Symptom Checklist for Young Children (TSCYC)	Briere, 2005[44]	PTSD, CTR, INT, CS, CSA	90	3–12	Caregiver	English, Spanish, Swedish	$230
Traumatic Events Screening Inventory (TESI) & TESI-Revised	Ford & Rogers, 1997[45]; Ippen et al, 2002[46]	TE, CS	16 or 24	0–18	Clinician, youth, &/or caregiver	English, Finnish, Portuguese, Spanish	Free
UCLA PTSD Reaction Index–Revised (UCLA PTSD RI-R)	Pynoos et al, 1999[47]	TE, PTSD, DIS, SS, CS	22	6–18	Youth	English, Arabic, Armenian, Chinese[e]	$1.30 per copy
Youth Outcome Questionnaire (Y-OQ) & Y-OQ Self-Report (Y-OQ-SR)	Burlingame et al, 2004[48]; Wells et al, 2003[49]	CTR, FI, INT, EXT, CS	64	4–17 12–18	Caregiver Youth	English, Dutch, French, Spanish, Swedish, Korean	$75 and up

Abbreviations: ATT, attachment/relationships; CS, cross settings; CSA, child sexual abuse; CTR, complex trauma response; DIS, postdisaster; EXT, externalizing; FI, functional impairment; INT, internalizing; PTSD, PTSD symptoms and/or diagnosis; SB, sexual behaviors; SS, school settings; STR, strengths; TE, trauma exposure.

[a] Many of these tools are included in the NCTSN Measures Review Database (www.nctsn.org/resources/online-research/measures-review). For additional measures specific to complex trauma, see www.nctsn.org/trauma-types/complex-trauma-types/complex-trauma/assessment.

[b] Korean, Russian, Spanish.

[c] Latvian, Lithuanian, Moldovan, Polish, Spanish, Swedish.

[d] Japanese, Latvian, Slovenian, Spanish, Swedish.

[e] Farsi/Persian, Filipino/Tagalog, French, German, Greek, Hebrew, Japanese, Norwegian, Russian, Spanish, Visayan, Nyanja.

Adapted from Crandal B, Conradi L. Review of child and adolescent trauma screening tools. San Diego (CA): Rady Children's Hospital, Chadwick Center for Children and Families; 2013; with permission.

observing, interpreting, and reporting the child's symptoms. It is important that clinicians make note of the discrepancies, looking for specific trends in the types of information that have been collected. For example, do the results from measures and behavioral observations suggest depressive symptoms, but the child is denying such symptoms? This information can then be shared with the child and family with specific questions designed to understand and make sense of the discrepant information, highlighting these issues and offering potential hypotheses. Therefore, although these discrepancies may present some challenges, they also provide an ideal opportunity to gain a greater understanding of the underlying issues, while also engaging the family in the treatment process by promoting discussion about these concerns.

CONSIDERATIONS FOR SELECTING AND IMPLEMENTING ASSESSMENT MEASURES

Before selecting measures to use for assessment purposes, there are several key questions that should be considered. **Table 2** highlights key questions for an agency or practitioner to consider when identifying and implementing assessment tools.

Table 2
Key questions to consider when implementing assessment tools

Domain	Question
Purpose	• What is the purpose of the tool? • Can it be used to facilitate decision-making or inform clinical practice?
Research	• What type of research has been conducted on the tool? • Does it have established reliability and validity and norms? • Has it been used with diverse (varied ethnic and racial) populations?
Language	• Is the tool available in the languages used by our clients?
Cost	• How can one obtain the measure? • Are certain qualifications required to order or administer the measure? • What is our budget? • What is the cost of the tool?
Administration and scoring	• How long does it take to administer? Are there specific time constraints in our setting? • Are there a range of formats we can use (eg, self-report, caregiver report or provider/clinician report)? • How is the measure scored? Do we need to work with information technology to create a system that scores and/or stores the information?
Feedback	• Are we able to provide feedback to the clinician or other staff in an efficient, understandable, and timely manner? • How is the information shared with the clinician? How is that information then shared with the child, caregivers, or family?
Staff education, training, and experience	• What staff do we have available to administer the tool? • What is their level of education and experience? • How much extra time is involved in completing the measure and then using the information for case and/or treatment planning purposes?
Measure change over time	• Does the measure track change over time and allow us to see if the child or adolescent has improved?

Similarly, Strand and colleagues[12] identify several considerations to take into account when selecting trauma-focused measures based on the needs of various settings or populations. They suggest looking at the degree to which the instrument is designed to measure history of trauma exposure as well as trauma-related symptoms; considering whether the measure focuses on PTSD or assesses complex trauma reactions more broadly; and considering whether it would make sense to include tools that focus specifically on one aspect of traumatic stress reactions (eg, dissociation) and/or a specific type of event (eg, sexual abuse). Furthermore, it is important to gather information on the properties of the tool (eg, reliability and validity) and determine in what settings or contexts it has been used (eg, clinic- or community-based, with ethnically diverse populations) to ensure it meets the needs in specific settings. Finally, it is useful to consider several practical issues including time to administer, cost, and the format of tools that would work in particular settings (eg, child report, provider report).[12]

The choice of assessment tools will sometimes depend on the type of events the child has experienced and his or her initial symptoms. For example, a survivor of sexual abuse may benefit from tools designed to assess more common reactions to sexual abuse (eg, attributions of shame/blame; dissociation; sexual behavior problems). Although the resources and capacity of staff at a given agency should always be taken into consideration, normed measures with solid psychometric properties should be used whenever possible. These tools are sometimes costly to purchase and administration may require specialized levels of training or licensure, but they can also allow for more reliable findings. There are times when the burden associated with specific types of techniques (eg, lengthy, diagnostic interview schedules) may actually outweigh the benefit. Finally, it may be that the initial trauma assessment identifies issues that may be more appropriately referred for a specialized assessment (eg, neuropsychological testing for cognitive processing issues, occupational therapy assessment for motor abnormalities).

The identification of specific measures that are useful, reliable, and valid; provide helpful information for both the clinician and families; translate readily into treatment planning; and do not add undue burden to the clinician or to the system is not without its share of challenges and barriers.[11] There is not one measure that universally meets the needs of all children who have been affected by trauma. Also, there is a cost-benefit analysis that systems need to conduct as they consider the integration of a tool in their agency practice. Although one tool may have sound psychometric properties, it may be cost-prohibitive or may require that providers have an advanced level of training and experience. On the other hand, another tool may be brief and easy for clinicians to complete but may not have solid psychometric properties or may not generate useful information to assist in treatment planning efforts. These factors are all important to consider in combination.

Factors for Consideration Across Contexts and Settings

Characteristics of each trauma assessment will also be informed by the settings and contexts in which it occurs, as well as by the level of trauma training of the staff completing the assessment. For instance, assessments in the context of disaster response will likely involve a targeted, triage-based, safety and services–deployment orientation in the short term;[14] whereas, over the longer term, they may take the form of a more in-depth trauma exposure and symptom-based assessment that is typical of an outpatient clinic setting. School-based trauma assessment may initially focus on manifestations of the trauma response most obviously related to difficulties with school behavior and achievement. However, to integrate these into a comprehensive picture of a child's overall trauma-related symptoms, clinicians in school-based settings may benefit from training on assessment that incorporates a wider "trauma lens."[15] In pediatric medical settings, a child's unique physical health care needs should be integrated with his or her mental health care needs, involving collaboration between medical social workers, psychological and/or psychiatric services, and physicians in the assessment process.

Developmental and Cultural Considerations

Selection of assessment tools and strategies needs to also be determined by specific developmental and cultural considerations. Exposure to trauma can have a pervasive impact across areas of development and functioning, and it is important to consider these effects in the context of a child's developmental stage. Manifestations of traumatic stress typically vary by developmental stages across trauma exposure types,[16] including specific to disaster-related responses[17]; thus, the process of assessment must also be sensitive to these developmental effects. The developmental stage of the child may also influence the reliability of his/her report. When working with young children, is it essential to keep in mind their more limited capacity to comprehend and accurately recount the timing of events. Likewise, adolescents may be more self-conscious or anxious about disclosing specific events or symptoms during an assessment, especially if they are unsure with whom the information will be shared.

Incorporating cultural sensitivity into the trauma assessment process is also necessary. Cultural factors need to be considered in how the assessment process is implemented and can also influence the ways that traumatic stress is experienced and expressed by youth.[18] Some considerations include determining the degree to which the child and family are acculturated to mainstream culture, as well as their preferred language for verbal communication, reading, and writing. For instance, a family may have culturally specific beliefs about certain types of trauma (eg, use of severe corporal punishment). Likewise, certain subcultures may have strong ideas about the types of information that are appropriate to be shared with people outside of their immediate family; this is essential to keep in mind during a trauma assessment. Efforts should be made to respect the child's and family's cultural beliefs and practices whenever possible during the assessment and treatment planning process. Furthermore, it is also beneficial for the family to have all aspects of the assessment conducted in their primary language.

Practical Considerations for Staff

Across all contexts and settings, effective trauma assessment relies on the skills of clinicians who have received adequate training in responding to child traumatic stress; in many cases, additional staff training and consultation on traumatic stress reactions can also provide the basis for improved assessment. In certain situations, it may be difficult for the clinician or other providers (eg, caseworkers) to listen and respond to a child's trauma history in a way that is supportive and encouraging to the child. Therefore, it is equally important for providers working with children and families exposed to trauma to be trained and attuned to their own potential symptoms of secondary trauma as well as related self-care strategies to support them in their work.[6] For these reasons, it is recommended that only staff with appropriate knowledge and training in child traumatic stress take an active role in conducting a trauma assessment.

Furthermore, although assessment can be a challenging and time-consuming process for staff, it may be particularly difficult for children and caregivers because they are often asked to share highly personal details within a relatively short amount of time. Thus, paying attention to the engagement of youth, caregivers, and other family members throughout the assessment process is important. Building trust and rapport with families, establishing a process that is safe, understandable, predictable, and confidential are important first steps; this can be done in a variety of ways and should meet the specific needs of each individual child/family. Limits on confidentiality should also be addressed up front and the child/family should be made aware of how assessment information and results will be solicited and shared. The order and flow of the assessment process can also help to set the child at ease. Whenever possible it is preferable to start with discussion of neutral topics or child/family strengths and to try and build some rapport; this is part of the initial engagement process that can occur within a short period of time (ie, in as little as a few minutes) and can be followed by collecting details about more challenging topics, including trauma experiences and reactions. This process can occur over the course of one or more sessions, as time allows, in a given agency setting. Finally, to be able to use assessment information in an effective way with caregivers and families, the clinician also needs to understand the meaning of scores on the measures and any limits to the information (eg, based on psychometric properties of the tools). **Box 1** lists practical tips for assessment.

APPLICATION OF TRAUMA ASSESSMENT INFORMATION IN CLINICAL PRACTICE

An enhanced focus has been placed on strategies to improve youth and caregiver engagement through both the assessment and the treatment process. The term "assessment translation" can be used to describe how to apply assessment information in a meaningful way to inform clinical practice. This section overviews how to use assessment to enhance engagement, guide treatment planning, and support the delivery of treatment services. Tips for translating assessment information and the use of available resources are also discussed in this section.

Despite the relatively robust relationship between trauma exposure and a range of symptoms and responses,[1,5,13] mental health services (including access to assessment and treatment) are generally underused and characterized by high rates of dropout with families engaged in services. To increase both access to and the quality of services for children and families impacted by trauma, several advances have been made within the child-trauma field. Some of these include considerable attention to reducing barriers to service utilization[19] by improving systems for screening and referral to qualified mental health professionals; increased awareness of the need to develop trauma-informed providers and agencies; and a proliferation of effective trauma-focused treatments for children exposed to trauma.[20–22]

Recent research has focused on overcoming many of the barriers to successful completion of treatment and identifying strategies to enhance clinical engagement. McKay and Bannon[23] have designed intensive engagement interventions that have effectively increased rates of service utilization and treatment completion.[24] Many of these efforts include critical strategies that can be integrated into both the assessment and the treatment process and include the following: (1) clarifying the need for child mental health treatment of both the caregiver and the provider; (2) maximizing the caregiver's investment and sense of efficacy in relation to help-seeking; (3) identifying attitudes about and previous experiences with mental health care that might discourage caregivers from bringing their children for services; and (4) developing strategies to overcome concrete (eg, transportation, scheduling, child care issues), contextual (eg, community violence), and agency (eg, wait list, parking) obstacles.

Moreover, with children and families exposed to trauma, it may be particularly helpful to provide psychoeducation about normal reactions to trauma; discuss the need for support and referral for services with caregivers who are also affected by the trauma; and collaborate with community partners (eg, child welfare, law enforcement, schools) to ensure access to community-based resources and services for children who need them the most. Because comprehensive assessment is a critical component of the intervention process, it also serves as a logical vehicle for clarifying the rationale for assessment and treatment, addressing concerns, sharing relevant information, communicating expectations, and demystifying the therapeutic process. This assessment can allow an important opportunity for initial engagement by sharing the purpose and benefits of the assessment process, including how fully understanding the child's needs and strengths will enable the clinician to best help the family. Some suggestions include providing a clear, nonthreatening rationale for the assessment and also being mindful to the timing of the assessment (eg, avoiding anniversaries of traumatic events if possible). This process can also help to facilitate a discussion of concrete, contextual, and agency level barriers that may interfere with the therapeutic process while generating ideas for how to address these issues.[23,24]

Using assessment information to engage families also extends to treatment planning, selection, and delivery. In particular, considering a range of perspectives in the assessment process (eg, youth, parent, teachers) and sharing feedback with families in a manner that is sensitive to their needs, validates their experiences, and highlights their strengths can instill a sense of hope. This can be reassuring that the impact of trauma on their lives is understood and can be addressed.[20] This reassurance also supports collaboration with the child and caregiver in generating treatment goals and targets and together monitoring changes or improvements over time. These steps are central to the process of engaging in collaborative treatment planning with family members and developing assessment-driven treatment goals that are responsive to needs.[10]

Challenges

There are a few challenges to using assessment information in clinical practice that are particularly heightened in the context of trauma. The first issue centers on the complex nature of child development when assessing for the range of needs following exposure to trauma. Given many of the developmental considerations noted previously, it is important to consider that children may lack the language to describe internal states, certain events, or experiences (eg, feelings of shame associated with sexual abuse), and their perceptions and reactions to traumatic events may be drastically different from that of adults. Furthermore, these perceptions of traumatic events can change as children develop and attain more complex and accurate language and knowledge for past traumatic events—making it common for children to have substantially delayed and varied reactions to trauma. For example, it is not uncommon for children who were sexually abused early in childhood to first develop PTSD in early adolescence when both language and knowledge related to sexual behavior matures.[25]

Another consideration relates to the secondary adversities, legal consequences, and system-level interventions (eg, family separation, divorce, incarceration, loss of resources, foster care placement) that may result from disclosure of the traumatic event. Similarly, children and caregivers may minimize, underestimate, or fail to disclose an event or related symptoms because of developmental, cultural, or contextual factors and/or fears regarding inadvertent consequences, which, in turn, may result in delays in identification of needs, assessment, and help-seeking. Finally, there are also challenges related to secondary traumatic stress and/or training that may affect a provider's ability and comfort level with administering, interpreting, and communicating assessment information in a way that will support the treatment process[6]; this is where further support, training, and consultation for providers is needed to help make the assessment process more meaningful and relevant for youth and families receiving services.

Resources

This section delineates several assessment resources that can be easily integrated into continuing education efforts, including training and consultation for providers regarding the assessment process. The following links (current at the time of publication) can connect the reader to valuable web-based resources. The first link is to the NCTSN Measures Review Database. As referenced previously, this includes descriptions (eg, psychometric properties, citations, reading level) of many of the measures referenced in this article, as well as other available measures that can enhance assessment and clinical care (http://www.nctsn.org/resources/online-research/measures-review). The next link is to the California Evidence-based Clearinghouse for Child Welfare Assessment Tools Web site (http://www.cebc4cw.org/assessment-tools/); this shares many of the characteristics of the NCTSN Measures Review Database. The Academy on Violence and Abuse Web site overviews the core competencies for training in trauma assessment and can be found along with other resources (http://www.avahealth.org/resources/resource_index/). Finally, the reader may benefit from additional trauma-focused resources on subpopulations of youth (eg, young children, adolescents, complex trauma, cultural/ethnic minorities, lesbian, gay, bisexual, transgender, and questioning youth, military families) and across service systems (schools, child welfare, juvenile justice); thus, the final 2 links are the NCTSN Learning Center (http://learn.nctsn.org/) and general NCTSN Web site (www.nctsn.org) with instructional videos, speaker series/Webinars, training curricula, tool kits, and fact sheets.

FUTURE DIRECTIONS AND CONCLUSIONS

There has been tremendous progress over the past several years in developing and refining existing tools and techniques for assessing the effects of child trauma, yet there are areas for future development and continued progress. Several tools have been established and successfully implemented to assess a range of key domains across settings, some with a broad focus and others with a more detailed assessment of specific domains.[3,6,11,12] Some existing gaps remain in types of tools for specific populations as well as "how-to" strategies to support the meaningful application of these tools in practice.[10,11] A focus on developing and refining trauma assessment tools that are developmentally sensitive and targeted to assessing age-specific outcomes across development is also a continued need.[12,26] This need includes designing tools that are feasible for use with young children[3,26] and those that capture the multiple and varied trauma responses among adolescents.[12] Furthermore, development of more detailed assessments of child strengths or resiliency factors—either separately or as part of a broader, comprehensive tool—is also a need. Especially in light of an increased focus on understanding the "multilevel" factors comprising resilience,[27] the range of strengths that also exist among youth with complex trauma responses,[5] and the potential importance of strengths as a moderator of risk behaviors among traumatized youth[13] are factors that support the importance of more fully assessing strengths and integrating them into the treatment planning process. Finally, despite the myriad of tools available, there still seem to be relatively few assessments that are psychometrically promising, free of charge, and accessible.[12]

With the release of the *Fifth Edition of the Diagnostic and Statistical Manual of Mental Disorders (DSM-5)*,[28] there are several new requirements for assessment tools that accurately assess for the revised PTSD diagnosis, which has undergone several important changes. Among these changes are several adjustments to the diagnostic criteria, and the addition of 2 new subtypes (ie, PTSD Preschool Subtype and PTSD Dissociative Subtype).[28] This not only requires adjustments to existing assessment tools but also training and education to support the accurate assessment of these clinical manifestations.

Finally, based on existing gaps identified in the literature and across practice settings, there seems to be a need for additional resources to support the use of trauma assessments in clinical practice settings.[10,11] As noted above, collaborating with caregivers and family members in the assessment process and using this information to guide effective treatment planning and engagement with families are of benefit to families and a critical part of treatment and services.[10,20] Nevertheless, challenges exist among providers as how to actually use assessment tools to support and facilitate engagement and subsequently translate assessment data in a meaningful way so that it is useful for caregivers and family members who are receiving trauma-informed services;[11] this seems to be an important area for continued development.

SUMMARY

The comprehensive assessment of trauma and its effects among children and adolescents is a critical part of trauma-informed treatment and service planning, family engagement, and intervention across settings. Using assessment strategies that are broad in assessing a range of exposures and domains of impact, targeted to the needs of clients and providers in a range of contexts and settings (eg, after disaster, school-based, or clinic settings), and sensitive to specific developmental effects and cultural factors are key to an effective assessment process. This process will likely require the use of several different tools and techniques (eg, structured measures, interviews, observations) with information gathered from a range of perspectives (as feasible) to have a thorough and accurate understanding of the child, caregiver, and family's needs and strengths that can be used to support the treatment process directly. It is recommended that assessment is (1) integrated into existing clinical practices in a given agency setting, identifying tools and strategies that are feasible for clinicians to complete both at the outset and over time; (2) gathered and shared at multiple time points and in a manner that is both sensitive and beneficial to the family; (3) used to guide collaborative treatment planning and goal setting with families; (4) used to target intervention strategies that address a child's and family's unique needs while highlighting and integrating strengths; and (5) used to monitor progress in treatment and identify any new needs that have emerged and may require adjustments to treatment or services or additional targeted interventions. If this comprehensive approach is implemented, the assessment process can then truly be used as a tool as it is intended: to facilitate engagement, communication, and strengths-building with family members, to foster communication and integrate services across all relevant providers and systems, and to support and empower the child in recovering from trauma and in continued growth and development.

REFERENCES

1. Briere J, Spinazzola J. Assessment of the sequelae of complex trauma. In: Courtois C, Ford J, editors. Treating complex traumatic stress disorders. New York: Guilford Press; 2009. p. 104–23.
2. Courtois C. Complex trauma, complex reactions: assessment and treatment. Psychother Theor Res Pract Train 2004;41(4):412–25. Available at: PsycINFO, Ipswich (MA). Accessed September 27, 2013.
3. Hawkins S, Radcliffe J. Current measures of PTSD for children and adolescents. J Pediatr Psychol 2006;31(4):420–30. Available at: PsycINFO, Ipswich (MA). Accessed September 27, 2013.
4. Kisiel C, Blaustein ME, Fogler J, et al. Treating children with traumatic experiences: understanding and assessing needs & strengths. In: Lyons JS, Weiner DA, editors. Behavioral health care: assessment, service planning, & total clinical outcomes management. Kingston (NJ): Civic Research Institute; 2009. p. 17.1–17.18.
5. Kisiel C, Fehrenbach T, Small L, et al. Assessment of complex trauma exposure, responses, and service needs among children and adolescents in child welfare. J Child Adolesc Trauma 2009;2(3):143–60.
6. Conradi L, Wherry J, Kisiel C. Linking child welfare and mental health using trauma-informed screening and assessment practices. Child Welfare 2011; 90(6):129–47. Available at: Consumer Health Complete - EBSCOhost, Ipswich (MA). Accessed September 24, 2013.
7. Hatfield D, Ogles B. The use of outcome measures by psychologists in clinical practice. Prof Psychol Res Pract 2004;35(5):485–91. Available at: PsycINFO, Ipswich (MA). Accessed September 27, 2013.
8. Lyons JS, Weiner DA. An introduction and overview of Total Clinical Outcomes Management and Communimetrics. In: Lyons JS, Weiner DA, editors. Behavioral health care: assessment, service planning, & total clinical outcomes management. Kingston (NJ): Civic Research Institute; 2009. p. 1-1–1-16.
9. Lambert M, Whipple J, Smart D, et al. The effects of providing therapists with feedback on patient progress during psychotherapy: are outcomes enhanced? Psychother Res 2001;11(1):49–68. Available at: PsycINFO, Ipswich (MA). Accessed September 27, 2013.
10. Lyons JS. Redressing the emperor: improving our children's public mental health care system. Westport (CT): Praeger; 2004. p. 127–77.
11. Ohan J, Myers K, Collett B. Ten-year review of rating scales. IV: scales assessing trauma and its effects. J Am Acad Child Adolesc Psychiatry 2002;41(12): 1401–22. Available at: PsycINFO, Ipswich (MA). Accessed September 27, 2013.
12. Strand V, Sarmiento T, Pasquale L. Assessment and screening tools for trauma in children and adolescents: a review. Trauma Violence Abuse 2005;6(1):55–78. Available at: CINAHL, Ipswich (MA). Accessed September 24, 2013.
13. Griffin G, Martinovich Z, Gawron T, et al. Strengths moderate the impact of trauma on risk behavior in child welfare. Resid Treat Child Youth 2009;26(2):105–18. Available at: PsycINFO, Ipswich (MA). Accessed September 24, 2013.
14. Speier A. Immediate needs assessment following catastrophic disaster incidents. In: Ritchie EC, Watson PJ, Friedman MJ, editors. Interventions following mass violence & disasters. New York: Guilford Press; 2006. p. 80–99.
15. Tishelman A, Haney P, O'Brien J, et al. A framework for school-based psychological evaluations: utilizing a 'trauma lens'. J Child Adolesc Trauma 2010;3(4): 279–302. Available at: Child Development & Adolescent Studies, Ipswich (MA). Accessed September 24, 2013.

16. Pynoos RS, Steinberg AM, Wraith R. A developmental model of childhood traumatic stress. In: Cicchetti D, Cohen DJ, editors. Developmental psychopathology, vol. 2: risk, disorder, and adaptation. Oxford (England): John Wiley & Sons; 1995. p. 72–95.

17. Dogan-Ates A. Developmental differences in children's and adolescents' post-disaster reactions. Issues Ment Health Nurs 2010;31(7):470–6. Available at: PsycINFO, Ipswich (MA). Accessed August 15, 2013.

18. Nader K. Culture and the assessment of trauma in youths. Cross-cultural assessment of psychological trauma and PTSD [e-book]. New York: Springer Science + Business Media; 2007. p. 169–96. Available at: PsycINFO, Ipswich (MA). Accessed August 15, 2013.

19. Owens PL, Hoagwood K, Horowitz SM, et al. Barriers to children's mental health services. J Am Acad Child Adolesc Psychiatry 2002;41(6):731–8.

20. Cohen JA, Mannarino AP, Deblinger E. Assessment strategies for traumatized children. In: Cohen JA, Mannarino AP, Deblinger E, editors. Treating trauma and traumatic grief in children and adolescents: a clinician's guide. New York: Guilford Press; 2006. p. 20–31.

21. Forbes D, Creamer M, Ursano R, et al. A guide to guidelines for the treatment of PTSD and related conditions. J Trauma Stress 2010;23(5):537–52. Available at: Academic Search Premier, Ipswich (MA). Accessed September 24, 2013.

22. Saunders BE, Berliner L, Hanson R, editors. Child sexual and physical abuse: guidelines for treatment (Revised report: April 26, 2004). Charleston (SC): National Crime Victims Research and Treatment Center; 2004. Available at: http://academicdepartments.musc.edu/ncvc/resources_prof/OVC_guidelines04-26-04.pdf. Accessed September 24, 2013.

23. McKay M, Bannon W. Engaging families in child mental health services. Child Adolesc Psychiatr Clin N Am 2004;13(4):905–21. Available at: PsycINFO, Ipswich (MA). Accessed September 24, 2013.

24. Gopalan G, Goldstein L, Klingenstein K, et al. Engaging families into child mental health treatment: updates and special considerations. J Can Acad Child Adolesc Psychiatry 2010;19:3.

25. Wondie Y, Zemene W, Reschke K, et al. The psychometric properties of the amharic version of the children's impact of traumatic events scale-revised: a study on child sexual abuse survivors in Ethiopia. J Child Adolesc Trauma 2012;5(4):367–78.

26. Stover C, Berkowitz S. Assessing violence exposure and trauma symptoms in young children: a critical review of measures. J Trauma Stress 2005;18(6):707–17. Available at: Academic Search Premier, Ipswich (MA). Accessed September 24, 2013.

27. Cicchetti D. Annual research review: resilient functioning in maltreated children - past, present, and future perspectives. J Child Psychol Psychiatry 2013;54(4):402–22. Available at: Academic Search Premier, Ipswich (MA). Accessed September 24, 2013.

28. American Psychiatric Association. Diagnostic and statistical manual of mental disorders. 5th edition. Arlington (VA): American Psychiatric Publishing; 2013.

29. Kisiel C, Lyons JS, Blaustein M, et al. Child and adolescent needs and strengths (CANS) manual: The NCTSN CANS Comprehensive – Trauma Version: a comprehensive information integration tool for children and adolescents exposed to traumatic events. Chicago, IL; Los Angeles (CA) & Durham (NC): Praed Foundation; National Center for Child Traumatic Stress; 2010.

30. Foa E, Johnson K, Feeny N, et al. The Child PTSD symptom scale: a preliminary examination of its psychometric properties. J Clin Child Psychol 2001;30(3): 376–84. Available at: PsycINFO, Ipswich (MA). Accessed January 31, 2014.
31. Jones RT, Fletcher K, Ribbe DR. Child's Reaction to Traumatic Events Scale-Revised (CRTES-R): a self report traumatic stress measure. Blacksburg (VA): Available from the author, Department of Psychology, Stress and Coping Lab, Virginia Tech University; 2002.
32. Friedrich WN. Child sexual behavior inventory: professional manual. Odessa (FL): Psychological Assessment Resources; 1997.
33. Saxe G, Chawla N, King L, et al. Child stress disorders checklist: a measure of ASD and PTSD in children. J Am Acad Child Adolesc Psychiatry 2003;42(8): 972–8. Available at: PsycINFO, Ipswich (MA). Accessed January 31, 2014.
34. Wolfe V, Gentile C, Michienzi T, et al. The children's impact of traumatic events scale: a measure of post-sexual-abuse PTSD symptoms. Behav Assess 1991; 13(4):359–83. Available at: PsycINFO, Ipswich (MA). Accessed January 31, 2014.
35. Saigh P, Yasik A, McHugh M, et al. The children's PTSD inventory: development and reliability. J Trauma Stress 2000;13(3):369–80. Available at: PsycINFO, Ipswich (MA). Accessed January 31, 2014.
36. Nader K, Kriegler JA, Blake DD, et al. Clinician-administered PTSD scale, child and adolescent version. White River Junction (VT): National Center for PTSD; 1996.
37. Scheeringa M, Haslett N. The reliability and criterion validity of the diagnostic infant and preschool assessment: a new diagnostic instrument for young children. Child Psychiatry Hum Dev 2010;41(3):299–312. Available at: PsycINFO, Ipswich (MA). Accessed January 31, 2014.
38. Hamada R, Kameoka V, Yanagida E, et al. Assessment of elementary school children for disaster-related posttraumatic stress disorder symptoms: the Kauai recovery index. J Nerv Ment Dis 2003;191(4):268–72. Available at: PsycINFO, Ipswich (MA). Accessed January 31, 2014.
39. Scheeringa MS, Zeanah CH. PTSD semi-structured interview and observational record for infants and young children. New Orleans (LA): Department of Psychiatry and Neurology, Tulane University Health Sciences Center; 1994.
40. Levendosky A, Huth-Bocks A, Semel M, et al. Trauma symptoms in preschool-age children exposed to domestic violence. J Interpers Violence 2002;17(2): 150–64. Available at: PsycINFO, Ipswich (MA). Accessed January 31, 2014.
41. Pelcovitz D, Habib M, DeRosa R, et al. Structured Interview for Disorders of Extreme Stress - Adolescent version (SIDES-A). Unpublished professional manual. 2005.
42. Pearlman LA. Trauma and attachment belief scale. Los Angeles (CA): Western Psychological Services; 2003.
43. Briere J. Trauma symptom checklist for children: professional manual. Lutz (FL): Psychological Assessment Resources; 1996.
44. Briere J. Trauma symptom checklist for young children: Professional manual. Lutz (FL): Psychological Assessment Resources; 2005.
45. Ford JD, Rogers K. Traumatic events screening inventory (TESI). Hanover (NH): National Center for PTSD; 1997.
46. Ippen CG, Ford J, Racusin R, et al. Traumatic events screening inventory - parent report revised. White River Junction (VT): National Center for PTSD; 2002.
47. Pynoos RS, Rodriguez N, Steinberg AM, et al. Reaction index – revised. Los Angeles (CA): Unpublished psychological test, University of California; 1999.

48. Burlingame G, Wells M, Lambert M, et al. Youth outcome questionnaire (Y-OQ). In: Maruish M, editor. The use of psychological testing for treatment planning and outcomes assessment: volume 2: instruments for children and adolescents. 3rd edition. Mahwah (NJ): Lawrence Erlbaum Associates Publishers; 2004. p. 235–73. Available at: PsycINFO, Ipswich (MA). Accessed January 31, 2014.
49. Wells MG, Burlingame GM, Rose PM. Youth outcome questionnaire self-report. Wilmington (DE): American Professional Credentialing Services; 2003.

Outcomes of Traumatic Exposure

Frederick J. Stoddard Jr, MD

KEYWORDS

- Childhood trauma • Posttraumatic sequelae • Resilience
- Trauma and stressor-related disorders

KEY POINTS

- Epidemiology of trauma exposure reveals that outcomes vary, from resilience to psychopathology, to developmental disability or death. Many factors influence outcomes.
- When psychopathologic outcomes are present, comorbidity is the rule.
- Infants and young children tend to be most susceptible, but older children and adolescents also have specific susceptibilities.
- Posttraumatic outcomes can be measured with broad screening and diagnostic instruments that assess longitudinal outcomes.
- DSM-5 includes a new category, Trauma and Stressor-Related Disorders, resulting from traumatic exposures. These ailments include attachment disorder, disinhibited social engagement disorder, adjustment disorder, acute stress disorder, posttraumatic stress disorder (PTSD), and PTSD for children 6 years and younger.
- Traumatic exposures are also associated with separation anxiety disorder, persistent complex bereavement disorder, mood disorders, disruptive behavior disorders, borderline personality, psychoses, somatoform disorders, and substance abuse disorders.
- Awareness of adverse outcomes underscores the importance of early socioeconomic, psychological, school, family, and psychopharmacologic interventions.
- Ethical considerations may influence triage, determination of those at most risk, allocation of services, and how to assess outcomes.
- Advocacy and public policy initiatives are essential to improving outcomes.

INTRODUCTION

Most children will not develop long-standing posttraumatic sequelae. When present, however, traumatic stress in children and adolescents is increasingly recognized globally as a problem affecting child health. Research that documents the scope of exposures and impact, and studies ways to mitigate the individual and social impacts of such widespread trauma, is expanding. This article examines outcomes of childhood traumatic exposure, including resilience, traumatic stress, depression, developmental

Department of Psychiatry, Harvard Medical School, Massachusetts General Hospital, 55 Fruit Street, SHC 610, Boston, MA 02114, USA
E-mail address: fstoddard@mgh.harvard.edu

Child Adolesc Psychiatric Clin N Am 23 (2014) 243–256
http://dx.doi.org/10.1016/j.chc.2014.01.004
1056-4993/14/$ – see front matter © 2014 Elsevier Inc. All rights reserved.

Abbreviations	
DSM-III	*Diagnostic and Statistical Manual of Mental Disorders. Third Edition*
ICD-9	*International Classification of Diseases. Ninth Revision*
PTSD	Posttraumatic stress disorder

pathology, and factors influencing such outcomes. In addition, the article provides extensive sources for further reference, and presents factors influencing response to trauma, nosology and evaluation, interventions, and ethical and public policy issues.

DEFINITIONS

Outcomes refer to individual or group health effects, including mental health effects, after traumatic events.

Psychological trauma is a stress that overwhelms one's ability to cope and reassert equilibrium.

Combined physical and psychological trauma refers to both forms of trauma affecting one individual.

Resilience is the ability to adapt successfully to severe or chronic stress.

Susceptibility in epidemiology refers to an individual who is at risk of a disease.

A disaster is an event that overwhelms a community's ability to cope.

LITERATURE REVIEW

This section is a concise, selective review of a huge and rapidly expanding, complicated body of knowledge informing our understanding of children's psychological responses to traumatic events.

Developmental trauma research has recently identified additional factors that influence posttraumatic outcomes, including:

- Genomics and epigenomics[1,2]
- Stage of biopsychosocial development
- Parental posttraumatic stress disorder (PTSD)[3]
- Socioeconomic and community susceptibility[4]
- Environmental impact
- Proximity
- Pain[5,6] and injury
- Prior trauma or disease, or disasters[7–9]
- Impact on family, social support, and treatment

Some historical impetus for understanding and treating the mental effects of trauma in children, adolescents, and adults, such as the addition of PTSD in the *Diagnostic and Statistical Manual of Mental Disorders Third Edition* (DSM-III),[10] derives from military psychiatry and lessons learned from the Vietnam War, which involved older adolescents as well as adults. Impetus also came from recognition of the enormous traumatic impacts of genocide, child abuse, and rape, and of the psychological effects of other injury or violence in the general population.

Several seminal writings set the stage for understanding child PTSD and developing treatments. In his study of survivors of Hiroshima, Robert Lifton[11] described the horror of atomic weapons and their lasting traumatic impacts on survivors, including children. His observations of reexperiencing, avoidance, and numbing, among other symptoms, helped form the basis of the criteria for PTSD. For children, Lenore Terr's[12] clinical observations and study of the children of Chowchilla who were kidnapped on a school bus provided key insights into the ongoing impact of trauma, including developmental manifestations of reexperiencing such as reenactments and posttraumatic play, as well as omen formation. Her series of studies are a major source informing current understanding of the symptomatology of PTSD in childhood and adolescence. Judith Herman[13] provided direction in the psychotherapy of victims of violence and trauma, especially women.

CLINICAL IMPACT OF TRAUMA IN CHILDREN

Mental trauma is evident in children who manifest acute emotional or psychological symptoms resulting from a broad range of experiences, many of which are described in this issue: "Mass Trauma: Disasters, Terrorism and War" by Chrisman; "School Intervention Related to School and Community Violence" by Jaycox and Stein; "Children's Exposure to Intimate Partner Violence" by MacMillan; "Child Sexual Abuse" by Murray; and "Complex Trauma" by Kliethermes. Children also develop traumatic responses to medical experiences, such as severe illness, burns, or other physical injuries.[8,14]

The National Traumatic Stress Toolkit[15] is especially helpful in providing guidance to health professionals to reduce retraumatization and assist working through traumatic experiences (http://nctsnet.org/nccts/nav.do?pid=typ_mt).

To illustrate the prevalence of physical and sexual abuse, a 2011 national survey reported that of 4503 children aged 1 month to 17 years, 41.2% of children and youth experienced a physical assault within that year, including 10.1% with an assault-related injury; in the subsample of 14- to 17-year-olds, 17.4% of girls and 4.2% of boys reported sexual assault during childhood.[16]

LONGITUDINAL RESPONSES TO TRAUMA

Trauma may result in immediate responses or delayed manifestations of psychological impact (eg, from rape or traumatic brain injury). Stress may result from a single event (eg, a single rape, a motor vehicle accident), or may be caused by continuous or repeated traumas that occur over time (eg, refugee trauma, extended surgical burn treatment, chronic child abuse).[17,18] Research indicates that 30% to 60% of child survivors of some serious disasters develop PTSD, and that about 40% of high school students have witnessed or experienced trauma or violence, with about 3% to 6% meeting PTSD criteria.[19]

OUTCOMES OF PSYCHOLOGICAL AND MENTAL TRAUMA

The varying impacts of childhood trauma are increasingly characterized more specifically. These effects range from initial distress and beneficial effects such as increased resilience[20] and posttraumatic growth, to adverse effects, particularly PTSD,[21] depression, and others. Clinically significant adverse posttraumatic outcomes as described in the DSM-5 or the *International Classification of Diseases Ninth Revision* (ICD-9) include:

- Reactive attachment disorder[22–24]
- Disinhibited social engagement disorder[25]
- Adjustment disorder
- Acute stress reaction
- Acute stress disorder
- PTSD

- New developmental subtype, PTSD in children ages 6 years and younger[26] (see also ICD-9)

Traumatic events have also been associated with separation anxiety, bereavement,[27] and prolonged grief[28,29]; major depression and other mood disorders; and long-term conditions such as disruptive behavior, borderline personality, and major psychotic, somatoform, and substance abuse disorders.[30]

Clinical outcomes have been investigated extensively, with many findings of long-term sequelae of childhood traumatic stress. These sequelae include persistence of posttraumatic symptoms, or alterations in developmental trajectories with impairments in affect regulation and behavioral control, with withdrawal or violence as possible manifestations. Moreover, learning disabilities result from an inability to maintain cognitive focus and executive functioning necessary for academic achievement, or even to relate within the school or home context. These posttraumatic symptoms or alterations in developmental trajectories may result in nonadherence (possibly oppositional or conduct-disordered) behaviors, which result in stigmatization and involvement of outside agencies in attempting to manage delinquent behavior, often including substance abuse. Not infrequently, this may result in disability from illnesses or disorders requiring sustained treatment, or death from somatic complications or behavioral dysregulation.[31]

OUTCOMES RESEARCH IN TRAUMATIZED CHILDREN
Prevalence of Psychological Trauma and Stress

The true prevalence of psychological trauma and stress in children and adolescents is difficult to determine, and may be higher than reported.[32,33] One meta-analysis reported the rate after trauma exposure as approximately 16%.[34] However, a large United States study found a lower lifetime prevalence rate of 4.7% among all adolescents,[35] with higher rates among females (7.3%) than males (2.2%).

Rates of PTSD among child and adolescent survivors of disasters vary widely, from 1% to 60%.[36] Some studies indicate that 30% to 60% of child disaster survivors may develop PTSD, and that about 40% of high school students have witnessed or experienced trauma or violence, with about 3% to 6% manifesting PTSD.[19] The rates vary, in part related to the type of disaster, proximity of exposure, and the degree and extent of the disaster's impact.

In preschool children PTSD may be chronic,[37] and among school-aged children data are mixed: from no long-term impact of a disaster[38] to high rates.[39] In adolescents and adults, PTSD symptoms and impairment may persist for decades (eg, Refs.[40,41]). A meta-analysis of risk factors for PTSD among children and adolescents aged 6 to 18 years[42] identified that factors relating to the experience of the event and posttrauma variables accounted for medium to large effect sizes in predicting PTSD.

WHAT CONSTITUTES CHILD AND ADOLESCENT TRAUMA?

Our understanding of what constitutes a traumatic experience continues to develop. Childbirth, a "normative" experience, is also a stressful event that is now being studied more extensively in adolescent girls as an event that may lead to negative psychological reactions in that population. Rates of PTSD in relation to childbirth vary from 2.8% to 5.6% at 6 weeks postpartum.[43,44] Stressful delivery, for example, preterm birth, significantly increases PTSD up to 24% to 77%. Childbirth PTSD may negatively affect the mother-infant relationship,[45] infant development, and the child's emotional and cognitive development.

Child and adolescent refugees from war zones are exposed to multiple traumas and losses. Although often resilient, many experience PTSD, depression, anxiety, and prolonged grief. There appears to be a dose-effect relationship between cumulative trauma and distress in these children.[46]

SUSCEPTIBILITY, COPING, ADAPTATION, AND RESILIENCE

There is increasing evidence that susceptibility, or risk of adverse outcomes after trauma exposure, varies widely owing to the many factors already described. As a result, there is much interest in understanding resilience factors, which influence the ability to adapt successfully to severe or chronic stress.[47,48] An individual's success in coping with the effects of traumatic events acutely, and adapting to their psychological and physical impacts over time, determines the degree of resilience after the trauma.

Although victims of many types of trauma, including sexual abuse, may lack symptoms consistent with all of the DSM criteria for PTSD, they may present with a set of symptoms similar to that of other trauma victims, which has been called complex trauma (see the article "Complex Trauma" by Kliethermes elsewhere in this issue). This concept[13,49] describes a persistent pattern of comorbidities observed in victims of sexual abuse and other types of interpersonal trauma, including problems in affect regulation, self concept, interpersonal relationships, somatization, and dissociation. Complex trauma was proposed for inclusion in DSM-5 but was not accepted owing to a lack of adequate evidence of construct validity.[50] While addressing complex effects of multiple trauma, modifications in the DSM-5 criteria for PTSD address some of these symptoms, and the focus on dimensionality in the DSM-5 enables clinicians to identify individuals who fall within the spectrum but do not meet the criteria.[51]

Children who are exposed to trauma may manifest subthreshold symptoms of PTSD or may manifest a range of other distressing symptoms of varying types, such as neurovegetative signs of sleep, eating, or interpersonal disturbance while displaying some but not all symptoms of PTSD (eg, avoidance and numbing but not arousal). In eliciting the details of the child's experience through both interview and play, and also from caregiver and other sources, a narrative of the child's experience may over time be understood, and be able to be explained to the child and caregiver if this is indicated and timely, so that the child may achieve some mastery of the experience. For some children, affective or behavioral symptoms will predominate, and psychotherapeutic and/or psychopharmacologic interventions may be necessary.

As already noted and referenced, reactive attachment disorder and other attachment problems are common in severely traumatized or abandoned young children. In addition to the aforementioned symptoms, other common manifestations of stress include disordered body image perceptions and impaired self concept, including blaming the self for traumatic experiences over which the child had no control. Traumatized adolescents have added vulnerabilities that may lead to posttraumatic symptomatology related to their sexuality, substance use, peer and school issues, disabilities, minority status, and susceptibility to abuse or to becoming victims of human trafficking.

TREATMENT PLANNING

Neurobiological considerations are central to the planning of appropriate care.[52] Identification of areas of strength and resilience as well as those of areas where the child is susceptible or vulnerable to preexisting or new dysfunction is essential. This approach can require specific educational or neuropsychological testing to reach a full understanding of the strengths and limitations of the child before planning care. An advantage of this approach is that goals and interventions may be better targeted to fit the capacities of the family and the child's own abilities, and areas identified for ongoing monitoring, such as improved attention in school, greater impulse control, reduced reexperiencing of intrusive traumatic memories, reduced depression, or improvement in areas of acknowledged strength.

In applying knowledge to practice, care of traumatized children and youth primarily must be collaborative with the caregivers, pediatric team, school personnel, and other involved agencies such as early childhood intervention, child protection services, youth services, probation officer, or substance abuse program.

It is important to be able to recognize trauma responses in children, including resilience, susceptibility or increased risk, and posttraumatic psychopathology. Psychosocial interventions that include school and family, in conjunction with psychotherapeutic and psychopharmacologic interventions based on the clinical evaluation, are critical components of care for children who are enduring, or have suffered severe stress.

Strategies informing therapeutic interventions include screening for distress, traumatic stress, other posttraumatic reactions, and protective and resilience factors. The reader is directed to articles in this issue focusing on therapeutic interventions: "Psychological and Pharmacologic Treatment of Youth with Posttraumatic Stress Disorder: An Evidence-Based Review" by Strawn and Keeshin; "Indicated and Selective Preventive Interventions" by Berkowitz; and "Universal Preventive Interventions for Children in the Context of Disasters and Terrorism" by Pfefferbaum. Specific therapeutic strategies include TARGET (Trauma-Focused, Patient-Centered, Emotional Self-Regulation Approach to Integrated Treatment for Posttraumatic Stress and Addiction: Trauma Adaptive Recovery Group Education and Therapy),[53] SPARCS (Structured Psychotherapy for Adolescents Responding to Chronic Stress),[54] ITCT-A (Integrative Treatment of Complex Trauma for Adolescents),[55] and TF-CBT (Trauma-Focused Cognitive Behavior Therapy),[28] discussed elsewhere in this issue.

SCREENING FOR POSTTRAUMA MENTAL EFFECTS

Screening, diagnostic evaluation, and DSM diagnoses assist in the identification of posttraumatic outcomes. Outcomes measures range from broad screening instruments to those that assess specific symptoms or diagnoses, as well as health, resilience, or emotional growth.

PHYSICAL EXAMINATION AND PSYCHIATRIC ASSESSMENT FOR POSTTRAUMA MENTAL EFFECTS

In most situations after trauma, a physical examination and comprehensive assessment are indicated if feasible. Among the key aspects of the comprehensive psychiatric assessment for impacts of trauma are taking the history of physical, psychosocial, and medical details of trauma, abuse, pain, injury, and alcohol or drug use; school/educational/child protective agency/health insurance status; and mental status examination evaluating appearance, orientation, mood especially pain, anxiety, depression, and specific bodily concerns or observed vulnerability; cognition, intellect (especially intellectual disability), judgment; and perceived adequacy and quality of relationships and psychosocial supports.

FAMILY AND SYSTEMS ISSUES

The impact of traumatic experiences on the family may resemble the impact on the child, such as a family witnessing and grieving the death of a loved one together. Although the impact of a traumatic experience on the family may exclude direct exposure of the child (eg, a severe burn to a sibling), the family's increased focus on the sibling can be indirectly traumatic to the child. Other family effects include the parents' own resilience and coping in aiding their children in contrast to their own PTSD adversely affecting their children; adaptive or adverse cultural coping with collective trauma; domestic violence; parental incarceration; and the overall family impact of caregivers who themselves cause trauma.

Systems issues are integral to intervention with traumatized children.[56] These approaches may include child psychiatric consultation or support of first responders, medical teams, and legal, emergency medical technician, police, or fire personnel. Other systems issues that affect families are Child Protective Services investigations, foster care, parent as perpetrator of neglect, domestic violence or sexual abuse, or complex infrastructure and community issues after disaster. The chronology of the impact of trauma or relief of trauma through systems is important. Commonly the impacts last for long periods, and systems initiatives to mitigate trauma may help both early and long after the event.

SELF CARE OF THOSE CARING FOR TRAUMATIZED CHILDREN

Few personal challenges are greater than working with severely traumatized children. Anticipating or responding to one's own needs for supervision, food, sleep, and companionship are essential, especially in emergency situations such as disasters. However, this applies equally to working in clinics, hospitals, and in the community with traumatized children and families.[57]

ETHICAL CONSIDERATIONS IN THE TREATMENT OF TRAUMATIZED CHILDREN

Ethical considerations of varying degrees of difficulty commonly arise in the care of traumatized children. Examples include issues arising in risk communication in anticipation of or following a disaster; whether quarantine may be indicated in an epidemic situation; how and when to safeguard abused or neglected children; when to use or not use selected treatments; how and when to choose medications, and which ones; how to be most effective with collaborative clinicians; and whether, and how, to relate to media representatives.

ADVOCACY AND PUBLIC POLICY INITIATIVES
Important Tools for Practice

Depending on the context and type of trauma, there are many different practical tools contained within the online therapeutic strategies cited at the end of Treatment Planning above for measuring the impacts of trauma exposure, including resilience, psychopathology, and developmental disability. Improved screening is enabling identification of the most affected children who are in need of care. Long-term outcomes measures are leading to recognition of the devastating long-term impacts of trauma on development and psychopathology. Awareness of potential adverse outcomes of exposure to trauma is making possible more systematic early social, psychological, and pharmacologic interventions. Ethical considerations include identification of those affected, who to treat, how to provide services, and how to assess outcomes.

FUTURE DIRECTIONS IN CHILD AND ADOLESCENT TRAUMA

Several areas in child and adolescent trauma are in need of future work:

- Greater collection of epidemiologic data in all trauma contexts to guide interventions
- Improved education of clinicians, educators, and parents worldwide on what can and should be done following children's exposure to complex traumatic events
- Further scientific research into the sociopsychological and neurobiological factors affecting trauma outcomes, particularly genomic and epigenomic factors
- New therapeutic and community resource directions to improve long-term outcomes in underserved areas
- Enhanced specialized psychiatric and related systems of care for complex trauma
- Broader training in and dissemination of evidence-based psychotherapeutic, psychopharmacologic, school and family prevention and treatment models
- Increased collaboration among systemic entities
- New advocacy and public policy initiatives to benefit traumatized children and adolescents worldwide

SUMMARY

In children and adolescents, recognition of outcomes after exposure to trauma is of increasing importance. Epidemiologic studies have helped to recognize the devastating long-term impacts of trauma on the lives of children and adolescents. Knowledge of outcomes informs current practice in targeting which children most need services to alleviate the devastating effects of exposure to major trauma. Infants and young children tend to be more susceptible to the adverse effects of trauma because of their dependency, but older children and adolescents are also susceptible in relation to adolescent development, sexuality, substances, school, peer issues, disabilities, minority status, and vulnerability to abuse or human trafficking. Improved screening measures, linked to adverse outcomes, are enabling identification of the most affected children in need of care. Long-term outcomes measures are leading to recognition of the devastating long-term impacts of trauma on development and psychopathology. Awareness of potential adverse outcomes of exposure to trauma is making possible more systematic early social, psychological, pharmacologic, family, school, and public policy interventions. Among future directions are broader training in, and dissemination of screening, psychotherapeutic, and school and family interventions. Ethical considerations include identification of those affected, who to treat, how to provide services both feasibly and optimally, and how to more effectively assess child and adolescent posttraumatic outcomes longitudinally.

REFERENCES

1. Banny AM, Cicchetti D, Rogosch FA, et al. Susceptibility to depression: a mediation model of the roles of child maltreatment, peer victimization, and serotonin transporter linked polymorphism region genetic variation among children from low socioeconomic status backgrounds. Dev Psychopathol 2013;25(3):599–614.
2. Ellis BJ, Boyce WT, Belsky J, et al. Differential susceptibility to the environment: an evolutionary-neurodevelopmental theory. Dev Psychopathol 2011;23(1):7–28.
3. Leen-Feldner EW, Feldner MT, Knapp A, et al. Offspring psychological and biological correlates of parental post-traumatic stress: review of the literature and research agenda. Clin Psychol Rev 2013;33(8):1106–33.

4. Boyce WT, Sokolowski MB, Robinson GE. Toward a new biology of social adversity. Proc Natl Acad Sci U S A 2012;109(Suppl 2):17143–8. http://dx.doi.org/10.1073/pnas.1121264109.

5. Sheridan RL, Stoddard FJ, Kazis LE, et al. Long-Term Post-Traumatic Stress Symptoms Vary Inversely with Early Opiate Dosing in Children Recovering from Serious Burns—Effects Durable At Four Years. 42nd Critical Care Conference of the Society of Critical Care Medicine (SCCM), San Juan, Puerto Rico, January 2013.

6. Stoddard FJ, White GW, Kazis LE, et al. Patterns of medication administration from 2001-2009 in the treatment of children with acute burn injuries: a multicenter study. J Burn Care Res 2011;32:519–28.

7. Bakker A, Maertens KJ, Van Son MJ, et al. Psychological consequences of pediatric burns from a child and family perspective: a review of the empirical literature. Clin Psychol Rev 2013;33(3):361–71.

8. Stuber M, Shemesh E, Saxe GN. Post-traumatic stress responses in children with in life threatening illness. Child Adolesc Psychiatr Clin N Am 2003;12:195–209.

9. Masten AS, Osofsky JD. Disasters and their impact on child development: introduction to the special section. Child Dev 2010;81:1029–39.

10. American Psychiatric Association. Diagnostic and statistical manual of mental disorders. 3rd edition. Washington, DC: American Psychiatric Association; 1980.

11. Lifton RJ. Survivors of Hiroshima. New York: Random House; 1967.

12. Terr LC. Children of Chowchilla: a study of psychic trauma. Psychoanal Study Child 1979;34:547–623.

13. Herman J. Trauma and recovery: the aftermath of trauma: from domestic violence to political terror. New York: Basic Books; 1992.

14. Stoddard FJ, Saxe G. Ten-year research review of physical injuries. J Am Acad Child Adolesc Psychiatry 2001;40(10):1128–45.

15. Stuber M, Kassam-Adams N, Kazak A, et al. The medical traumatic stress toolkit. CNS Spectr 2006;11(2):137–42.

16. Finkelhor D, Turner HA, Shattuck A, et al. Violence, crime and abuse exposure in a national sample of children and youth: an update. JAMA Pediatr 2013;167(7):614–21.

17. Stoddard FJ. Care of infants, children and adolescents with burn Injuries. In: Lewis M, editor. Child and adolescent psychiatry. 3rd edition. Baltimore (MD): Lippincott Williams & Wilkins; 2002. p. 1188–208.

18. Spies G, Afifi TO, Archibald SL, et al. Mental health outcomes in HIV and childhood maltreatment: a systematic review. Syst Rev 2012;1:30. http://dx.doi.org/10.1186/2046-4053-1-30 [review].

19. Kaminer D, Seedat S, Stein DJ, et al. Post-traumatic stress disorder in children. World Psychiatry 2005;4:121–5.

20. Rutter M. Resilience as a dynamic concept. Dev Psychopathol 2012;24:335–44.

21. Chen LP, Murad MH, Paras ML, et al. Sexual abuse and lifetime diagnosis of psychiatric disorders: systematic review and meta-analysis. Mayo Clin Proc 2010;85:618–29.

22. Rutter M, O'Connor TG. Are there biological programming effects for psychological development? Findings from a study of Romanian adoptees. Dev Psychol 2004;40:81–94.

23. van Ijzendoorn MH, Sagi-Schwartz A. Cross-cultural patterns of attachment: universal and contextual dimensions. In: Cassidy J, Shaver PR, editors. Handbook

of attachment: theory, research, and clinical applications. New York: Guilford; 2009. p. 713–34.

24. Zeanah CH, Smyke AT, Koga SF, et al. Attachment in institutionalized and community children in Romania. Child Dev 2005;76:1015–28.

25. Gleason MM, Fox NA, Drury S, et al. Validity of evidence-derived criteria for reactive attachment disorder: indiscriminately social/disinhibited and emotionally withdrawn/inhibited types. J Am Acad Child Adolesc Psychiatry 2011;50: 216–31.e3.

26. American Psychiatric Association. Diagnostic and statistical manual of mental disorders. 5th edition. Washington, DC: American Psychiatric Association; 2013.

27. Kaplow JB, Layne CM, Pynoos RS, et al. DSM-V diagnostic criteria for bereavement-related disorders in children and adolescents: developmental considerations. Psychiatry 2012;75:243–66.

28. Cohen JA, Mannarino AP, Deblinger E. Treating trauma and traumatic grief in children and adolescents. New York: Guilford Press; 2006.

29. Cohen JA, Mannarino AP, Staron VR, et al. A pilot study of modified cognitive-behavioral therapy for childhood traumatic grief (CBT-CTG). J Am Acad Child Adolesc Psychiatry 2006;45:1465–73.

30. Subica AM, Claypoole KH, Wylie AM. PTSD's mediation of the relationships between trauma, depression, substance abuse, mental health, and physical health in individuals with severe mental illness: evaluating a comprehensive model. Schizophr Res 2012;136:104–9.

31. Deans KJ, Thackeray J, Askegard-Giesmann JR, et al. Mortality increases with recurrent episodes of nonaccidental trauma in children. J Trauma Acute Care Surg 2013;75(1):161–5.

32. Fletcher KE. Childhood posttraumatic stress disorder. In: Mash EJ, Barkley RA, editors. Child psychopathology. New York: Guilford Press; 1996. p. 242–76.

33. Cohen JA, Scheeringa MS. Post-traumatic stress disorder diagnosis in children: challenges and promises. Dialogues Clin Neurosci 2009;11:91–9.

34. Alisic E, Zalta AK, van Wesel F, et al. PTSD rates in trauma-exposed children and adolescents: a meta-analysis. Br J Psychiatry, in press.

35. McLaughlin KA, Koenen KC, Hill ED, et al. Trauma exposure and posttraumatic stress disorder in a national sample of adolescents. J Am Acad Child Adolesc Psychiatry 2013;52(8):815–30.e814. http://dx.doi.org/10.1016/j.jaac.2013.05.011.

36. Wang CW, Chan CL, Ho RT. Prevalence and trajectory of psychopathology among child and adolescent survivors of disasters: a systematic review of epidemiological studies across 1987-2011. Soc Psychiatry Psychiatr Epidemiol 2013;48(11):1697–720. http://dx.doi.org/10.1007/s00127-013-0731-x.

37. Scheeringa MS, Wright MJ, Hunt JP, et al. Factors affecting the diagnosis and prediction of PTSD symptomatology in children and adolescents. Am J Psychiatry 2006;163(4):644–51.

38. McFarlane AC, Van Hooff M. Impact of childhood exposure to a natural disaster on adult mental health: 20-year longitudinal follow-up study [Research Support, Non-U.S. Gov't]. Br J Psychiatry 2009;195(2):142–8.

39. McLaughlin KA, Koenen KC, Hill ED, et al. The Aberfan disaster: 33-year follow-up of survivors [Research Support, Non-U.S. Gov't]. Br J Psychiatry 2003;182: 532–6.

40. O'Toole BI, Catts SV, Outram S, et al. The physical and mental health of Australian Vietnam veterans 3 decades after the war and its relation to military service, combat, and post-traumatic stress disorder [Research Support, Non-U.S. Gov't]. Am J Epidemiol 2009;170(3):318–30.

41. Yule W, Bolton D, Udwin O, et al. The long-term psychological effects of a disaster experienced in adolescence: I: the incidence and course of PTSD [Research Support, Non-U.S. Gov't]. J Child Psychol Psychiatry 2000;41(4): 503–11.
42. Trickey D, Siddaway AP, Meiser-Stedman R, et al. A meta-analysis of risk factors for post-traumatic stress disorder in children and adolescents. Clin Psychol Rev 2012;32(2):122–38.
43. Goutaudier N, Séjourné N, Rousset C, et al. Negative emotions, childbirth pain, perinatal dissociation and self-efficacy as predictors of postpartum posttraumatic stress symptoms. J Reprod Infant Psychol 2012;30(4):352–62.
44. Wijma K, Soderquist J, Wijma B. Posttraumatic stress disorder after childbirth: a cross sectional study. J Anxiety Disord 1997;11(6):587–97. pii:S0887-6185(97) 00041-8.
45. Ballard CG, Stanley AK, Brockington IF. Post-traumatic stress disorder (PTSD) after childbirth. Br J Psychiatry 1995;166(4):525–8.
46. Mollica RF, Poole C, Son L, et al. Effects of war trauma on Cambodian refugee adolescents' functional health and mental health status [Research Support, Non-U.S. Gov't]. J Am Acad Child Adolesc Psychiatry 1997;36(8):1098–106.
47. Charney DS. Psychobiological mechanisms of resilience and susceptibility: implications for successful adaptation to extreme stress. Am J Psychiatry 2004; 161:195–216.
48. Rutter M. Implications of resilience concepts for scientific understanding. Ann N Y Acad Sci 2006;1094:1–12.
49. van der Kolk B, Pelcovitz D, Roth S, et al. Dissociation, affect dysregulation and somatization: the complexity of adaptation to trauma. Am J Psychiatry 1996;153: 83–93.
50. Resick PA, Bovin MJ, Calloway AL, et al. A critical evaluation of the complex PTSD literature: implications for DSM-5. J Trauma Stress 2012;25:241–51.
51. Stoddard FJ, Simon NM, Pitman RK. Trauma- and stressor-related disorders. In: Hales RE, Yudofsky S, Roberts L, editors. American Psychiatric Publishing textbook of psychiatry. 6th edition. American Psychiatric Press, in press.
52. Saxe G, Ellis BH, Kaplow J. Collaborative treatment of traumatized children and teens: the trauma systems therapy approach. New York: Guilford; 2007.
53. Ford J, Russo E. Trauma-focused, present-centered, emotional self regulation approach to integrated treatment for posttraumatic stress and addiction: trauma adaptive recovery group education and therapy. Am J Psychother 2006;60(4):335–55.
54. DeRosa R, Pelcovitz D. Igniting SPARCS of change: structured psychotherapy for adolescents responding to chronic stress. In: Ford J, Pat-Horenczyk R, Brom D, editors. Treating traumatized children: risk, resilience and recovery. New York: Routledge; 2009. p. 225–9.
55. Briere J, Lanktree C. Integrative treatment of complex trauma for adolescents (ITCT-A) treatment guide. 2nd edition. Los Angeles, CA: University of Southern California; 2013. Available at: http://www.attc.usc.edu.
56. Kantor E, Beckert D. Preparation and systems issues. Integrating into a disaster response. In: Stoddard FJ, Pandya A, Katz CL, editors. Disaster psychiatry: readiness, evaluation, and treatment. Arlington, VA: American Psychiatric Press; 2011. p. 3–18.
57. Merlino JP. Rescuing ourselves: self care in the disaster response community. In: Stoddard FJ, Pandya A, Katz CL, editors. Disaster psychiatry: readiness, evaluation, and treatment. Arlington, VA: American Psychiatric Press; 2011. p. 35–48.

RECOMMENDED READINGS

Binder EB, Bradley RG, Liu W, et al. Association of FKBP5 polymorphisms and childhood abuse with risk of post-traumatic stress disorder symptoms in adults. JAMA 2008;299:1291–305 [the more traumatic events the greater the intensity of PTSD symptoms].

Chemtob CM, Pat-Horenczyk R, Madan A, et al. Israeli adolescents with ongoing exposure to terrorism: suicidal ideation, post-traumatic stress disorder, and functional impairment. J Trauma Stress 2011;24(6):756–9. http://dx.doi.org/10.1002/jts.20708.

DeBellis MD, Keshavan MS. Sex differences in brain maturation in maltreatment-related pediatric post-traumatic stress disorder. Neurosci Biobehav Rev 2003; 27:103–17.

DeBellis MD, Keshavan MS, Clark DB, et al. A.E. Bennett Research Award: developmental traumatology: Part II. Brain development. Biol Psychiatry 1999;45:1271–84.

De Bellis MD, Woolley DP, Hooper SR. Neuropsychological findings in pediatric maltreatment: relation of PTSD, dissociative symptoms, and abuse/neglect indices to neurocognitive outcomes. Child Maltreat 2013;18(3):171–83.

De Young AC, Kenardy JA, Cobham VE. Trauma in early childhood: a neglected population. Clin Child Fam Psychol Rev 2011;14(3):231–50.

Fergusson DM, McLeod GF, Horwood LJ. Childhood sexual abuse and adult developmental outcomes: findings from a 30-year longitudinal study in New Zealand. Child Abuse Negl 2013;9:664–74.

Gilbert R, Wisom CS, Browne K, et al. Burden and consequences of child maltreatment in high income countries. Lancet 2009;373:68–81.

Harville E, Xiong X, Buekens P. Disasters and perinatal health: a systematic review. Obstet Gynecol Surv 2010;65(11):713–28.

Hilyard KL, Wolfe DA. Child neglect: developmental issues and outcomes. Child Abuse Negl 2002;26(6–7):679–95.

Huang MC, Schwandt ML, Ramchandani VA, et al. Impact of multiple types of childhood trauma exposure on risk of psychiatric comorbidity among alcoholic inpatients. Alcohol Clin Exp Res 2012;36(6):1099–107. http://dx.doi.org/10.1111/j.1530-0277.2011.01695.x.

International classification of diseases. Ninth revision (ICD-9). National Center for Health Statistics. Classification of diseases and injuries. 2002. Available at: ftp://ftp.cdc.gov/pub/Health_Statistics/NCHS/Publications/ICD-9/ucod.txt.

Jonson-Reid M, Kohl PL, Drake B. Child and adult outcomes of chronic child maltreatment. Pediatrics 2012;129(5):839–45.

Kazis LE, Liang MH, Lee A, et al. The development, validation, and testing of a health outcomes burn questionnaire for infants and children 5 years of age and younger: American Burn Association/Shriners Hospitals for Children. J Burn Care Rehabil 2002;23(3):196–208.

Kendler KS, Bulik CM, Silberg J, et al. Childhood sexual abuse and adult psychiatric and substance abuse disorders in women. Arch Gen Psychiatry 2000;57:953–9.

Kolassa IT, Kolassa S, Ertl V, et al. The risk of post-traumatic stress disorder after trauma depends on traumatic load and the catechol-O-methyltransferase Val158-Met polymorphism. Biol Psychiatry 2010;67:304–8.

Leenarts LE, Diehle J, Doreleijers TA, et al. Evidence-based treatments for children with trauma-related psychopathology as a result of childhood maltreatment: a systematic review. Eur Child Adolesc Psychiatry 2013;22(5): 269–83.

Lustig S, Kia M, Ellis H, et al. Review of child and adolescent refugee mental health. J Am Acad Child Adolesc Psychiatry 2004;43:24–36.

Maniglio R. The impact of child sexual abuse on health: a systematic review of reviews. Clin Psychol Rev 2009;29:647–57.

Maniglio R. Child sexual abuse in the etiology of depression: a systematic review of reviews. Depress Anxiety 2010;27:631–42.

Marsac ML, Hildenbrand AK, Kohser KL, et al. Preventing post-traumatic stress following pediatric injury: a randomized controlled trial of a web-based psycho-educational intervention for parents. J Pediatr Psychol 2013;38(10): 1101–11.

McLean CP, Rosenbach SB, Sandra Capaldi S, et al. Social and academic functioning in adolescents with child sexual abuse-related PTSD. Child Abuse Negl 2013;37(9):675–8.

Mehta D, Klengel T, Conneely KN, et al. Childhood maltreatment is associated with distinct genomic and epigenetic profiles in post-traumatic stress disorder. Proc Natl Acad Sci U S A 2013;110(20):8302–7.

Melnyk BM, Feinstein N, Alpert-Gillis L, et al. Reducing premature infants' length of stay and improving parents' mental health outcomes with the COPE NICU program: A randomized clinical trial. Pediatrics 2006;118(5):e1414–27.

Meyer W, Blakeney P, Thomas CR, et al. Prevalence of major psychiatric illness in young adults who were burned as children. Psychosom Med 2007;69:377–82.

Navon M, Nelson D, Murphy JM. Innovations in pediatric preventative behavioral health care. Psychiatr Serv 2001;52:800–4.

National Child Traumatic Stress Network (NCTSN) toolkit for health care. Providers. Available at: http://nctsnet.org/nccts/nav.do?pid=typ_mt.

Norrholm SD, Jovanovic T, Olin IW, et al. Fear extinction in traumatized civilians with post-traumatic stress disorder: relation to symptom severity. Biol Psychiatry 2011; 69:556–63.

Palusci VJ, Covington TM. Child maltreatment deaths in the U.S. National Child Death Review Case Reporting System. Child Abuse Negl 2013. pii:S0145-2134(13) 00245-7.

Panter-Brick C, Goodman A, Tol W, et al. Mental health and childhood adversities: a longitudinal study in Kabul, Afghanistan. J Am Acad Child Adolesc Psychiatry 2011;50(4):349–63.

Rheingold AA, Zinzow H, Hawkins A, et al. Prevalence and mental health outcomes of homicide survivors in a representative US sample of adolescents: data from the 2005 National Survey of Adolescents. J Child Psychol Psychiatry 2012;53(6): 687–94. http://dx.doi.org/10.1111/j.1469-7610.2011.02491.x.

Saxe GN, Miller A, Bartholomew D, et al. Incidence of and risk factors for acute stress disorder in children with injuries. J Trauma 2005;59(4):946–53.

Scheeringa MS, Zeanah CH, Cohen JA. PTSD in children and adolescents: toward an empirically based algorithm [Review Validation Studies]. Depress Anxiety 2011; 28(9):770–82. http://dx.doi.org/10.1002/da.20736.

Sheridan RL, Lee A, Kazis L, et al. Impact of family characteristics on pediatric injury recovery. J Burn Care and Research 2008;29(2):S65.

Stoddard FJ, Pandya A, Katz CL, editors. Disaster psychiatry: readiness, evaluation and treatment. Washington, DC: American Psychiatric Press Inc; 2011.

Stoddard FJ, Sheridan RL, Martyn JA, et al. Pain management. Chapter 23. Ritchie EC, editor. Combat and operational behavioral health. In: Lenhart MK, editor.

The textbooks of military medicine. Washington, DC: Department of the Army, Office of The Surgeon General, Borden Institute; 2011. p. 339–58.

Terr LC. Too scared to cry: psychic trauma in childhood. New York: Basic Books; 1990.

Tol WA, Song S, Jordans MJ. Annual research review: resilience and mental health in children and adolescents living in areas of armed conflict—a systematic review of findings in low- and middle-income countries. J Child Psychol Psychiatry 2013; 54(4):445–60.

Trickett PK, Noll JG, Putnam FW. The impact of sexual abuse on female development: lessons from a multigenerational, longitudinal research study. Dev Psychopathol 2011;23:453–76.

Zatzick DF, Grossman DC, Russo J, et al. Predicting post-traumatic stress symptoms longitudinally in a representative sample of hospitalized injured adolescents. J Am Acad Child Adolesc Psychiatry 2006;45(10):1188–95.

Mass Trauma: Disasters, Terrorism, and War

Allan K. Chrisman, MD[a,b,c],*, Joseph G. Dougherty, MD[d,e]

KEYWORDS

- Child development • Children • Disasters • Mental health • Terrorism
- Mass trauma • War

KEY POINTS

- Mass-exposure events, such as disaster, terrorism, and war, have unique impacts on children.
- Effective conceptual approaches must balance risk and resilience from a developmental perspective.
- Models of mass trauma effects and exposures include exposure dose, cumulative risk, determinants, and moderators.
- Children are a special needs population particularly vulnerable to the impact of mass trauma due to a lack of experience, skills, and resources to independently meet their mental and behavioral health needs.
- The National Commission on Children and Disaster's Report recommends a greater focus on the disaster mental and behavioral health needs of children throughout planning, training, exercises, and response and recovery effort.
- Higher-intensity exposures lead to worse outcomes.
- Parental and social support are critical protective factors as moderators of negative outcomes in children exposed to mass trauma.

Disclosures: Allan K. Chrisman: Doris Duke Foundation; North Carolina Pediatric Society Foundation; this project was supported in part by salary from the Mid-Atlantic Mental Illness Research, Education and Clinical Center, Department of Veterans Affairs (VISN 6 MIRECC) of the Department of Veterans Affairs Office of Mental Health Services; Joseph G. Dougherty has no disclosures to report. The views expressed in this article are those of the authors and do not necessarily reflect the official policy or position of the Department of the Army, Navy, Defense, or the US Government.

[a] Division of Child and Adolescent Psychiatry, Department of Psychiatry and Behavioral Sciences, Duke University Medical Center, Durham, NC, USA; [b] Duke Child and Family Study Center, 2608 Erwin Road Lakeview Pavilion, Suite 300, Durham, NC 27705, USA; [c] Mental Health Service Line, Department of Veterans Affairs Medical Center, Durham, NC 27705, USA; [d] National Capital Consortium Child and Adolescent Psychiatry Fellowship, Uniformed Services University of the Health Sciences School of Medicine, 4301 Jones Bridge Road, Bethesda, MD 20814, USA; [e] Walter Reed National Military Medical Center, 8901 Wisconsin Avenue, Bethesda, MD 20889, USA
* Corresponding author. Duke Child and Family Study Center, 2608 Erwin Road Lakeview Pavilion, Suite 300, Durham, NC 27705.
E-mail addresses: allan.chrisman@dm.duke.edu; allan.chrisman@va.gov

Abbreviations	
CBT	Cognitive behavioral therapy
CHASM	Community Health and Service Missions
PFA	Psychological first aid

INTRODUCTION

Mass trauma experiences that have an impact on children and adolescents include natural disasters, human-made disasters (including intentional [ie, terrorism] and unintentional [ie, chemical and nuclear accidents] disasters), and wars. Increasingly, there are several factors that have evolved to create a frequency and severity of mass trauma not previously seen. These factors include the rapid growth of populations, globalization of communication and commerce, industrialization of underdeveloped countries, and rapid changes in weather patterns spawning major storms. These challenges are often superimposed on global regions already destabilized by conflict and warfare. Consequently, millions of children every year are exposed to mass trauma both directly and through the indirect effects on families, communities, and societies. This article focuses on the large groups and populations of children and families who are affected by mass trauma within a relatively short period of time.

Important to an understanding of the psychological effects of mass trauma are the definitions of the following terms—disaster, primary and secondary stressors, acute and chronic stress reactions, resilience, and cumulative risk.[1]

According to the World Health Organization,[2] *disaster* is defined as a severe ecological and psychosocial disruption that greatly exceeds the coping capacity of the community. Disasters are dynamic events that have phases (preimpact, impact, and postimpact) and can be subdivided into natural disasters or human-made intentional and unintentional disasters.[3]

There are *primary and secondary stressors* that result from disasters that can contribute to both acute and chronic stress reactions. Primary stressors are part of the direct exposure to harm or threat of harm during the disaster impact and secondary stressors occur as consequences of the disaster impact (ie, adversities in the aftermath, such as loss of home, school or injury, or the need to relocate). In a majority of cases, recovery is the naturally expected outcome of acute stress responses (which include regressed or disrupted behavior, tearfulness, sleep or appetite problems, and other signs of distress) after a disaster when adequate support is available. *Resilience* according to the UNISDR is the ability of a system, community or society exposed to hazards to resist, absorb, accommodate to and recover from the effects of a hazard in a timely and efficient manner.[4]

In the wake of disaster, resilience indicates the ability to rapidly restore to predisaster levels of function and psychological equilibrium. For children, this requires a host of family/parent and community/social support at a developmentally appropriate level. Given this reliance on external support, children's resilience is more variable and dependent on their caretakers. In contrast, chronic stress reactions often result in pathologic outcomes and in children are manifested by anxiety, depressed mood, interpersonal and social problems, and diminished performance at school. Such chronic traumatic responses can lead to loss of developmental and psychosocial gains.[5]

Cumulative risk refers to the added challenge resulting from the accumulation of multiple traumatic experiences. An individual has an increasing risk of subsequent emotional and behavioral problems and negative adaptation with increasing trauma exposures. A dose-response effect occurs with repeated exposure to traumatic events because a child is more likely to experience posttraumatic stress symptoms with higher exposure.[1]

Bearing in mind these important definitions, attention is focused on the *National Commission on Children and Disasters 2010*[6,7] report to the President and Congress, which highlights the unique vulnerability and needs of children in disasters. These findings include the following:

- Children may experience long-lasting effects, such as academic failure, post-traumatic stress disorder (PTSD), depression, anxiety, bereavement, and other behavioral problems, such as delinquency and substance abuse.
- Children are more susceptible to chemical, biologic, radiological, and nuclear threats and require different medications, dosages, and delivery systems than adults.
- During disasters, young children may not be able escape danger, identify themselves, and make critical decisions.
- Children are dependent on adults for care, shelter, transportation, and protection from predators.
- Children are often away from parents, in the care of schools, childcare providers, Head Start, or other child congregate care environments, which must be prepared to ensure children's safety.
- Children must be expeditiously reunified with their legal guardians if separated from them during a disaster.
- Children in disaster shelters require age-appropriate supplies, such as diapers, cribs, baby formula, and food.

VULNERABLE PEDIATRIC POPULATIONS
Disaster

In order to effectively intervene with child populations in times of disaster, child-specific risks and vulnerabilities must be recognized by responders and planners. Within the general population of children are those with special needs who deserve unique attention as the most vulnerable to secondary stressors associated with violence, abuse, and opportunistic crimes. They require a priority for intervention and referral. These special needs children include "those exposed to maltreatment or poverty; children from minority backgrounds; refugee and immigrant children; children from families with limited language proficiency; children residing in foster care homes, halfway houses, shelters for domestic violence, and youth hostels; homeless and runaway children; children confined to juvenile detention centers; and children with medical illnesses, developmental disabilities, mobility challenges, and psychiatric disorders".[7] The special needs category cannot be fully predefined, however, prior to a disaster. Often individual children and families are directly impacted by the disaster and consequent adversities, leaving them with special needs.[1]

War and Terrorism

Beyond disasters, children and their families are faced with a significant rise in war and terrorism as a common occurrence in their lives. As Williams[8] summarized in his 2007 review, "Children and families are now in the front line of war, conflict and terrorism as a consequence of the paradigm shift in the nature of warfare and the growth of terror as a weapon." The impact of these traumas is both direct and indirect along with youth being both victims and perpetrators of violence (child soldiers). In addition, recent US participation in combat efforts has exposed a large population of American children to war through the experience of their service member parents.

Pine and colleagues[9] described terrorism as "a form of undeclared war that often targets the civilian population as well as, or instead of, the military... combination of targeted hate and random violence that is particularly frightening. Terrorism combines 2 threats: deliberate harm to a child's community and random harm to children and their families. These characteristics pose special challenges to the emotional balance of a community, and they require unique responses from communities and care providers." Despite these unique features of terrorism, there are many common elements to other traumas, which are discussed in this article.[9]

This article uses a risk and resilience framework informed by developmental systems theory and the related core principles of contemporary developmental psychopathology to discuss the impact of mass trauma on children. Specific features of each traumatic event and degree of life threat and physical injury in turn form children's reactions to disasters, war, and terrorism and also are discussed. Impact on children is complex because mass trauma events occur across a timeline and in a complex array of contextual factors at multiple levels.

REVIEW
Epidemiology

Although children and adolescents, as discussed previously, are a special needs population particularly vulnerable to disaster, exposure to some form of trauma during childhood has been documented in epidemiologic studies of general populations as more common than most investigators realize. Mass trauma, often including multiple forms of trauma exposure both direct and indirect, poses the greatest risk for the development of serious mental health disorders and associated impairments.

Disasters

The frequency of natural disasters is also noted to be rising. The number of natural disasters around the world has increased by more than 4 times in the past 20 years, according to a report released by the British charity Oxfam.[10] Additionally the United Nations Office for Disaster Risk Reduction notes that between the years 2000 and 2012 there were 2.9 billion people affected by and 1.2 million people killed by natural disasters. Earthquakes and storms are the major causes of these casualties. A yearly average of 790 disasters between 2001 and 2011 was noted.[11] High estimates of psychiatric symptom prevalence have been reported in studies of children and adolescents exposed to various types of disasters that affected entire communities. In a representative sample of 2030 US children aged 2 to 17, 13.9% reported lifetime exposure to disaster, and 4.1% reported experiencing a disaster in the past year.[12]

Two years after Hurricane Katrina, 14.9% of children and adolescents had a serious emotional disturbance, with 9.3% estimated to have serious emotional disturbance directly attributable to the hurricane.[13] This is in contrast to prevalence estimates of serious emotional disturbance at 4.4% to 7.47% in studies of communities across the country.[14] Kelly and colleagues report that 13% of children exposed to Hurricane Katrina had posttraumatic stress symptoms at 3 to 7 months in the immediate aftermath of the disaster. The presence of these symptoms right after the hurricane was also a predictor of the presence of chronic symptoms at 14 to 17 months after impact of the study. The hurricane was also found a direct contributor to the symptoms even in the presence of a history of previous trauma.[14]

The Great East Japan Earthquake (the Tohoku earthquake) has been described as "an unprecedented triple disaster: an earthquake followed by a devastating tsunami and, finally, the destruction of a major nuclear power plant with the leaking of large amounts of radiation... Children and adolescents younger than 19 years accounted for 6.5% of the deaths, and there were 229 survivors younger than 18 years who lost both their parents in the disaster and 1295 who lost one of their parents."[15] Analysis of more than 11,000 Japanese children's traumatic symptom questionnaire responses after the 2011 Great East Japan Earthquake and Tsunami revealed that children whose houses were damaged or who experienced separation from family members had higher scores than children who did not experience environmental damage. Likewise, many children who experienced evacuation or bereavement had elevated trauma symptom scores. Although such findings may not be surprising given the nature of items assessed, investigators speculated that collecting information about environmental damage experienced by children and correlating this with stress questionnaire scores may result in a more accurate prediction of who may have an elevated risk for developing PTSD.[16]

War

Unfortunately, mass trauma seems to be rapidly escalating on a global basis. The scope of the impact of war on children is immense. As reported in the UNICEF publication, *Machel Study 10-Year Strategic Review: Children and Conflict in a Changing World*,[17] "Globally, it is estimated that over one billion children live in countries or territories affected by armed conflict – almost one sixth of the total world population. Of these, some 300 million are under the age of five. They suffer from both the direct consequences of conflict, as well as the long-term effects on their development and well-being." "They are not only caught in the crossfire, they are often the intended targets of violence, abuse and exploitation," said UNICEF Executive Director Ann M. Veneman.[18] "Over the past decade, children have been the victims of attacks on schools and hospitals, and they continue to be killed or maimed by landmines and other explosive devices. In conflict zones, their vulnerabilities often increase because violence claims their first line of defense: that is their parents."[18] Current reports by the United Nations are that more than a million children have been displaced from the civil conflict in Syria to refugee camps.[19] In a review by Wilson and Thomson[20] of the epidemiology of international terrorism from 1994–2003 data for 21 "established market economy" countries and 18 "former socialist economies of Europe", a total of 32 international terrorist attacks causing fatalities were identified over the 10-year period. During this decade, no statistical trend in the number of attacks was found but the number of deaths per attack (severity) increased.[21]

In a recent study sponsored jointly by Bahçeşehir University, New York University, and the Norwegian Institute of Public Health, *Bahçeşehir Study of Syrian Refugee Children in Turkey*[22] evaluated 301 of 1000 children attending school. The Syrian child refugees reported a variety of direct and indirect war related experiences (ie, bombing, shooting, and social upheaval prior to coming to the refugee camp). After having spent an average of half a year in the Islahiye refugee camp in Gaziantep, the Syrian refugee children showed the following findings:

- "On the positive side: 71% of the girls and 61% of the boys had strong close relationships they trusted for help and support (experiences from other studies have shown that strengthening parents' potential for care and supportive relationships with their offspring may be the most valuable intervention in a refugee camp context).
- 74% of the children had experienced the death of somebody they cared strongly about, and 50% had been exposed to 6 or more traumatic events.
- The mental health problems associated with the war experiences were very serious—60% had symptoms of depression, 45% PTSD, 22% aggression, and

65% psychosomatic symptoms—to a degree that seriously reduced the children's level of functioning. Of course, many children suffered from 2 or more of these mental health problems."

The role of children in war has been a major source of added concern that has more recently been highlighted by the United Nations Children and Armed Conflict section. It is estimated that between 250,000 and 300,000 children are functioning as soldiers at any given time.[23] A vast majority of wars being fought today are intrastate conflicts in the poorest areas of the world.[24] It is in these wars that children are widely used as soldiers.[25] Historically, children currently defined as younger than age 18 have always been used as soldiers, and many historical accounts of battles and armies have amply documented this. Even the American Civil War had an estimated 100,000 boys in the Union Army.[7] The Coalition to Stop the Use of Child Soldiers estimated in 2008 that there were 300,000 child soldiers in global armed conflicts.[26] Since Western countries have actively banned the use of child soldiers in their armies, the role of children in armed conflicts has shifted to the developing countries, where the laws against the recruitment and use of children in armed conflict are ignored and where "societal chaos" exists. Consequently the role and experience of these child soldiers are both of perpetrators and victims, further compounding the trauma scenario.

Children of contemporary US military families are also a special population effected by war. Of all potential stressors in the life of a child, parental deployment to a combat zone is considered by some investigators among the most stressful.[27] Children of deployed US service members have been studied to assess the potential impact of such experiences on military families. After the initial Persian Gulf War in 1990–1991, a study of children whose parents had deployed indicated higher levels of self-reported depressive symptoms compared with a control group of children of nondeployed parents.[28] Nevertheless, when compared with community samples of nondeployed parents, elevations in clinically significant or pathologic psychological symptoms were not noted, suggesting an inherent resiliency in this child population. In another study of children of parents who deployed as part of the first Persian Gulf War, increased tearfulness, disciplinary challenges in the home setting, and attention-seeking behaviors in children were noted.[29]

Since 2001, more than 2 million Americans have deployed to Iraq and Afghanistan, with more than 45% of these service members having children.[30] A study of children ages 3 and 5 years old with a deployed parent revealed increased externalizing scores compared with same-aged peers without a deployed parent after controlling for a caregiver's stress and depressive symptoms.

Terrorism

Exposure to terrorism is now an everyday threat with more frequent occurrence in the United States. Examples of recent terrorist attacks studied include those on the Murrah Federal Building on April 19, 1995, and the World Trade Center and Pentagon on September 11, 2001. Six months after the September 11 attack, a survey of a random sample of more than 8000 New York City children in grades 4 through 12 six months showed that 28.6% of the children had 1 or more anxiety/depressive disorders.[31] Developmental analysis of the findings showed that younger children (6–11 years) were more likely to present with anxiety, problems concentrating, social isolation, and withdrawal, whereas older children (12–17 years) were more likely to exhibit numbing, avoidance reactions, and substance abuse.[32]

The overarching dynamic to the epidemiology of these areas of mass trauma is the confluence/interplay of these catastrophes taken together. All too often there is a simultaneous occurrence of major weather disasters in war zones, which often has the effect of restricting efforts for international aid organizations to deliver medical supplies, food, and supplies to those in dire need.

Phenomenology

Mass trauma's main effect is best understood in terms of groups of individuals/families and populations. Individual stress reactions and trauma effects are addressed elsewhere in other articles in this issue by Harriet Macmillan, Laura Murray, and Matthew Kliethermes. The developmental level of children and associated family functioning along with the intensity of primary and secondary stressors are important factors in determining the impact of mass trauma on groups and populations. The disruption of family functioning (ie, daily household activities, social support of parents, or loss of family members) results in a loss of family resilience. The loss of family support network has been shown to effect adult parenting and in turn a child's distress. The role of media exposure to coverage of mass trauma has been shown in studies by Pfefferbaum[33] and Schuster[21] to play a role in the development of stress reactions in children who were not directly affected by the trauma.

In contemporary US military families, parental deployment was shown to have a cumulative effect on 6- to 12-year-old children that extended beyond the deployment period, with increased risks for depression, anxiety, and externalizing symptoms noted after their return.[34] Similar findings have been observed with adolescents contending with parental deployment to combat zones. Among adolescents experiencing parental deployment to Iraq, perceived stress levels (in addition to elevated measured heart rates) were noted compared with civilian controls of adolescents without a deployed parent.[29] In a separate study, after controlling for family and service-member characteristics, 11- to 17-year-old children were noted to have more emotional difficulties compared with national samples. Older youth and girls of all ages reported significantly more school, family, and peer-related difficulties with parental deployment.[35] Likewise, factors, such as length of parental deployment and poorer mental health of the nondeployed parent, were associated with a greater number of challenges for adolescents both during deployment and during subsequent reintegration. In an analysis of children with a currently deployed parent, the most significant predictor of child psychosocial functioning was the parental level of stress.[36]

Such findings are not reflected only in studies of children of American service members. A survey of British families contending with the deployment of a father to Iraq indicated 61% of wives reporting "negative changes" in their children's behaviors, including issues, such as "tantrums, displays of aggression, sleeping problems, enuresis, being more emotionally upset, general insecurity, and fixations with death."[35]

Clinical Outcomes

The topics of exposure to mass violence and children's exposure to conflict, war, and terrorism and children as combatants have been increasingly reported and studied.[37] As discussed previously, the types of exposure can be direct or indirect, both as perpetrators and victims. Despite their distress, "Children are, inevitably, in the process of developing resilience when and if they are engaged in violent and disastrous circumstances."[8] Studies investigating risk and resilience in populations of children who experienced mass trauma have found a set of factors that have been associated with better neurobiological and psychosocial outcomes. Called *promotive factors* (predictors of better outcomes under high- as well as low-risk conditions) and *protective factors* (particularly relevant under high-risk conditions), these include an array of elements, "such as self-control and problem-solving skills, close relationships with competent caregivers or good schools and safe neighborhoods", which depend "to a large extent on fundamental human adaptive systems embedded in individuals, relationships, families, friends, communities, and cultures."[37] These findings are particularly important because there are also vulnerability factors for children, which may include genetic predispositions to anxiety and depression when exposed to trauma (ie, gene-environment interaction).[38] Gender differences have also been noted in reviews of disaster studies, with adolescent girls more likely to manifest posttraumatic stress symptoms then boys.[30,37,39,40] **Box 1** displays individual, family, and community factors that enhance resilience in children and adolescents.

Early researchers found that "trauma exposure could have lasting effects on children, though often the effects were short term; that loss and injury to loved ones had greater effects than material losses; and that parent availability, function, and support played significant roles in the responses of children."[37]

Disaster

A review of children's reactions to disaster is well described by the National Child Traumatic Stress Network Web site (http://www.nctsn.org/) as follows: "Children react differently, during and after an act of terrorism or other crisis, depending on their age, developmental level, and prior experiences. Some will respond by withdrawing, while others will have angry outbursts. Still others will become agitated or irritable. Parents should attempt to remain sensitive to each child's reactions." **Box 2** displays typical reactions children might exhibit after any act of terrorism or other disaster.

Shannon and colleagues[41] did a large-scale survey of school-aged children 3 months after Hurricane Hugo, which struck the United States on the evening of September 21, 1989. The findings of this study highlighted the reliable and strong variations in the expression of posttraumatic symptoms, symptom clusters, and presence or absence of the posttraumatic stress syndrome in children affected by a large-scale disaster. Children's reactions were found dependent on a race, gender, and age. African American children were more likely than were white or other minority children to report that they experienced anhedonia, attentional difficulties, and omen formatio, and engaged in hazardous or reckless behavior. Female children were more likely than male children to experience symptoms associated with emotional processing and emotional reaction to the trauma. In contrast, male children were more likely than female children to experience symptoms related to cognitive or behavioral factors. Within the adolescent groups, age was not strongly related to the experience of bad dreams, repetitive thoughts of the trauma, psychological distress associated with thoughts and/or reminders of the trauma, behavioral avoidance, or fear of reoccurrence. In contrast, the experience of repetitive images, emotional isolation or detachment, and guilt was related to age even within the adolescent group.

Grouped by age group, examples of potential psychological responses to trauma noted in the literature are listed in **Box 3**.

War and Terrorism

War and terrorism pose particular challenges to understanding the impact of mass trauma on children. In contrast to natural disasters or unintentional human accidents, intentional acts of violence, destruction, and psychological terror tend to have a more severe and lasting effect. It is estimated that more than 300,000 children (40% girls) are child soldiers around the world. Their roles include fighters or noncombatant purposes, including sexual. Studies of former child soldiers reveal that injuring or killing others and rape are common and can have a particularly toxic effect on their long-term psychosocial adjustment. One study by Betancourt and associates found the

---

Box 1
Factors that enhance resilience in children and adolescents

Individual protective factors

The capacity to recognize opportunities in adversity

Ability to elaborate problem solving and emotional coping skills

Good social skills with peers and adults

Personal awareness of strengths and limitations

Feeling of empathy for others

Internal locus of control—a belief that one's efforts can make a difference

Sense of humor

Positive self-concept

Self-reliance

Cognitive flexibility

Positive emotions (optimism, sense of humor, interests, joy)

Ability to interact positively with others

Active coping

Physical exercise

Religion

Family protective factors

Positive family ambience

Good parent-child relationships

Parental harmony

A valued social role in the household

Community protective factors

Strong social support networks

Supportive extended families

A close relationship with unrelated mentor

Good peer relationships

Community influences that offer positive role models

Positive school experiences

Valued social role, such as a job or volunteering

Membership in a religious or faith community

Extracurricular activities

Adapted from Shaw JA, Espinel Z, Shultz JM. Children: stress, trauma & disaster. Tampa (FL): Disaster Life Support Publishing; 2007.

---

degree of the maladjustment far outweighed the protective effects of community reintegration.[42]

Remarkably, "most child survivors of war who participated in long-term follow-up studies report no significant relationships between adverse experiences during the

Box 2
Typical reactions children might exhibit after an act of terrorism or other disaster

- Fear and worry about their safety or the safety of others, including pets
- Fear of separation from family members
- Clinging to parents, siblings, or teachers
- Worry that another attack will come
- Increase in activity level
- Decrease in concentration and attention
- Withdrawal from others
- Angry outbursts or tantrums
- Aggression to parents, siblings, or friends
- Increase in physical complaints, such as headaches and stomachaches
- Change in school performance
- Changes in sleep patterns
- Changes in appetite
- Lack of interest in usual activities, even playing with friends
- Regressive behaviors, such as baby talk, bedwetting, or tantrums
- Long-lasting focus on the attack, such as talking repeatedly about it or acting out the event in play
- Increase in risky behaviors for teens, such as drinking alcohol, using substances, harming themselves, or engaging in dangerous activities

From the National Child Traumatic Stress Network. Earthquakes: Children's reactions. Available at: http://www.nctsn.org/trauma-types/natural-disasters/earthquakes#q3. Accessed December 16, 2013.

war and enduring patterns of emotional distress."[43] Furthermore, the presence of psychological distress associated with PTSD symptoms developed later was not correlated with disability or psychosocial impairments. The protective factors found to moderate the impact of war adversities for children include "a strong bond between the primary caregiver and the child; the mother's mental health; the availability of additional caregivers, such as grandparents and older siblings; the social support of members in the community who are exposed to the same hardships, especially teachers and peers, a shared sense of values; a religious belief that finds meaning in suffering; the assumption of responsibility for the protection and welfare of others; an internal locus of control, and the use of humor and altruism as defense mechanisms."[43]

Terrorism has unique features, which create complicated scenarios of harm. The objectives of terrorists vary. **Box 4** lists some of these objectives.

Terrorism has also been characterized as using "targeted hatred and random violence" to create the threats of "deliberate harm to a child's community and of random harm to children and their families," which "pose special challenges to the emotional balance of a community, and they require unique responses from communities and care providers."[9] Beyond these specific features, terrorism has many that are common to other forms of trauma. The potential effect on the psychological health of children is related to "(1) the degree of exposure to the event (victim, member of victimized group; victim of event's consequences (eg, famine following war), friend

Box 3
Potential psychological responses by age group

Preschool children

Sleep and appetite disturbance

Fear of the dark

Separation anxiety

Nightmares

Regressive behaviors

Hypervigilence

Behavioral reenactments

Clinging/dependent behavior

School-age children

Re-experiencing symptoms

Disorganized or confused behaviors

Somatic complaints

Arousal symptoms

Disruptive symptoms

Anxiety symptoms

Decreased academic perfomance

Adolescents

Anxiety

Depression

Guilt, anger, fear, disillusionment

Fears of a foreshortened future

Flight into pleasurable activity

Substance abuse

Adapted from Shaw JA, Espinel Z, Shultz JM. Children: stress, trauma & disaster. Tampa (FL): Disaster Life Support Publishing; 2007.

Box 4
Objectives of terrorists

Creating mass anxiety, fear, and panic

Fostering a sense of helplessness and hopelessness

Demonstrating the incompetence of the authorities

Destroying a sense of security and safety

Provoking inappropriate reactions from individuals or the authorities (eg, repressive and/or incompetent legislation or the excessive use of violence against suspect individuals and organizations)[44]

From Alexander DA, Klein S. The psychological aspects of terrorism: from denial to hyperbole. J R Soc Med 2005;98(12):557–62; with permission.

killed; witness to horrific events; exposure through media); (2) the amount of family support available during the experience and in the aftermath (parents killed, parents psychologically unavailable, parents supportive); (3) the amount of life disruption (orphan refugee, refugee with family, home and/or school damaged, little effect on home/school life); and (4) the amount of social disorganization (social order collapses into chaos, emergency systems overwhelmed, or work effectively)."[9]

Using a developmental resilience framework, Pine and colleagues[9] gave the following fundamental principles for understanding the impact of terrorism on children:

Principle 1: The nature of the threat must be considered—children, like adults, show a dose gradient in response to direct threat. More severe reactions occur in response to events that threaten basic security (eg, a parent is killed, injured, or terrified), body, and self-integrity (eg, a child is tortured, raped, or injured, or threatened with such) and to threats perpetrated by human design rather than natural disaster (for children old enough to understand). Secondary exposure via media and rumors is an increasing concern for children because of the degree of exposure to media among children in modern societies and the intensity of the live coverage that is now commonplace. Perceived exposure is important; studies find high symptom levels in children and adolescents who believed they had been exposed to a toxin but had not.

Principle 2: Developmental timing of the terrorism will influence child and family reactions, protections, and developmental sequelae—younger children are protected from full psychological exposure to terrorism by their cognitive immaturity; most adolescents, on the other hand, are capable of apprehending the full horror of such events. Children gauge threats based on caregiver responses, a propensity termed, *social referencing*...separation can be more stressful to children than the traumatic event itself.

Principle 3: The experiences and consequences for children in the context of terrorism are mediated and moderated by family, peer, and school systems and particularly by the quality of relationships in these systems—effective adults function as highly adaptable protective systems for children in their care.

Principle 4: Individual differences in vulnerabilities and capabilities influence child responses and recovery patterns—children functioning well prior to the experience and who have more resources available during the experience manage well under extenuating circumstances, reflecting fundamental human adaptive systems. Children lacking such protections may face the highest need for intervention.[9]

Family Issues

The impact of disaster, terrorism, and war can affect both the cohesiveness and resiliency of families. A family's ability to maintain unity in the face of disaster may be predictive of the potential for the development of a child's psychopathology, regardless of the nature of the trauma. Predictors of a child's response to a disaster include variables, such as their family's structure, cohesiveness, communication patterns, parental response to the disaster, and overall family level of functioning after the significant event.[1] In brief, an intact family (or body of caregivers) in the face of overwhelming trauma affords a certain degree of protection. Family/caregiver cohesion may have a profoundly positive impact on a child's progress through developmental stages, because a young child may be unable to integrate a new or shocking experience into his or her schema and may rely on a parent or caregiver to provide a safe environment, an age-appropriate interpretation of a confusing or unfamiliar event, and an appropriate degree of reassurance. Such an approach may decrease the ultimate development of child psychopathology, regardless of the type of disaster is experienced by the family. Given these issues, a child's geographic separation from parents in the midst of natural disaster or military conflict or due to sudden refugee status can present both acute and chronic stressors that may lead to psychopathology if reunification with primary caregivers cannot be effected in a timely manner. In a refugee population, the degree of family support and maternal well-being have been shown predictive of a child's long-term emotional response.[40]

It is well known that children often reflect parental responses and attitudes to a disastrous or traumatic event. Factors that influence a child's short-term or long-term maladaptive response to such an event include disaster-related parental psychopathology, negative family emotional tone, a distressed family environment, parental overprotectiveness, reversal of dependency role, and excessive parental prevention of regressive behaviors.[45] Likewise, children with their own past history of trauma may experience a re-emergence of previous PTSD symptoms in the face of a new trauma, such as a disaster.[46] In some families, parental unawareness of these issues may lead in increased difficulties for such children.

It is well established that for traumatized children, the level of exposure to an acutely dangerous event predicts risk for the development of subsequent psychiatric symptoms.[47] This association has been noted along the full spectrum of trauma, from war to human-made and natural disasters to abuse. Regardless of which type of trauma a child experiences, families contending with either elevated degrees of social disruption or elevated psychiatric symptoms in care-giving adults have an increased risk for development of child psychiatric symptoms.[47]

A child's reaction to stressors is influenced by the effects of the traumatic event on the family.[5] Children's responses to the stressors of war or significant natural disasters (for instance, hurricanes, flooding, or earthquakes) may be influenced by the fact that their parents are often contending with the same immediate, stressful environment and possible losses (such as the loss of home, the death of a family member, the need to suddenly relocate, the destruction of a school, or the loss of a pet). Parents in mass trauma are often participants or victims in the disaster itself, which can have a distinct impact on children and their ability to be cared for. This dynamic is often absent when a child experiences individual trauma, which may not directly affect a parent or caretaker.[40]

Systems Issues

Community and social supports for children and families are essential for protection and resilience in recovery from mass trauma. Consequently postdisaster community health is considered essential for resilience of families. It "depends in part on the effectiveness of organizational responses, and ultimately the purpose of disaster management is to ensure the safety and well-being of the public."[48] The concept of community resilience was introduced by Norris and colleagues[48] in 2008 in an extensive review of multiple disciplines' literature that concluded with a definition of resilience as "a process linking a set of adaptive capacities to a positive trajectory of functioning and adaptation after a disturbance," with emphasis on "the process linking resources (adaptive capacities) to outcomes (adaptation)." A model of community resilience (a process linking a set of networked adaptive capacities to a positive trajectory of functioning and adaptation in constituent populations after a disturbance) based on Dohrenwhend's[49] earlier psychosocial model of stress and updated to include contemporary models of stress was created. In this model, "resilience occurs when resources are sufficiently robust, redundant, or rapid to buffer or counteract the effects of the stressor such that a return to functioning, adapted to the altered environment, occurs. For human individuals and communities, this adaptation is manifest in well-ness. Vulnerability occurs when resources were not sufficiently robust, redundant, or rapid to create resistance or resilience, resulting in persistent dysfunction. The more severe, enduring, and surprising the stressor, the stronger the resources must be to create resistance or resilience."[48]

Incorporating these principles, Pfefferbaum and colleagues,[50] in the American Academy of Child and Adolescent Psychiatry Practice Parameter on Disaster Preparedness, includes the following information: "Disaster System of Care-The disaster system of care is built on existing systems. It includes both a public health component, which emphasizes resilience focusing on identifying those in need of services, and a clinical component, which is designed to treat posttraumatic stress or maladaptive emotional and behavioral responses that result from the disaster and secondary adversities. Mental and behavioral health considerations should be integrated into public health, medical, and pediatric disaster management.

In developing an effective response system to considerable disasters, there are select groups in the child and adolescent population that should be taken into consideration. Children with developmental or intellectual disabilities, residents of group homes or foster homes, those with severe psychiatric illness, those for whom sudden separation from psychotropic medication may result in acute decompensation, pregnant youth who may have already less than ideal access to prenatal services, children with communicative difficulties (including those who are not primary English speakers and therefore may have difficulty expressing needs in times of disaster), and those of lower socioeconomic class who may have contended with considerable stress prior to the onset of a calamity should not be overlooked in the disaster planning process.

Another unique system that continues to evolve serves the needs of US military families and children. In response to extensive American military combat deployments over the past 12 years, robust behavioral health interventions have been developed and refined across the military health care system. In implementation of such programs on military installations, in medical and behavioral health clinics, through educational and outreach programs in military communities, in schools serving military children, and through programs targeting active duty, guard, and reserve components, both preventive and treatment approaches have been utilized.

Continued optimization of support services to military families remains essential, particularly in light of increased child maltreatment rates noted during periods of deployment of select populations. In a study of families of enlisted soldiers in the US Army with substantiated reports of child maltreatment, rates were elevated when soldiers were on combat-related deployments.[17] Increased levels of child neglect were noted during 2 large-scale deployments of US Army troops both during the initial Persian Gulf War (1991) and during the early years of US deployments to Iraq and Afghanistan (2002–2004), whereas national rates of child neglect showed little change.[11]

Community Response Strategies

Community resilience relies on a public health approach to the well-being of a population of people. It has been adapted by many governmental agencies in the United States[51,52] and abroad (ie, United Kingdom *Strategic National Framework on Community Resilience* https://www.gov.uk/government/uploads/system/uploads/attachment_data/file/60922/Strategic-National-Framework-on-Community-Resilience_0.pdf).

Schreiber and colleagues[53] report in a recent article that no strategy or concept of operations linking best practices for disaster response is currently in place. They note, however, that the National Children's Disaster Mental Health Concept of Operations,[54] which details the essential elements needed for an interoperable, coordinated response for the mental health needs of children by local communities, counties, regions, and states to better meet the needs of children affected by disasters and terrorism incidents, is a new effort to redress this deficiency.

The Department of Health and Human Services noted in the *2011 Update on Children and Disasters: Summary of Recommendations and Implementation Efforts*[55] that the National Disaster Medical System has begun training all personnel (approximately 7200) in psychological first aid (PFA) so they may be better able to address the emotional and behavioral health needs of disaster responders and survivors, including children. The US Public Health Service Commissioned Corps includes PFA training in its entire field training activities, including its Community Health and Service Missions (CHASM) initiative. Recent CHASM missions have specifically incorporated emergency preparedness for children, including day care and childcare facility preparedness. An example also cited for a strategic therapeutic response was as follows.

In response to the Joplin, Missouri, tornado disaster of May 2011, the Administration for Children and Families, along with the state of Missouri and community-based groups, created the Joplin Child Care Task Force, which consolidated federal, state, local, and nonprofit efforts to provide emergency childcare and to reconstitute the childcare infrastructure of the community. Through the efforts of this task force, 510 of the 670 childcare slots needed were immediately provided through a coordinated referral system. The Joplin experience provides an important model for other communities that experience severe damage to childcare systems due to disasters.

On October 29, 2012, Superstorm Sandy made landfall in New Jersey, resulting in more than 60% of the population being without power as well as gas shortages. Superstorm Sandy was responsible for 697 childcare provider closures and 86 Head Start center closures spanning the states of Connecticut, New Jersey, and New York. This severe disruption of the government offices and community's childcare capacity jeopardized the recovery of thousands of families with children. Shortly after the disaster, partners formed the New Jersey State–led Children's Task Force and New York Children's Task Force to address children's and families' needs caused by Superstorm Sandy's disruption of the community's infrastructure. The task forces' purpose was to identify issues and needs of children and families in the state; to develop immediate, short-term, and long-term needs of children and families impacted by the storm; and to coordinate response and actions across federal, state, local, and nongovernmental organization partners. Among several activities provided were the movement of families out of congregate care shelters to housing by providing targeted services for families with children in the Federal Emergency Management Agency Transitional Sheltering Assistance program and coordination of behavioral health resources and expertise to mitigate possible behavioral health issues that arose, to build resilience for the future and to prepare for future disasters.[24]

Challenges

Schreiber and colleagues[53] note that significant deficiencies exist in the community response to "mental health needs of children and families across the continuum of disaster phases (ie, preparedness, response, and recovery)," which is a national challenge. They comment, "Both the National Advisory Committee on Children and Terrorism and the National Commission on Children and Disasters have concluded that more must be done to specifically address the mental health needs of children in the context of disasters and terrorism."

Given that the community response to a disaster is a complicated quilt of local, state, and federal agencies and both governmental and nongovernmental agencies, the coordination of agency responses and adequate resourcing of these agencies is a major challenge. The reliance in many instances on citizen volunteers further complicates this challenge. Adequate training in a designated role as a mental health responder in itself requires an additional commitment beyond the usual scope of practice for community providers. This poses a not insignificant challenge at all levels of preparedness, response, and recovery.

Community resilience may be further improved by "matching of interventions and services to specified mental health outcomes (eg, psychiatric illness vs disaster-related distress) for exposed and unexposed groups, encouraging the use and integration of appropriate assessment and referral, and evaluating the effectiveness of the interventions and services offered."[56]

IMPORTANT TOOLS FOR PRACTICE

Participation in a disaster response does not equate to the direct application of clinical skills to a traumatized group of individuals. As discussed previously, the role of a mental health clinician is to participate in a disaster system of care that is careful organized and coordinated and provides supportive responses that emphasize the basic care and protection of the most vulnerable (ie, children and families). There are dizzying arrays of unproved techniques of intervention promoted at times of disasters, which can cause more harm than good if applied inappropriately. The American Academy of Child and Adolescent Psychiatry has published a Practice Parameter on Disaster Preparedness,[50] which has well-researched and evidence-based rated principles for child mental health clinicians to follow. Many of these principles are reviewed in this article.

In addition to this important document, there is an excellent resource provided by the National Child Traumatic Stress Network, which gives an updated review of empirically supported treatments and promising practices. The following link contains fact sheets linked from this page, which describe some of the clinical treatment and trauma-informed service approaches implemented by National Child Traumatic Stress Network centers, with the common goal of reducing the impact of exposure to traumatic events on children and adolescents: http://www.nctsn.org/resources/topics/treatments-that-work/promising-practices.

Of the ones listed, the following have been adapted by many national disaster response agencies:

PFA is an evidence-informed approach for assisting children, adolescents, adults, and families in the aftermath of disaster and terrorism. In addition to the English-language edition of the *Psychological First Aid Field Operations Guide*, there are versions in Spanish, Japanese, and Chinese. Developed by Melissa Brymer at the National Child Traumatic Stress Network, it is now in its second edition and can be fully accessed at http://www.nctsn.org/content/psychological-first-aid.

The core actions
- Contact and engagement
- Safety and comfort
- Stabilization
- Information gathering: current needs and concerns
- Practical assistance
- Connection with social supports
- Information on coping
- Linkage with collaborative services

Along with the several language translations, National Child Traumatic Stress Network members have worked to develop PFA adaptations for community religious professionals, Medical Reserve Corps members, and staff at facilities for families and youth who are experiencing homelessness.

- PFA for Schools
- PFA Field Operations Guide for Community Religious Professionals
- PFA Medical Reserve Corps Field Operations Guide
- PFA for Families Experiencing Homelessness
- PFA for Youth Experiencing Homelessness

Online training is available for free at http://learn.nctsn.org/course/category.php?id=11.

Skills for Psychological Recovery

Skills for psychological recovery (SPR) is a skills-training intervention designed to accelerate recovery and increase self-efficacy. SPR utilizes several core skill sets that have been found helpful in a variety of posttrauma situations. Research suggests that a skills-building approach is more effective than supportive counseling. SPR differs from mental health treatment in that it does not assume pathology but places emphasis on helping a survivor regain a sense of control and competence. Although SPR was not designed to address severe psychopathology, it may be augmented by specific services that do so. Unlike PFA, SPR requires training and certification to ensure compliance with this more complex intervention.[57] Online training sponsored by the International Society for Traumatic Stress Studies was done on February 6, 2013, and a recording is available.[58] Key components of SPR can be found in **Box 5**.

FUTURE DIRECTIONS

Wright and colleagues,[59] in their review of resiliency research of the past 40 years, commented that a robust database has been developed that has provided a strong

---

Box 5
Key components of SPR

Gathering information and prioritizing assistance help identify a survivor's primary concern and suggest an action plan.

Building problem-solving skills teaches survivors to break a problem into manageable components and identify the steps to addressing the problem.

Promoting positive activities offers a structured, behavioral means to reduce depression by increasing positive or meaningful activities.

Managing reactions assists in managing distress via several skills, such as breathing retraining, writing about one's experiences, and identifying and planning for triggers and reminders.

Promoting helpful thinking helps identify the common maladaptive appraisals made after a disaster/emergency and to rehearse more adaptive, helpful appraisals.

Rebuilding healthy social connections teaches people to access and enhance social and community supports in a practical way.

From Pennsylvania State University. Skills for Psychological Recovery. Available at: http://www.militaryfamilies.psu.edu/programs/skills-psychological-recovery. Accessed December 16, 2013. The information from the fact sheet was excerpted from www.nctsn.org and Forbes D, Fletcher S, Wolfgang B, et al. Practitioner perceptions of Skills for Psychological Recovery: A training programme for health practitioners in the aftermath of the Victorian bushfires. Aust N Z J Psychiatry 2010;44(12):1105–11.

knowledge of adaptive systems and processes that are associated with resilience, including risk and protective factors. The focus on psychological and interpersonal areas is now shifting to address biologic and cultural levels in a "fourth wave of research." The goals remain the same—learn the mechanisms of risk reduction and key ingredients of successful interventions to promote resilience among vulnerable children and their families. This requires elucidation of the conditions for effective interventions, noting the strategic and cost-effective targets and timing for interventions while exploring natural reparative processes. This requires integrative approaches, which span systems and disciplines. Despite the awareness that resilience in youth is dependent on others and has multiple levels of influence that interact synergistically, there is a lack of knowledge for proved models of clinical intervention that incorporate the biologic, psychological, interpersonal, and cultural elements. This integrative approach would apply the increasing levels of knowledge about resilience in development to populations of vulnerable children and their communities in mass trauma. Policy decisions on when, where, and how to make strategic plans for effective interventions to promote positive adaptations in communities impacted by mass trauma are increasingly crucial to the increasing demands for global relief efforts.

In a recent editorial, Asarnow[60] raised the issue of building stress resistance and resilience in war- and trauma-exposed communities. She noted the urgent need for data to inform public health and clinical programs to maximize program effectiveness. Commenting on a study by Wolmer and colleagues[13] using a controlled trial for teacher-based, resilience-focused intervention (a step forward in the development of an evidence-based practice), she noted that there is a lack of effectiveness trials to inform community practice.

In addition to the need for more rigorous research to inform the development of prevention and intervention practices after mass trauma, the public health approach taken by the community resilience metaphor proposed by Norris and colleagues[48] has focused attention on the need to incorporate a population-based approach to mitigate vulnerabilities, reducing negative health consequences, and rapidly restoring community functioning. This is now considered a cornerstone of national health security[51] in the United States, the United Kingdom,[61,62] and Australia.[63]

Finally there is recognition of the need to study the long-term consequences of exposure to mass trauma during war. To meet this objective, "longitudinal studies that recruit representative samples, establish the cultural relevance and validity of the instruments used, and provide input from multiple informants are needed."[43] Further study of military families to determine the impact of parental deployment through repeated and/or extended absences in harm's way is also needed to help determine the effectiveness of programs designed to provide support.

SUMMARY

Mass trauma, encompassing disasters, war, and terrorism, can destroy all dimensions of a child's ecology, causing both direct and indirect lasting effects for individuals, families, and whole communities. There are now overlapping forms of mass trauma, such as the triple disasters recently in Great East Japan Earthquake—earthquake followed by a devastating tsunami and, finally, the destruction of a major nuclear power plant. Even in these circumstances, research informs that an important modifiable predictor of child outcomes is adult reactions and behaviors. Parents' own anxieties can have a profound impact on their children by exacerbating their fears.[9]

Beyond the realm of natural disasters, the most toxic environment for children subjected to mass trauma is one where a prolonged exposure to war and terrorism undermines a civil society. Examples of this are notable in Belfast, Mozambique, and refugee camps in the many civil war arenas today. In these circumstances, the recruitment of children into armed conflict further threatens to traumatize generations.

In the face of these mass traumas, a series of consensus recommendations have been developed to address the need to protect and intervene with vulnerable populations of children (themselves at risk as a group). Due to the dearth of empirically supported evidence to recommend specific interventions for populations exposed to mass trauma, a group of international experts concluded that there are 5 empirically supported intervention and prevention principles to guide practices and programs at the early to midterm stages of disaster recovery. These are aimed at promoting (1) a sense of safety, (2) calming, (3) a sense of self- and community efficacy, (4) connectedness, and (5) hope.[64]

A child's social ecology is a central feature of resilience, which has been linked to a community resilience model.[48] In a recent publication on this topic, Noffsinger and colleagues[39] note, "The Macro system affects disaster response and recovery indirectly through intangible cultural, social, economic, and political structures and processes. Children's responses to adversity occur in the context of these dynamically interconnected and interdependent nested environments, all of which endure the burden of disaster."

In keeping with this approach, Masten and Narayan[37] recently recommended "training of all disaster-response personnel on special needs and issues of children; recognition of parents, teachers, and care providers as first responders who also need training; avoiding separation of children from caregivers and reuniting separated families; careful monitoring of media exposure in children; and rapid restoration of routines, schools, and opportunities to play or socialize with peers."

Focusing more specifically on individual children, Pine recommended identifying and monitoring children at high risk for psychiatric symptoms after exposure to trauma. A trial of cognitive behavioral therapy (CBT) for children manifesting trauma-related anxiety and mood symptoms is also recommended. A lack of response to CBT for anxiety or mood symptoms or the presentation of other psychiatric symptoms is an indication for the use of other treatments, including the use of psychotropic medications that have proved efficacy for the treatment of these symptoms/disorders.[45,65]

The role of psychotropic medications in the treatment of children and adolescents in a mass trauma recovery period is limited. A literature review in 2010 concluded, "extant data do not support the use of SSRIs [selective serotonin reuptake inhibitors] as first-line treatments for PTSD in children and adolescents. There is limited evidence that the brief use of antiadrenergic agents, second-generation antipsychotics, and several mood stabilizers may attenuate some PTSD symptoms in youth."[66] The appropriate use of psychotropic medications for continued treatment of previously diagnosed psychiatric disorders is the most likely indicated use. Extreme caution is urged for the use of these agents in a mass trauma circumstance.[65]

REFERENCES

1. Shaw JA, Espinel Z, Shultz JM. Care of children exposed to the traumatic effects of disaster. 1st edition. Washington, DC: American Psychiatric Publishing; 2012. p. 243.
2. Organization, W.H. Glossary of humanitarian terms-relief web. 2008. Available at: http://www.who.int/hac/about/definitions/en/index.html.
3. Shaw JA. Children exposed to war/terrorism. Clin Child Fam Psychol Rev 2003; 6(4):237–46.

4. Reduction, U.N.I.S.f.D., 2009 UNISDR Terminology on Disaster Risk Reduction. UN Editor. UN; 2009. p. 24. Available at: www.unisdr.org/publications.
5. Pine DS, Cohen JA. Trauma in children and adolescents: risk and treatment of psychiatric sequelae. Biol Psychiatry 2002;51(7):519–31.
6. National Commission on Children and Disasters. 2010 Report to the President and Congress. AHRQ Publication No. 10-M037, October 2010. Rockville, MD: Agency for Healthcare Research and Quality; 2010. Available at: http://www.ahrq.gov/prep/nccdreport/.
7. Pfefferbaum B, Shaw JA. Practice parameter on disaster preparedness. J Am Acad Child Adolesc Psychiatry 2013;52(11):1224–38.
8. Williams R. The psychosocial consequences for children of mass violence, terrorism and disasters. Int Rev Psychiatry 2007;19(3):263–77.
9. Pine DS, Costello J, Masten A. Trauma, proximity, and developmental psychopathology: the effects of war and terrorism on children. Neuropsychopharmacology 2005;30(10):1781–92.
10. Gutierrez D. Natural disasters up more than 400 percent in two decades. 2008. Available at: naturalnews.com.
11. United Nations Office for Disaster Risk Reduction (UNISDR). 2013 disaster impacts, 2000–2012-graphic. United Nations Office for Disaster Risk Reduction (UNISDR); 2013. p. 2013.
12. Becker-Blease KA, Turner HA, Finkelhor D. Disasters, victimization, and children's mental health. Child Dev 2010;81(4):1040–52.
13. Wolmer L, Hamiel D, Laor N. Preventing children's posttraumatic stress after disaster with teacher-based intervention: a controlled study. J Dev Behav Pediatr 2011;50(4):340–8.e2.
14. Kelley ML, Self-Brown S, Le B, et al. Predicting posttraumatic stress symptoms in children following Hurricane Katrina: a prospective analysis of the effect of parental distress and parenting practices. J Trauma Stress 2010;23(5):582–90.
15. Hayashi K, Tomita N. Lessons learned from the Great East Japan Earthquake: impact on child and adolescent health. Asia Pac J Public Health 2012;24(4):681–8.
16. Usami M, Iwadare Y, Kodaira M, et al. Relationships between traumatic symptoms and environmental damage conditions among children 8 months after the 2011 Japan earthquake and tsunami. PLoS ONE 2012;7(11):e50721.
17. UNICEF, O.o.t.S.R.o.t.S.-G.f.C.a.A.C.i.c.w. Machel study 10-year strategic review: Children and conflict in a changing world; 2009.
18. Bennett A. Ten years on, the Machel study cites continued abuse against children in conflict. UNICEF; 2013. p. 1.
19. Nebehay S. A million Syrian child refugees is a "shameful milestone": U.N., P. Char, Editor. 2013.
20. Wilson N, Thomson G. The epidemiology of international terrorism involving fatal outcomes in developed countries (1994–2003). European Journal of Epidemiology 2005;20(5):375–81.
21. Schuster MA, Stein BD, Jaycox L, et al. A national survey of stress reactions after the September 11, 2001, terrorist attacks. N Engl J Med 2001;345(20):1507–12.
22. Özer S, Şirin S, Oppedal B. Bahçeşehir study of Syrian refugee children in Turkey. 2013.
23. Rosen DM. Child soldiers: A reference handbook contemporary world series. Santa Barbara, California, USA: 2012. ABC-CLIO. 323.
24. Families, A.f.C.a., O.o.H.S. Emergency, and P.a. Response, Children and Youth Task Force in Disasters Guidelines for Development. 2013. p. 14.

25. Rosen DM. Child soldiers, international humanitarian law, and the globalization of childhood. Am Anthropol 2007;109(2):296–306.
26. Soldiers, T.C.t.S.t.U.o.C. Child Soldiers Global Report 2008. 2008. p. 15.
27. Chartrand MM, Frank DA, White LF, et al. Effect of parents' wartime deployment on the behavior of young children in military families. Arch Pediatr Adolesc Med 2008;162(11):1009–14.
28. Chandra A, Lara-Cinisomo S, Jaycox LH, et al. Children on the homefront: the experience of children from military families. Pediatrics 2010;125(1):16–25.
29. Flake EM, Davis BE, Johnson PL, et al. The psychosocial effects of deployment on military children. J Dev Behav Pediatr 2009;30(4):271–8. http://dx.doi.org/10.1097/DBP.0b013e3181aac6e4.
30. Kronenberg ME, Hansel TC, Brennan AM, et al. Children of Katrina: lessons learned about postdisaster symptoms and recovery patterns. Child Dev 2010; 81(4):1241–59.
31. Costello EJ, Messer SC, Bird HR, et al. The prevalence of serious emotional disturbance: a re-analysis of community studies. J Child Fam Stud 1998;7(4): 411–32.
32. McLaughlin KA, Fairbank JA, Gruber MJ, et al. Serious emotional disturbance among youths exposed to Hurricane Katrina 2 years postdisaster. J Am Acad Child Adolesc Psychiatry 2009;48(11):1069–78.
33. Pfefferbaum B. The impact of the Oklahoma City bombing on children in the community. Mil Med 2001;166(Suppl 12):49–50.
34. Lester P, Peterson K, Reeves J, et al. The long war and parental combat deployment: effects on military children and at-home spouses. J Am Acad Child Adolesc Psychiatry 2010;49(4):310–20.
35. Dandeker C, French C, Birtles C, et al. Deployment experiences of British Army wives before, during and after deployment: satisfaction with military life and use of support networks, in King's College London (United Kingdom) Department of War Studies; 2006.
36. Shaw J. Children, adolescents and trauma. Psychiatr Q 2000;71(3):227–43.
37. Masten AS, Narayan AJ. Child development in the context of disaster, war, and terrorism: pathways of risk and resilience. Annu Rev Psychol 2012;63: 227–57.
38. Cicchetti D. Resilience under conditions of extreme stress: a multilevel perspective. World Psychiatry 2010;9(3):145–54.
39. Noffsinger MA, Pfefferbaum B, Pfefferbaum RL, et al. The burden of disaster: Part I. Challenges and opportunities within a child's social ecology. Int J Emerg Ment Health 2012;14(1):3–13.
40. Wright MO, Masten AS, Narayan AJ. Chapter 3: resilience processes in development: four waves of research on positive adaptation in the context of adversity. In: Handbook of resilience in children. Springer; 2013. p. 370.
41. Shannon MP, Lonigan CJ, Finch AJ Jr, et al. Children exposed to disaster: I. Epidemiology of post-traumatic symptoms and symptom profiles. J Am Acad Child Adolesc Psychiatry 1994;33(1):80–93.
42. Betancourt TS, Brennan RT, Rubin-Smith J, et al. Sierra Leone's former child soldiers: a longitudinal study of risk, protective factors, and mental health. J Am Acad Child Adolesc Psychiatry 2010;49(6):606–15.
43. Werner EE. Children and war: risk, resilience, and recovery. Dev Psychopathol 2012;24(2):553–8.
44. Alexander DA, Klein S. The psychological aspects of terrorism: from denial to hyperbole. J R Soc Med 2005;98(12):557–62.

45. Frankenberg E, Friedman J, Gillespie T, et al. Mental health in Sumatra after the tsunami. Am J Public Health 2008;98(9):1671–7.
46. Almqvist K, Broberg AG. Mental health and social adjustment in young refugee children 3 1/2 years after their arrival in Sweden. J Am Acad Child Adolesc Psychiatry 1999;38(6):723–30.
47. Gibbs DA, Martin SL, Kupper LL, et al. Child maltreatment in enlisted soldiers' families during combat-related deployments. JAMA 2007;298(5):528–35.
48. Norris FH, Stevens SP, Pfefferbaum B, et al. Community resilience as a metaphor, theory, set of capacities, and strategy for disaster readiness. Am J Community Psychol 2008;41(1–2):127–50.
49. Dohrenwend BS. Social stress and community psychology. Am J Community Psychol 1978;6(1):1–14.
50. Pfefferbaum B, Shaw JA. Practice parameter on disaster preparedness. J Am Acad Child Adolesc Psychiatry 2013;52(11):1224–38.
51. Chandra A, Acosta J, Meredith LS, et al. Understanding community resilience in the context of National Health Security: a literature review. Santa Monica (CA): RAND Corporation; 2010.
52. Security, U.D.o.H. Children in disasters guidance. 2012.
53. Schreiber M, Pfefferbaum B, Sayegh L. Toward the way forward: the national children's disaster mental health concept of operations. Disaster Med Public Health Prep 2012;6(2):174–81.
54. Services, U.D.o.H.a.H. HHS disaster behavioral health concept of operations. 2011. p. 48.
55. Group, T.C.s.H.I.L.o.D.C.W. 2011 update on children and disasters: summary of recommendations and implementation efforts. In: H.a.H. Services, editor. 2012.
56. North CS, Pfefferbaum B. Mental health response to community disasters: a systematic review. JAMA 2013;310(5):507–18.
57. Forbes D, Fletcher S, Wolfgang B, et al. Practitioner perceptions of skills for psychological recovery: a training programme for health practitioners in the aftermath of the Victorian bushfires. Aust N Z J Psychiatry 2010;44(12):1105–11.
58. Studies, T.I.S.f.T.S. Online trauma training webinars: skills for psychological recovery Josef I. Ruzek, PhD-director of the Dissemination and Training Division of the National Center for PTSD. 2013.
59. Wright MD, Masten A, Narayan A. Resilience processes in development: four waves of research on positive adaptation in the context of adversity. In: Goldstein S, Brooks RB, editors. Handbook of resilience in children. Springer; 2013. p. 15–37.
60. Asarnow JR. Promoting stress resistance in war-exposed children. J Am Acad Child Adolesc Psychiatry 2011;50(4):320–2.
61. Balaban V. Psychological assessment of children in disasters and emergencies. Disasters 2006;30(2):178–98.
62. Governments, T.C.o.A, editor. National strategy for disaster resilience. Australia: Companion Booklet, Co; 2012. p. 40.
63. Baren JM, Mace SE, Hendry PL. Children's mental health emergencies-part 3: special situations: child maltreatment, violence, and response to disasters. Pediatr Emerg Care 2008;24(8):569–77.
64. Ungar M, Ghazinour M, Richter J. Annual research review: what is resilience within the social ecology of human development? J Child Psychol Psychiatry 2013;54(4):348–66.
65. Shibley HL, Stoddard FJ Jr. Child and Adolescent Psychiatry Interventions. In: Stoddard FJ, Pandya AA, Katz CL, editors. Disaster psychiatry: readiness,

evaluation, and treatment. Washington, DC: American Psychiatric Pub; 2011. p. 287–312.

66. Strawn JR, Keeshin BR, DelBello MP, et al. Psychopharmacologic treatment of posttraumatic stress disorder in children and adolescents: a review. J Clin Psychiatry 2010;71(7):932–41.

School Intervention Related to School and Community Violence

Lisa H. Jaycox, PhD[a],*, Bradley D. Stein, MD, PhD[b],
Marleen Wong, PhD[c]

KEYWORDS

- School • Community • Violence • Intervention

KEY POINTS

- Schools have a long history of responding to crises that occur on their campuses.
- The role of schools has expanded to include responding to community-wide disasters, community violence, and other traumatic events.
- School-based trauma interventions focus on both mental health and academic outcomes.
- Schools circumvent several key barriers in access to mental health services, and can reach vulnerable, underserved youth.
- Interventions in schools tend to be less intense and have less family involvement than clinic-based interventions.
- Best practices for emergency planning and crisis intervention for schools are widely disseminated.
- Early interventions show promise in the school setting for both immediate and longer-term recovery.
- Good evidence is building for the effectiveness of cognitive behavior techniques for longer-term trauma recovery in schools.

INTRODUCTION

With high numbers of children exposed to community and school violence, schools are uniquely positioned to help with their recovery. Schools have long been tasked not only with educating children, but with detecting and reducing barriers to learning. With many salient traumatic events directly affecting school children in recent years, from school shootings to hurricanes and tornadoes, there are more and more calls

The authors have contributed to the development of two of the interventions mentioned in this paper: Cognitive-Behavioral Intervention for Schools, and Psychological First Aid for Schools: Listen, Protect, Connect.
[a] RAND Corporation, 1200 South Hayes Street, Arlington, VA 22202, USA; [b] RAND Corporation, 4570 Fifth Avenue, Suite 600, Pittsburgh, PA 15213, USA; [c] School of Social Work University of Southern California, 669 West 34th Street, MRF 214-MC0411, Los Angeles, CA 90089, USA
* Corresponding author.
E-mail address: jaycox@rand.org

Child Adolesc Psychiatric Clin N Am 23 (2014) 281–293
http://dx.doi.org/10.1016/j.chc.2013.12.005

Acronyms	
EMHE	Emergency Management for Higher Education
LAUSD	Los Angeles Unified School District
LEAs	Local Education Agencies
OESE	Office of Elementary and Secondary Education
SERV	School Emergency Response to Violence
TA	Technical assistance

for schools to serve as agents of healing. Schools have long served as the most common source of mental health care for students in need,[1-3] but schools' role in healing from trauma has continued to evolve and expand. This article describes the role of schools in healing from trauma and disaster, and discusses the existing interventions as well as areas for growth and further development.

CLINICAL PRACTICE APPLICATIONS
Phenomenology

The unique role of schools
Schools can play a critical role in meeting the emotional needs of children exposed to traumas, violence, and disasters that occur at both an individual and community level. On any given day, almost 60 million people, more than 1 out of every 5 Americans, participate in education in a K to 12 school.[4,5] However, the opportunity for schools to help communities better support traumatized children in their midst extends beyond just the individuals on school campuses. In many communities, schools serve as a setting for town hall meetings, to gather and discuss a range of pressing community issues, and parents and others responsible for children often look to schools to help them best meet the needs of their children, and often seek direction from schools about how best to support children and adolescents in times of crisis.

As a result, there is a long history of schools playing a central role in responding to community-wide disasters and traumatic events. Following the 1995 bombing of the Murrah Federal Building in Oklahoma City, the Oklahoma City Public School District screened thousands of students and provided psychological support services to many students and school staff.[6-8] In the aftermath of the September 11, 2001 attacks on the World Trade Center and the Pentagon, schools were also active in providing services to students. In New York City, more than half of the students who received counseling in the months following September 11, 2001 received it through schools,[9] whereas nearly two-thirds of parents responding to a national survey reported that their children's schools had been actively engaged in helping children and families cope with the psychological effects of the September 11 attacks.[10] Many parents reported that schools provided counseling services for children, and even more parents reported that their children's schools provided information and materials to guide them in helping their children cope or conducted special school assemblies and classroom programs.[10]

In the Gulf States region following Hurricane Katrina, most schools perceived a need to support their own affected students and displaced students who enrolled in their school, and many found ways to implement programs, despite considerable barriers in funding, training, and capacity. Many professionals working in schools discussed the need for more infrastructure and support around their individual efforts in schools.[11,12] Moreover, many of the professionals best poised to help with the response (both inside schools and in community settings) reported being overly burdened and personally stressed by the hurricanes and aftermath, limiting their ability to extend additional resources to implement new programs or services.[11–13] As a result, a key finding of studies following Katrina was that the schools most successful in delivering postdisaster interventions were those already trained and ready to do so.[13] However, what also emerged from this work was that the affected children had exposure to traumas that they experienced both before and after the hurricane, many of which were unrelated to the hurricane that contributed to their symptoms and impaired functioning.[14] This recognition has led to ongoing use of trauma-focused strategies in affected schools to deal with ongoing violence and trauma exposure beyond the disaster.[15]

There are several advantages to intervening with traumatized children through schools. One of the most fundamental is the enhanced access to interventions that can be achieved through schools compared with many other venues. An example of this comes from a study following Hurricanes Katrina and Rita; disasters that affected mental health but also disrupted community infrastructure for months and years, making access to mental health services challenging. In this project, symptomatic children exposed to the hurricanes and other traumatic events were identified in New Orleans schools, and then randomized to receive intervention either in their school in groups, or in the clinic in parent-child dyads.[16] After randomization, 98% of those randomized to the school-based intervention began it, whereas only 37% of those randomized to the clinic-based intervention attended their intake session, despite offers of carfare, babysitting, and flexible appointment scheduling. All students benefited from the services they received, making the case for providing a variety of services in schools so that more children can be served. In particular, such school-based interventions may have the most benefit for students from poor and minority families, who are exposed to high rates of community violence on an ongoing basis.[17] These families have clear need for support, but they are the least likely to benefit from the existing mental health system.[18] Intervening in schools can circumvent many barriers to mental health treatment, such as logistical and financial barriers as well as stigma. For instance, mental health support services in schools rarely include lengthy diagnostic assessments and thus minimize labeling students with a mental health disorder. School-based social workers can support and intervene with students both as part of their routine activities in a school, as well as providing more intensive treatment after receiving parental consent. Thus, school-based services enable many students to receive professional support for mental health problems without diagnostic labels, insurance claims, or coordination of complex schedules and competing demands. The direct access to the child in schools is likely one of the reasons that school-based mental health services are seen as a key way to reduce disparities.[19]

As part of the fabric of a community, individuals working in community schools are also likely to be more attuned than individuals working in many other settings to recent or historical events in a community. Such events could complicate a child's recovery from an individual or community-wide traumatic event. For example, communities with large numbers of recent immigrant students may have large numbers of students who experienced additional traumas during the process of immigration (eg, violence, arrests, separation from caregivers), which might complicate efforts to address more recent traumas.[20] Working with students every day, individuals in schools may also be more likely than individuals working in other settings to be attuned to a child's developmental issues and challenges, as well as the family context in which each child lives. Such familiarity with children and their families can allow school interventions to make more nuanced modifications to best meet the needs of an individual child than is often possible for children receiving services in which they are not as well known. Leveraging schools also fits well within the principle of using the natural environment to facilitate recovery.[21–23]

Clinical outcomes in school-based interventions

As described later in this article, there are an increasing number of evidence-based and promising school interventions for traumatized students.[24] These interventions often target symptoms of posttraumatic stress disorder,[25] but often also target depressive symptoms, anxiety, as well as behavior problems and functioning (eg, Refs.[26–34]). A challenge in the school setting is in obtaining valid, clinically meaningful assessment data without lengthy clinical assessments. Using a diagnostic or in-depth clinical assessment is often impractical or infeasible in schools, and does not fit with the intent of many school programs of avoiding the stigma of formal mental health treatment. Thus, many school programs rely on self-reported, parent-reported, or teacher-reported problems and include a range of students with moderate to severe symptoms or behavioral problems. From the educators' perspective, school interventions for traumatized students are ideally also associated with improved academic performance, and evaluations of some interventions have found such effects. In a study evaluating academic outcomes related to the Cognitive Behavioral Intervention for Trauma in Schools program, students who participated in the intervention earlier in the school year showed superior grades in some courses in the spring.[35] However, grades are accrued over the school year on a different schedule than most studies, making it difficult to interpret change as a function of intervention, and markers such as absenteeism or discipline referrals have low base rates and variability, making it difficult to detect change.

Family issues

As discussed earlier, working in school has some key advantages in reducing barriers and accessing students. Another aspect of this direct access to intervening with the child is that families are less likely to engage in the intervention than they would be in a specialty mental health setting. In our own work with a group-based, trauma-focused intervention in schools, it is common for only about a fifth to a quarter of parents to engage in the intervention in person, and for only about three-quarters to engage with the interventionists via telephone. However, our school partners tell us that in some of the most disadvantaged schools, these rates of parental involvement are high compared with parent involvement in other activities such as parent-teacher conferences and Parent-Teacher Association meetings. Even these low levels of parent involvement produce the improvements in student mental health found in our studies to date,[34] and significant improvements were observed in a school-based intervention when we held no parent meetings in our work in posthurricane New Orleans.[18] Creative efforts to engage parents through informational meetings, routine letters home, telephone and text communications, and finding ways to meet families' other needs (eg, providing meals, babysitting, or addressing other family needs such as managing child behavior problems) can be used to augment group-based interventions in schools.

The History of School Preparedness and Crisis Intervention Strategies/Educational Policy and Funding in the National Context

A brief examination of critical incidents that have occurred in American schools over the past 150 years reveals that school safety and the need for school interventions related to school and community violence and other traumatic events have not historically been recognized as essential among educators, the US Department of

Education, and the American public. Fatal events caused by fires, gas explosions, and even a 1927 school massacre (killing 38 children and 7 adults, and injuring 45 others) perpetrated by a disturbed school board member in Bath, Michigan, were viewed as isolated, atypical occurrences for which counseling was unavailable.

Crisis intervention strategies, particularly those directed toward mental health, were limited by the knowledge and science of the times, leaving individual schools and school districts to create their own strategies based on existing community resources. For example, in February 1984, a school shooting occurred at the 49th Street Elementary School in South Los Angeles. At that time little was known among educators about the effects of school shootings on educators and students. Child psychiatrists Pynoos and Eth[36,37] assisted the administrators and school mental health professionals of the Los Angeles Unified School District (LAUSD) with the assessment of psychological trauma based on their work on children as witnesses to violence.

The LAUSD's response was to create the first district-wide crisis intervention team in the nation, which evolved into a model for schools across the country. A 2-tiered system of school-based and regional crisis teams were developed across the 1000 schools of the district. A policy crisis intervention bulletin described the need to identify and train multidisciplinary crisis team members comprising the school principal, who led the team, and school social workers, school psychologists, nurses, counselors, school police, and support staff such as the custodian and the school secretary. The school site team was the first level of response for life events such as the accidental death or serious injury of students or staff. The school crisis team focused its efforts on alleviating the distress of students and teachers, by encouraging students to remain in school in an enhanced environment of social and emotional supports. The district-level team was requested by the principal of the school when events overwhelmed the resources and training of the school site team. Comprising experienced school mental health professionals and regional administrators, this team helped to organize a response after a high-profile event drawing the attention of media, particularly in the aftermath of gang-related shootings or incidents of mass injury and many deaths caused by a bus crash.

School crisis management and recognition of the need for school-based trauma interventions at the national level began in the recent past The watershed event that prompted policy and congressional funding for school-based trauma interventions was the 1999 shooting at Columbine High School in Littleton, Colorado, after which the public's perception was that schools were not safe and that school shootings could happen anywhere. Following Columbine, the Department of Education engaged in several initiatives that provided funding for school-based trauma services. Terrorist events also drove the need for a national-level crisis intervention response. In 1995, the Department's Office of Safe and Drug-Free Schools (OSDFS) engaged in a sustained response to the needs of the Oklahoma Public Schools after the bombing of the Murrah Office Building, followed by funding and assistance with the development of recovery services in the New York Board of Education schools after September 11, 2001. Both incidents were alarming to the US public, and it was made clear in the 2004 terrorist attack on a secondary school in Beslan, Russia, that children in schools could be the intended targets of terrorism.

In 2001, the US Department of Education OSDFS created Project SERV (School Emergency Response to Violence), which provided funding for response and recovery services and programs in schools, broadening funding eligibility to include not only a school shooting or an act of terrorism but also a district experiencing a student suicide cluster.

As it became apparent that training of school personnel was also needed, the US Department of Education in 2003 furthered efforts to provide some standards for emergency response and preparedness by creating the Emergency Response and Crisis Management Grant Program, now called Readiness and Emergency Management for K-12 Schools (REMS). Through a competitive grant process, local education agencies (LEAs) representing a district, cluster of schools, or regional districts submitted an all-hazards plan that identified likely crisis and disaster scenarios including active shooters and acts of terrorism, as well as the resources available to respond and recover from those hazards. The grants were required to address all phases of preparedness and response including mitigation, loss prevention, response, continuity of operations, and recovery (operational, business, and specific school-based crisis interventions that addressed psychological recovery). In 2007, the department provided assistance to Virginia Tech University in the aftermath of a student-perpetrated school shooting in which an undergraduate student shot and killed 32 people and wounded 17 others before committing suicide. It became evident that colleges and universities needed a special set of emergency response and preparedness protocols and strategies on open campuses where most students were adults. In response to secondary education needs, in 2008 the department established the Emergency Management for Higher Education (EMHE) grant program, patterned after the K to 12–focused REMS grants. Schools or universities were funded if their proposals showed the best evidence of in-depth assessment of current resources and proposed use of evidence-based or evidence-informed interventions and response capabilities in addition to corresponding future plans for improvement and training in the selected interventions.

Because of budget cuts in 2011, the OSDFS was closed and some programs were moved into a new Office of Safe and Healthy Students within the Office of Elementary and Secondary Education. The funding for REMS and EMHE was not available to schools and colleges when the tragedy at Sandy Hook Elementary School occurred on December 14, 2012. However, prompted by the President's call to action in 2013 to reduce gun violence ("The Time is Now"), the White House, the Office of Safe and Healthy Students, and its REMS Technical Assistance Center, along with several federal partners, released 2 guides for emergency operations plans, one for K to 12 schools and another for higher education (available at the REMS Web site at http://rems.ed.gov/EOPGuides). School intervention strategies for students traumatized by school and community violence are identified in those guides. Funding is available to implement trauma interventions for students through SERV, which schools may submit at any time after critical traumatic events disrupt the learning environment of the school.

Impact of Trauma on Educators as a Workforce Issue

The crisis intervention programs described earlier have been widely disseminated across the United States, and are primarily used to respond to single-incident, discrete events such as a shooting, accident, suicide, or other sudden death of a teacher or student. However, recent widespread disasters and more extreme crisis events, such as the shootings at Sandy Hook or Hurricane Katrina, have brought to the forefront the need to attend not only to the affected students and staff but also to the helper professionals engaged in the healing process. For instance, the Department of Education actively supported the school districts in the Gulf States affected by Hurricane Katrina/Rita, and long-term support efforts were redoubled in 2010 after the Deep Water Horizon oil spill put renewed stress on many youth just as schools and communities were making progress in their recovery from the hurricanes.

Disaster-weary educators who were also victims of both the natural and human-made disasters began to experience the effects of compassion fatigue and secondary trauma, as seen in our own work with school-based clinicians in the months after the hurricanes.[11–13] Increasing attention on secondary stress for educators involves not only this type of extreme disaster scenario but also the everyday experience of educators in inner city schools who experience traumatic events, both themselves and through their students, on a daily basis.

Therapeutic Strategies

Early interventions

The predominant early intervention strategy in schools is Psychological First Aid, a concept that can be traced to an article published by the American Psychiatric Association in 1954 and that acknowledged the need for an acute intervention to alleviate human stress "of a severity and quality not generally encountered ... due to the 'forces of nature or from enemy attack'."[38] Since that time, many researchers and health organizations, including the National Institute of Mental Health,[39] the Institute of Medicine,[40] and the US Department of Health and Human Services,[41] have supported the idea that early, brief, and focused intervention can reduce the social and emotional distress of children and adults after traumatic events. However, research on the effectiveness of this approach has lagged behind its dissemination, in large part because of the challenges and ethics of testing interventions in a group of acutely affected children.

Two different versions of Psychological First Aid are currently being disseminated. Psychological First Aid for Schools[42] provides guidelines for sheltering students and ways in which to intervene in mass casualty events. The training is intensive and is appropriate to mental health professionals with experience in providing trauma-focused interventions. A second version, Psychological First Aid for Schools: Listen, Protect, Connect[43] (http://www.ready.gov/sites/default/files/documents/files/PFA_SchoolCrisis.pdf) is a model developed for use by teachers, administrators, and other schools staff who interact with students on a daily basis, including educational aides, school secretaries, and custodians. Training for this model can be provided within a brief period of time, building on many of the routine communication approaches school staff use with students.

The two versions of Psychological First Aid contain several common components, including protecting survivors from further physical or psychological harm, identifying and providing support for those most distressed, reestablishing social supports, and keeping families together and facilitating reunion with loved ones. Within the school setting, teachers, administrators, and other school staff are directed to actively work to help students in order to restore social and emotional equilibrium and order to the learning environment. Strategies include reuniting friends, teachers, and returning students to school; providing information and linkage with local resources on school campuses; and returning students to school and familiar routines. School nurses, school psychologists, and school social workers have important tasks as well, including facilitating communication among families, students, and community agencies; educating those affected about the expectable psychological responses to stressful and traumatic events, and basic coping tools; listening patiently in an accepting and nonjudgmental manner and conveying genuine compassion; identifying basic practical needs and ensuring that these are met; encouraging participation in normal daily routines; facilitating use of positive means of coping; and referring to locally available support mechanisms or to trained clinicians as appropriate.

Strategies for long-term recovery

After the acute posttrauma phase and stabilization, there are several types of school interventions that can be used to help in the longer-term recovery process. School buy-in to the inclusion of such interventions is based on achieving educational objectives that include increasing student self-regulation of behavior and emotion and returning the student in an improved cognitive, social, and emotional state, and therefore more ready to learn. Although most students recover in the weeks and months following traumatic events, a significant minority continue to have anxiety and depressive symptoms. Such children may benefit from a range of school-wide or curricular interventions, indicated for students at risk or with increased symptoms or functional problems, as well as from treatments for children with post-traumatic stress disorder or related problems that are delivered at school.[24,44] Programs developed specifically for schools are more common, such as early interventions or group interventions for students with exposure to trauma and increased symptoms or concerns that put them in an at-risk category. In these cases, it is necessary to determine who might benefit from such a program through a screening process to identify the at-risk or symptomatic group.

Although school programs stem from different theoretic underpinnings, most of those developed to date use cognitive behavior techniques that incorporate psychoeducation, relaxation skills, affective modulation skills, cognitive coping skills, trauma narrative, in vivo mastery of trauma reminders, conjoint sessions for parents, and enhancing safety.[45] These types of techniques have the advantage of being easily taught in a group format for use in schools, and there are several that have been developed and tested.[24] Some school interventions also include techniques stemming from psychodynamic theory or crisis intervention models, but these are less common and less well tested at present.

School group-based interventions differ from clinic-based interventions in several ways. For example, cognitive behavior therapy in clinics is usually delivered in individual or parent-child sessions, whereas school interventions are predominantly delivered in groups, making them less intensive than individual or dyadic therapy. In particular, interventions for trauma typically include some kind of focus on trauma processing, and, for children exposed to multiple severe traumas, this can take some time. Shorter, group-based interventions in schools often allow for only limited processing of the trauma. In addition, as reviewed earlier, parents tend to be less involved, or not involved at all, in school-based interventions, compared with clinic-based interventions. However, the advantage of delivering services in schools is the ability to efficiently provide services to larger numbers of youth through the reduction of stigma and barriers such as cost, transportation, and scheduling that interfere with receipt of care in clinical settings. An array of services, from the less intense group-based interventions to the more intense individual or dyadic therapy models, would ideally be offered in schools, so that students could be matched with an appropriate service according to their level of need, degree of parental involvement, and preferences.

An extensive literature review as part of the International Society for Traumatic Stress Studies treatment guidelines shows that much work is being done to develop trauma-focused interventions for schools, both internationally in conflict-torn regions and in the United States to respond to disasters, violence, and loss. However, evaluation of such programs is lagging behind their dissemination, with only a few rigorous studies conducted to date,[24] and only a handful of studies using experimental or quasi-experimental designs to test intervention effects. A recent meta-analysis reported medium to large effects across 19 studies, with 16 of those studies using cognitive behavior techniques.[25] These techniques included elements such as psychoeducation, relaxation training, safety planning, cognitive restructuring, coping with loss, reduction of anxiety related to trauma reminders, construction of a trauma narrative, and problem solving.

Thus, although cognitive behavioral programs show positive effects in the school setting, several other approaches have been developed but remain untested. Conducting rigorous studies of school interventions for trauma or violence is challenging,[46] because the research designs need to account for the real-world school conditions as well as complex ethical and logistical issues related to children and violence exposure. However, the benefits of evaluating school-based interventions in their natural environment, namely schools, increase the likelihood that those same effects will be observed once they are disseminated.[47,48]

Challenges

Despite the developing evidence of the effectiveness of the growing number of school-based interventions related to trauma, a range of challenges must be addressed in efforts to further develop and evaluate such interventions.

First is intervention timing. In the immediate aftermath of a school crisis or community disaster, school officials, parents, and the public are receptive to crisis intervention efforts, but it is often premature to implement many of the effective mental health programs. For such interventions, weeks or months must pass to determine which students and staff will recover on their own and who will need more support. In our own work, it often is not until a year or so later that a school is ready to begin intervention efforts, and at that time the funding streams and public attention have sometimes turned away. A long-term view of recovery is advantageous, so that the groundwork is laid early on for future intervention efforts to support the significant minority of students who will be in need of support a year, 2 years, or more after the event.

A second challenge is one of competing priorities, with schools' mission being education, not mental health. Underperforming schools often have the dual problems of routine trauma and violence exposure and student underachievement, and have to balance the expenditure of limited funding across these two priorities. Many of the interventions for longer-term recovery require removing students from class for small group interventions, cutting into precious instructional time.

In addition, engaging parents is extremely challenging in the school setting, particularly for older children. Despite the advantage of being able to work directly with students, parental participation in the recovery process is seen as a key element.[45]

FUTURE DIRECTIONS

From the challenges and issues discussed earlier in the article stem some natural avenues for future improvement and enhancement of school-based trauma intervention efforts:

- Translate and align intervention objectives with the mission, goals, and objectives of education.
- Evaluate the effectiveness of existing crisis intervention and early interventions.
- Include plans for long-term recovery in disaster and crisis planning, in terms of funding, training, and capacity building.
- Develop capacity for trauma intervention before school crisis or trauma, so that the long-term recovery efforts are prepared and ready to be used.

- Collect information about academic functioning and performance as part of research on intervention effectiveness, and communicate these results with education policy makers.
- Find novel and engaging ways to include parents in intervention efforts, perhaps through emerging technologies such as social media, texting, and web-based tools.

SUMMARY

Schools offer the opportunity for intervention efforts related to student trauma, capitalizing on the natural environment and reduced stigma to leverage recovery. Such programs can be divided into different phases: crisis intervention, early intervention, and selective interventions for longer-term recovery. Although best practices for crisis intervention have been developed and rolled out nationally, interventions for early and longer-term recovery tend to be disseminated in a piecemeal fashion without the benefit of organized training and funding. Dissemination has most typically occurred following specific community-wide or school crises, or in inner city schools where violence exposure is endemic. Evaluations of program effectiveness have focused on the longer-term recovery interventions, and those that contain cognitive behavior elements have been the best tested to date. Future directions include research that measures educational gains, improvements in attendance, and reduction in behaviors associated with expulsion and suspension.

REFERENCES

1. Burns BJ, Costello EJ, Angold A, et al. Children's mental health service use across service sectors. Health Aff 1995;14(3):147–59.
2. US Department of Health and Human Services. Mental health: a report of the surgeon general: executive summary. Rockville (MD): US Department of Health and Human Services, Substance Abuse and Mental Health Services Administration, Center for Mental Health Services, National Institutes of Health, National Institute of Mental Health; 1999. Available at: http://mentalhealth.about.com/library/sg/blsummary.htm.
3. US Department of Health and Human Services, US Public Health Service. Mental health: culture, race and ethnicity: a report of the surgeon general. Rockville (MD): US Department of Health and Human Services, Substance Abuse and Mental Health Services Administration, Center for Mental Health Services; 2001. Available at: http://www.ncbi.nlm.nih.gov/books/NBK44243/.
4. US Census Bureau. Annual estimates of the resident population for selected age groups by sex for the United States, States, Counties, and Puerto Rico Commonwealth and Municipios: April 1, 2010 to July 1, 2012. 2013. Available at: http://factfinder2.census.gov/faces/tableservices/jsf/pages/productview.xhtml?pid=PEP_2012_PEPAGESEX&prodType=table. Accessed September 18, 2013.
5. Center for Education Reform. K-12 facts. 2010. Available at: http://www.edreform.com/2012/04/k-12-facts/. Accessed September 18, 2013.
6. Pfefferbaum B, Nixon SJ, Krug RS, et al. Clinical needs assessment of middle and high school students following the 1995 Oklahoma City bombing. Am J Psychiatry 1999;156(7):1069–74.
7. Pfefferbaum B, Call JA, Sconzo GM. Mental health services for children in the first two years after the 1995 Oklahoma City terrorist bombing. Psychiatr Serv 1999;50(7):956–8.

8. Pfefferbaum B, Doughty DE, Reddy C, et al. Exposure and peritraumatic response as predictors of posttraumatic stress in children following the 1995 Oklahoma City bombing. J Urban Health 2002;79(3):354–63.

9. Stuber J, Fairbrother G, Galea S, et al. Determinants of counseling for children in Manhattan after the September 11 attacks. Psychiatr Serv 2002;53(7):815–22.

10. Stein BD, Jaycox L, Elliott M, et al. The emotional and behavioral impact of terrorism on children: results from a national survey. Appl Dev Sci 2004;8(4):184–94.

11. Dean K, Langley A, Kataoka S, et al. School-based disaster mental health services: clinical, policy, and community challenges. Prof Psychol Res Pract 2008;39(1):52–7.

12. Kataoka S, Nadeem E, Wong M, et al. Improving disaster mental health care in schools: a community-partnered approach. Am J Prev Med 2009;37(6S1):S225–9.

13. Jaycox LH, Tanielian T, Sharma P, et al. Schools' mental health responses following Hurricanes Katrina and Rita. Psychiatr Serv 2007;58(10):1339–43.

14. Langley AK, Cohen JA, Mannarino AP, et al. Trauma exposure and mental health problems among school children 15 months post-Hurricane Katrina. J Child Adolesc Trauma 2013;6(3):143–56.

15. Cohen JA, Jaycox LH, Mannarino AP, et al. Treating traumatized children after Hurricane Katrina: Project Fleur-de Lis™. Clin Child Fam Psychol Rev 2009; 12(1):55–64.

16. Jaycox LH, Cohen JA, Mannarino AP, et al. Children's mental health care following Hurricane Katrina: a field trial of trauma-focused psychotherapies. J Trauma Stress 2010;23(2):223–31.

17. Stein BD, Jaycox LH, Kataoka SH, et al. Prevalence of child and adolescent exposure to community violence. Clin Child Fam Psychol Rev 2003;6(4):247–64.

18. Kataoka SH, Zhang L, Wells KB. Unmet need for mental health care among U.S. children: variation by ethnicity and insurance status. Am J Psychiatry 2002; 159(9):1548–55.

19. Garrison EG, Roy IS, Azar V. Responding to the mental health needs of Latino children and families through school-based services. Clin Psychol Rev 1999; 19(2):199–219.

20. Stein BD, Kataoka S, Jaycox L, et al. Theoretical basis and program design of a school based mental health intervention for traumatized immigrant children: a collaborative research partnership. J Behav Health Serv Res 2002;29(3): 318–26.

21. Amaya-Jackson L, Reynolds V, Murray MC, et al. Cognitive-behavioral treatment for pediatric posttraumatic stress disorder: protocol and application in school and community settings. Cognit Behav Pract 2003;10(3):204–13.

22. National Child Traumatic Stress Network, National Center for PTSD. Psychological first aid: field operations guide. 2nd edition. 2006. Available at: http://www.nctsn.org/content/psychological-first-aid. Accessed January 10, 2014.

23. Macy RD. Community-based trauma response for youth. New Dir Youth Dev 2003;98:29–49.

24. Jaycox LH, Stein BD, Amaya-Jackson LM. School-based treatment for children and adolescents. In: Foa EB, Keane TM, Friedman MJ, et al, editors. Effective treatments for PTSD: practice guidelines from the International Society of Traumatic Stress Studies. New York: Guilford Publications; 2008. p. 327–45.

25. Rolfsnes ES, Idsoe T. School-based intervention programs for PTSD symptoms: a review and meta-analysis. J Trauma Stress 2011;24(2):155–65.

26. Berger R, Pat-Horenczyk R, Gelkopf M. A school-based intervention for the prevention and treatment of elementary students' terror-related distress in Israel: a quasi-randomized controlled trial. J Trauma Stress 2007;20(4):441–51.

27. Goenjian AK, Pynoos RS, Karayan I, et al. Outcome of psychotherapy among pre-adolescents after the 1988 earthquake in Armenia. Am J Psychiatry 1997; 154:536–42.
28. Goenjian AK, Walling D, Steinberg AM, et al. A prospective study of posttraumatic stress and depressive reactions among treated and untreated adolescents 5 years after a catastrophic disaster. Am J Psychiatry 2005;162:2302–8.
29. Khamis V, Macy R, Coignez V. Impact of the classroom/community/camp-based intervention program on Palestinian children: USAID report on Palestinian Children. 2004.
30. Kataoka SH, Stein BD, Jaycox LH, et al. A school-based mental health program for traumatized Latino immigrant children. J Am Acad Child Adolesc Psychiatry 2003;42(3):311–8.
31. Layne CM, Pynoos RS, Cardenas J. Wounded adolescence: school-based group psychotherapy for adolescents who sustained or witnessed violent injury. In: Shafii M, Shafii SL, editors. School violence: assessment, management, prevention. Arlington (VA): American Psychiatric Association; 2001. p. 163–86.
32. March JS, Amaya-Jackson L, Murray MC, et al. Cognitive-behavioral psychotherapy for children and adolescents with posttraumatic stress disorder after a single-incident stressor. J Am Acad Child Adolesc Psychiatry 1998;37(6):585–93.
33. Saltzman WR, Pynoos RS, Layne CM, et al. Trauma- and grief-focused intervention for adolescents exposed to community violence: results of a school-based screening and group treatment protocol. Group Dyn 2001;5(4):291–303.
34. Stein BD, Jaycox LH, Kataoka SH, et al. A mental health intervention for schoolchildren exposed to violence: a randomized controlled trial. JAMA 2003;290(5): 603–11.
35. Kataoka S, Jaycox LH, Wong M, et al. Effects on school outcomes in low-income minority youth: preliminary findings from a community-partnered study of a school-based trauma intervention. Ethn Dis 2011;21(3 Suppl 1):S1-71-7.
36. Eth S, Pynoos R. Psychiatric interventions with children traumatized by violence. In: Schetky H, Benedek EP, editors. Emerging issues in child psychiatry and the law. New York: Brunner/Mazel; 1985. p. 285–309.
37. Pynoos RS, Eth S. Special intervention programs for child witnesses to violence. In: Lystad M, editor. Violence in the home: inter-disciplinary perspectives. New York: Brunner/Mazel; 1986. p. 193–216.
38. Everly GS, Phillips SB, Kane D, et al. Introduction to and overview of group psychological first aid. Brief Treatment and Crisis Intervention 2006;6(2):130–6.
39. National Institute of Mental Health. Mental health and mass violence: evidence-based early psychological interventions for victims/survivors of mass violence. A Workshop to Reach Consensus on Best Practices. NIH Publication No. 02–5138. Washington, DC: US Government Printing Office; 2002.
40. Institute of Medicine. Preparing for the psychological consequences of terrorism: a public health strategy. Washington, DC: The National Academies Press; 2003.
41. New Freedom Commission on Mental Health. Achieving the promise: transforming mental health care in America. Final Report (No. SMA-03-3832). Rockville (MD): US Department of Health and Human Services; 2003.
42. Brymer M, Taylor M, Escudero P, et al. Psychological first aid for schools: field operations guide. 2nd edition. Los Angeles (CA): National Child Traumatic Stress Network; 2012.
43. Schreiber R, Gurwitch M, Wong M. Listen, protect, connect. The Advertising Council and US Department of Homeland Security, and The National Center for School Crisis and Bereavement; 2006. Available at: www.ready.gov.

44. Jaycox LH, Stein BD, Amaya-Jackson LM, et al. School-based interventions for child traumatic stress. In: Evans SW, Weist M, Serpell Z, editors. Advances in school-based mental health interventions, vol. 2. Kingston (NJ): Civic Research Institute; 2007. p. 16.1–16.19.
45. Cohen JA, Mannarino AP, Deblinger E. Treating trauma and traumatic grief in children and adolescents. New York: Guilford Press; 2006.
46. Jaycox LH, McCaffrey DF, Ocampo BW, et al. Challenges in the evaluation and implementation of school-based prevention and intervention programs on sensitive topics. Am J Eval 2006;27(3):320–36.
47. Chorpita BF, Yim LM, Dorkervoet JC, et al. Toward large-scale implementation of empirically supported treatments for children: a review and observations by the Hawaii Empirical Basis to Services Task Force. Clin Psychol Sci Pract 2002; 9(2):165–90.
48. Weisz JR, Donenberg GR, Han SS, et al. Bridging the gap between laboratory and clinic in child and adolescent psychotherapy. J Consult Clin Psychol 1995; 63(5):688–701.

Children's Exposure to Intimate Partner Violence

Harriet L. MacMillan, MD, MSc, FRCPC[a,b,]*, C. Nadine Wathen, PhD[c]

KEYWORDS

- Intimate partner violence • Child abuse • Spouse abuse • Mental disorders
- Child welfare

KEY POINTS

- Children's exposure to IPV is common and associated with impairment similar to other types of maltreatment.
- There is no evidence to support universal IPV screening; however, clinicians should be alert to signs and symptoms of IPV exposure among children and their caregivers, and include questions regarding IPV and safety at home in their assessments, which should be conducted individually to ensure safety of children and their caregivers.
- The evidence for reducing children's exposure to IPV by reducing IPV itself is limited.
- Mother-child and child-focused therapies for children exposed to IPV show promise in improving mental health outcomes.
- Clinicians working with children at risk of or exposed to IPV must ensure there is close collaboration among health care and child protection professionals.

Disclosure: Drs H.L. MacMillan and C.N. Wathen receive funding from the Canadian Institutes of Health Research (CIHR) Institute of Gender and Health (IGH) and Institute of Neurosciences, Mental Health and Addictions (INMHA) to the PreVAiL Research Network (a CIHR Center for Research Development in Gender, Mental Health and Violence across the Lifespan – www. PreVAiLResearch.ca). H.L. MacMillan holds the Chedoke Health Chair in Child Psychiatry at McMaster University in Hamilton, Ontario, Canada.

[a] Department of Psychiatry and Behavioural Neurosciences, Offord Centre for Child Studies, McMaster Children's Hospital, Hamilton Health Sciences, McMaster University, 1280 Main Street West, Hamilton, Ontario L8S 4K1, Canada; [b] Department of Pediatrics, Offord Centre for Child Studies, McMaster Children's Hospital, Hamilton Health Sciences, McMaster University, 1280 Main Street West, Hamilton, Ontario L8S 4K1, Canada; [c] Faculty of Information & Media Studies, The University of Western Ontario, 1152 Richmond Street, North Campus Building, Room 254, London, Ontario N6A 5B7, Canada
* Corresponding author. Department of Psychiatry and Behavioural Neurosciences, Offord Centre for Child Studies, McMaster Children's Hospital, Hamilton Health Sciences, McMaster University, 1280 Main Street West, Hamilton, Ontario L8S 4K1, Canada.
E-mail address: macmilnh@mcmaster.ca

Child Adolesc Psychiatric Clin N Am 23 (2014) 295–308
http://dx.doi.org/10.1016/j.chc.2013.12.008
1056-4993/14/$ – see front matter © 2014 Elsevier Inc. All rights reserved.

Acronyms	
IPV	Intimate partner violence
NatSCEV	National Survey of Children's Exposure to Violence
PTSD	Posttraumatic-stress disorder
WHO	World Health Organization
WPV	Witnessing partner violence

DEFINITION

The phrase "intimate partner violence" (IPV) is defined as "physical, sexual or psychological harm by a current or former partner or spouse. This type of violence can occur among heterosexual or same-sex couples and does not require sexual intimacy."[1] Although much of the literature has focused on women's exposure to IPV, it has become increasingly recognized over the past decade that children's exposure to IPV is a type of child maltreatment; this includes any incident of violent or threatening behavior or abuse between adults who are, or have been, intimate partners or family members.[2] It is important to underscore that IPV is not limited to physical aggression, such as hitting, kicking, and beating. It also encompasses emotional abuse, which includes such behaviors as intimidation; controlling actions, such as isolation from family and friends; and financial control or abuse. Much of the literature refers to children's exposure as "witnessing" IPV, but it is now understood that the impairment for children is associated with awareness that a caregiver is being harmed or is at risk of harm (ie, it occurs even without direct observation by a child of the violence). For this reason, we use the term "exposure" rather than "witnessing," except when referring to specific studies that focus on witnessing.

Dating violence is a type of IPV that occurs between two people in a close relationship, but in the literature, this usually involves adolescents as victims and perpetrators.[3] This article addresses children's exposure to IPV generally, and does not specifically address dating violence. We focus on children's (from infants through to adolescents up to the age of 18 years) experiences of violence between caregivers, rather than between peers.

EPIDEMIOLOGY
Prevalence

The prevalence of children's exposure to IPV is difficult to determine contemporaneously. As is the case for other types of child maltreatment, it is well recognized that official reports of children's experiences of IPV, for example to child welfare agencies, underestimate the extent of exposure. One of the most comprehensive approaches to estimating children's exposure to violence generally, the National Survey of Children's Exposure to Violence (NatSCEV), conducted most recently in 2011 (NatSCEV II), included questions about witnessing partner assault.[4] The study involved a cross-sectional national telephone survey with a target sample of more than 4500 children, aged infant to 17 years (if the selected child was younger than 10 years, the interview was conducted with the caregiver who was most familiar with the child's daily activities). Approximately one-sixth (17.3%) of the sample had witnessed an assault between parental partners in their lifetime, and 6.1% had witnessed such an assault in the past year. We also have prevalence data about IPV exposure in childhood through studies in which adults provide retrospective self-reports of their experiences. A review of US community studies conducted in 2000 estimated a yearly prevalence of 10% to 20%.[5]

Most of our global estimates of children's exposure come from considering women's experiences of IPV. Although men also experience IPV, much less is known about their exposure. It is also now recognized that bilateral violence, sometimes referred to as "common couple violence," can occur. Much of the research examining the extent of IPV has focused on women, because it is clear that repeated coercive, sexual, and severe physical violence are perpetrated predominantly against women by men.[6] For example, a recent systematic review based on data from 66 countries found that one in seven homicides globally are committed by an intimate partner; this figure is six times higher for female victims than for males.[7] IPV against women varies internationally, but is universally high; a comparative survey that included almost 25,000 women from 15 sites in 10 countries found a lifetime prevalence of physical or sexual violence, or both, ranging from 15%, primarily in developed countries, to 71% in developing countries,[8] although many other factors also play a role.

Risk and Protective Factors

Most of the knowledge about risk factors associated with IPV falls into the category of correlate (an association between a specific variable, such as poverty, and an increased likelihood of occurrence of IPV) rather than causal risk factors, where there is a demonstrated temporal and causal relationship between an antecedent variable and IPV as an outcome. As outlined by the World Health Organization (WHO), it is useful to consider the "ecological model" when summarizing risk factors for violence (in this case, IPV), because it is possible to include factors from multiple domains of influence.[9] The ecological model uses four levels to organize a framework of risk factors for increasing risk of IPV victimization and/or perpetration: (1) individual (biologic and personal history factors); (2) relationship (with peers, partners, and family members); (3) community (contexts in which social relationships are embedded, such as schools and neighborhoods); and (4) societal (larger factors, such as gender inequality, societal norms, and economic or social polices).[10]

Table 1 summarizes the risk factors for IPV[9]; those factors that show the strongest association with IPV are highlighted in bold. Most factors associated with exposure to, and perpetration of, IPV that have been identified to date are at the individual level; there is the least amount of knowledge about societal-level factors.[9] Such information is important, as are the data about protective factors (see below), because this can inform the development of interventions (programs and policies) to reduce the occurrence of IPV, and in turn, children's IPV exposure.

Much more research to date has been conducted on identifying risk factors, compared with protective factors. There is some evidence, however, to suggest that the following factors are protective in reducing the risk of IPV[9]: (1) women with higher levels of education (secondary school or higher) are less likely to experience IPV, (2) men with higher levels of education are less likely to perpetrate IPV, (3) healthy parenting during childhood, (4) having a supportive family, (5) living within an extended family or family structure, (6) belonging to an association, and (7) women's ability to recognize risk of experiencing sexual violence.

These factors are all those that influence the risk of IPV generally, rather than focus specifically on the issue of children's risk of exposure to IPV. One of the issues central to children's well-being is the overlap between experiences of IPV and co-occurrence with other types of child maltreatment. Using the 2008 NatSCEV dataset, Hamby and colleagues showed that there is a close association between "witnessing partner violence (WPV)" and other types of family violence.[11] The odds ratios indicating strength of association between WPV and other types of family violence ranged

Table 1
Risk factors for intimate partner violence

Perpetration by Men	Victimization of Women
INDIVIDUAL LEVEL	
DEMOGRAPHICS	
• Young age	• Young age
• Low socioeconomic status/income	• Low socioeconomic status/income
• Low education	• **Low education**
• Unemployment	• Separated/divorced marital status
	• Pregnancy
EXPOSURE TO CHILD MALTREATMENT	
• Intraparental violence	• **Intraparental violence**
• **Sexual abuse**	• **Sexual abuse**
• Physical abuse	
MENTAL DISORDER	
• **Antisocial personality**	• Depression
SUBSTANCE USE	
• **Harmful use of alcohol**	• Harmful use of alcohol
• **Illicit drug use**	• Illicit drug use
• **Acceptance of violence**	• **Acceptance of violence**
• **Past history of being abusive**	• **Exposure to prior abuse/victimization**
RELATIONSHIP LEVEL	
• Educational disparity	• Educational disparity
• **Multiple partners/infidelity**	• Number of children
RELATIONSHIP QUALITY	
• **Marital dissatisfaction/discord**	• **Marital dissatisfaction/discord**
• Gender role disputes	
• Marital duration	
COMMUNITY LEVEL	
• Acceptance of traditional gender roles	• Acceptance of traditional gender roles
NEIGHBORHOOD CHARACTERISTICS	
• High proportion of poverty	• High proportion of poverty
• High proportion of unemployment	• High proportion of unemployment
• High proportion of male literacy	• High proportion of female literacy
• Acceptance of violence	• Acceptance of violence
• High proportion of households that use corporal punishment	• Low proportion of women with high level of autonomy
	• Low proportion of women with higher education
• Weak community sanctions	• Weak community sanctions
SOCIETAL LEVEL	
	• **Divorce regulations by government**
	• **Lack of legislation on intimate partner violence within marriage**
	• **Protective marriage law**
• Traditional gender norms and social norms supportive of violence	• Traditional gender norms and social norms supportive of violence

Adapted from World Health Organization/London School of Hygiene and Tropical Medicine. Preventing intimate partner and sexual violence against women: taking acting and generating evidence. Geneva (Switzerland): World Health Organization; 2010; with permission.

from 3.88 to 9.15, even after controlling for demographic factors. Among the youth who had witnessed IPV in the past year, 33.9% had experienced other types of maltreatment; the proportion for lifetime exposure was more than half (56.8%). As highlighted by the authors, the same perpetrator had often assaulted multiple family members. NatSCEV I findings showed that children exposed to IPV and one or more types of other child maltreatment tend to experience more severe maltreatment compared with those children who do not witness partner violence. For example, among those youth who were physically abused, the injury rate among WPV children was 59.9% compared with 34% among non-WPV youth. For those youth who experienced neglect, the illness rate was 38.6% among WPV youth; this was more than double the rate experienced by non-WPV youth (17.4%).

Impairment

In past decades, the prevailing view about harm associated with children's exposure to IPV emphasized risk of physical abuse of the child occurring inadvertently as a result of physical IPV between caregivers. It is now recognized that a broad range of adverse outcomes are associated with exposure to IPV in childhood, including an increased risk of emotional and behavioral problems, such as anxiety disorders, post-traumatic stress disorder (PTSD), externalizing conditions, substance abuse, difficulties in relationships with peers, school-related problems,[2,12-18] and physical impairment. In extreme cases, children face acute physical harm, and even death, with up to 20% of filicide (especially paternal) cases involving a history of IPV[19]; children suffer significant loss and harm in the context of interparental domestic homicide.[20] Four meta-analyses conducted during the past decade that reviewed the literature on the effects of IPV among children (referred to as domestic violence in the reviews) warrant discussion.[15-18] Wolfe and colleagues[15] conducted a meta-analysis based on 41 studies published between 1985 and 2003 and determined that children exposed to IPV experienced more emotional and behavioral difficulties than their peers, but there were too few studies to examine educational and cognitive outcomes. Kitzmann and colleagues[16] examined 118 studies, published between 1978 and 2000, of the psychosocial outcomes of children exposed to IPV and concluded that children exposed to violence had significantly worse outcomes compared with those without such histories, and that the outcomes of exposed children did not differ significantly from those who were physically abused, or from a third group who experienced both IPV and physical abuse. Furthermore, children's exposure to IPV showed similar associations with internalizing and externalizing problems.

A subsequent meta-analysis by Evans and colleagues[17] included 60 studies published between 1990 and 2006 that evaluated the association between exposure to physical IPV and child psychosocial outcomes. The findings showed a relationship between childhood exposure and internalizing, externalizing, and trauma symptoms in children. There was notable consistency across the meta-analyses by Evans and colleagues[17] and Kitzmann and colleagues[16] with regard to the significant relationship between children's exposure to IPV and a broad range of emotional and behavioral symptoms. A fourth meta-analysis by Chan and Yeung[18] evaluated 37 studies published between 1995 and 2006 and focused on family violence, which included interparental violence; it notably found variation in strength of relationship between exposure and outcome: PTSD, internalizing, and externalizing problems seemed to have a stronger association with exposure to family violence compared with interpersonal relationship problems, competence, and perceptions or cognitions related to family violence (eg, self-blame).

Although most of these findings are based on cross-sectional studies, there is increasing evidence from longitudinal studies that the impairment associated with IPV exposure in childhood can extend into adulthood and become part of an intergenerational cycle of violence. These children are more likely to have subsequent problems parenting, and to maltreat their own children.[21] In addition, children who have experienced IPV are at increased risk of having violent dating and intimate relationships as adults, either as victims or as perpetrators.[22]

When considering the broad range of types of impairment experienced by children exposed to IPV, it is important to emphasize the increased risk of PTSD. Interestingly, in 2003, Wolfe and colleagues[15] described emerging evidence for the link between IPV exposure and PTSD in children, and noted that the dearth of studies precluded drawing any firm conclusions. In 2008, Evans and colleagues[17] identified "trauma symptomatology" as being the strongest outcome in their meta-analysis, although this outcome was limited to only six studies. One of the challenges in determining the association between IPV exposure in childhood and PTSD (and with other types of trauma), is the difficulty in diagnosing PTSD in children, especially young children.[12] Previously, the Diagnostic and Statistical Manual (DSM)-IV PTSD criteria did not take into account the variation in symptom presentation across development, but with the advent of DSM-V,[23] there is a new PTSD subtype "for children 6 years and younger." In DSM-IV, there was a requirement for three avoidance/numbing symptoms in young children, whose capacity to express such experiences verbally is only emerging.[24] The DSM-V criteria now include one or more symptoms that indicate either persistent avoidance or negative changes in cognitions and mood and presence of one or more intrusive symptoms with two or more symptoms showing alterations in reactivity and arousal. It is hoped that these changes to DSM-V will lead to a greater recognition of PTSD symptoms in children, including those associated with exposure to IPV.[25] This is particularly important, given that there are evidence-based approaches to responding to children with a history of IPV exposure and PTSD symptoms, as discussed further next.

STRATEGIES FOR IDENTIFYING AND ADDRESSING IPV IN THE CLINICAL SETTING

The key areas of intervention for clinicians working with children fall into four main areas: (1) identification and assessment, (2) prevention, (3) treatment, and (4) systems issues. These are briefly reviewed next, highlighting the important issues and evidence to be considered when providing care to children who are at risk for, or have been exposed to, IPV. This summarizes our recent review of this topic.[26]

Identification and Assessment

As with other types of child maltreatment, there is no evidence to justify universal screening of children for exposure to IPV.[27] It is also true that screening women in health care settings, including those that provide care to children, for IPV is not warranted. As outlined in the recent WHO guidelines on responding to IPV and sexual violence against women, there is no evidence to support such screening.[28] Two large randomized controlled trials, one in the United States and one in Canada, demonstrate that universal screening of women presenting to health care settings does not reduce subsequent violence or improve their life quality or health outcomes.[29,30] However, as with IPV generally, it is important for clinicians to be alert to the signs and symptoms that children exposed to IPV may exhibit, and any indicators of IPV among their caregivers. Despite the lack of evidence for universal screening, assessment of children for emotional and behavioral problems needs to include evaluation of their exposure to all types of child maltreatment, including IPV. This specific history-taking is part of the diagnostic assessment for these conditions.

During interviews with children and parents as part of a diagnostic assessment for emotional or behavioral problems, each child and caregiver must be interviewed separately. Safety of the child and a caregiver who has been abused is paramount, and discussing violence in the home in the presence of the abuser may increase the risk of further, potentially escalated, violence. It is important when asking any patient about IPV, even a general question about violence in the home, to do so with no one else present; overhearing any discussion about IPV by an abusive partner or parent could put the individual at risk.

Even very young children can provide important information about their family and adverse experiences, once they are speaking in sentences.[31] General questions for the child about various exposures, including IPV, should be included, in addition to questions about exposure to other types of maltreatment, given the frequent co-occurrence as outlined previously. It is important that such questions be tailored to a child's age and developmental stage. Examples of general questions that can identify children's exposure to IPV include the following: (1) discussion of how people in the family get along, including questions about relationships and roles; (2) inquiry about family members' safety (for example "do you feel safe at home?" and "what about other people in your family, are they safe in your home?"), specifically asking about the child, each parent, and all siblings; (3) asking the child about any worries he or she might have generally, or about any family members; and (4) general inquiry about how much "yelling, hitting, pushing" happens in the home, including discussion of what happens when "someone gets in trouble." Further information regarding inquiring about children's exposure to violence as part of history-taking during a diagnostic assessment can be found in the chapter by MacMillan and colleagues.[32]

It is not uncommon for clinicians to interview parents together in taking their child's history about exposure to adverse experiences; however, this creates a situation of potential risk and these interviews should be conducted individually. When asking individual caregivers about IPV, the clinician needs to be prepared to respond if IPV is disclosed, including showing support and inquiring about immediate safety. A meta-analysis of qualitative studies of women's experiences and expectations when the issue of IPV is raised within a clinical setting concluded that patients want confidentiality ensured and do not want to be pressured to disclose.[33] In those jurisdictions where disclosure of IPV can lead to mandatory reporting, it is important that patients be advised about the limits on confidentiality before being asked about experiences of IPV.

The initial clinical response when IPV is disclosed by a child's caregiver should include validation of the experience (eg, everyone deserves to feel safe at home), expression of support, and affirmation that violence is not acceptable.[33] The clinician should have some knowledge about appropriate community- and hospital-based referral services. The assessment should include an evaluation of safety, which includes at a minimum asking if it is safe for the caregiver and his or her child to return home. The following are examples of safety considerations as outlined in a recent summary of IPV: "(1) Has the frequency or severity of the violence increased? (2) Is the partner or ex-partner obsessed with the patient? (3) How safe does she (he) feel? (4) Does the partner or ex-partner have a weapon or access to one? (5) Has she (he) been threatened with a weapon? Although a general discussion of gun violence is beyond the scope of this section, having firearms in the home is associated with an increased risk for homicide associated with IPV. Another predictor of domestic homicide is threats of deadly violence."[6] An excellent resource for responding to disclosures of IPV is the recently released WHO guidelines,[28] which offer specific patient-centered, safety-oriented responses, based on the best available evidence.[34]

Disclosures of IPV should be reported to child protection authorities in those regions where such reporting is mandatory. It is important to be familiar with regional child protection legislation; not all states have specific reporting requirements for children exposed to IPV.[35] When health care providers are unclear about whether specific behaviors between caregivers warrant reporting to a child protection agency, an agency intake worker can be contacted and the case discussed anonymously, before making a decision about reporting. This is important, because with a few exceptions (eg, concern that a caregiver may flee with the child), the parent who discloses that his or her child is being exposed to IPV should be informed that a report is being made.[31] Ideally such a report can be made jointly with the nonoffending parent, but sometimes the IPV is committed by both parents, and in such cases the report needs to be made separately from the caregivers.

Prevention

Efforts aimed at primary prevention of IPV through educational programs have generally focused on changes in attitude, knowledge, skills, or self-reports of dating (relationship) violence. No studies to date have measured physical or emotional health. A recent meta-analysis assessed the efficacy of interventions aimed at preventing dating or relationship violence in adolescents and young adults.[36] The authors concluded that there was no evidence that the interventions were effective in improving attitudes, behaviors, or skills related to relationship violence or reducing episodes of relationship violence; there was a small improvement in knowledge about relationships. However, given that there was substantial heterogeneity between the studies, and when those studies considered at high risk of selection bias were excluded, the only remaining study showed no effect on knowledge, the overall conclusion was no evidence of effect for the interventions.

Although the best way to prevent children's exposure to IPV is by preventing or ending the IPV itself, there is limited evidence evaluating IPV interventions in adequate and generalizable samples[37,38]; promising work in the area of advocacy-based interventions requires replication in larger and more diverse samples,[39,40] and the effectiveness of shelters and other services that assist women and children to reduce or escape violence also requires timely study. Similarly, evidence regarding interventions for common couple violence or female-perpetrated IPV is weak, and although there is some US-based evidence that such approaches as permanent restraining orders against abusive partners may prevent recurrent abuse, programs for abusive partners have had mixed but generally negative (ie, in some cases, men become more abusive, or better at avoiding the consequences of abuse perpetration, after participating in these kinds of programs) results.[41]

Treatment

As with other types of abuse and neglect exposure among children, the broad range of health problems associated with experiences of IPV in childhood show little specificity.[42] Furthermore, not all children exposed to IPV experience impairment. IPV is an exposure, not a symptom or disorder; it is essential that children who have experienced IPV (and their caregivers) undergo a thorough diagnostic assessment to determine whether the child has any symptoms or disorders that would benefit from intervention. It is also crucial that any assessment of a child include an evaluation of whether exposure to IPV or other types of maltreatment is ongoing. Too often this is considered the responsibility of the child protection agency, and the clinician misses an important opportunity to assess the child's ongoing risk. Treatment needs should not simply be determined based on exposure, but take into account the child's needs for treatment of mental health conditions, and requirements for ongoing protection and access to appropriate educational and recreational activities. Recent clinical trial–level evidence provides promise regarding specific interventions for children exposed to IPV, as discussed next.

Child-parent psychotherapy in dyads including an abused mother and IPV-exposed preschooler was evaluated by Lieberman and colleagues,[43] who demonstrated significant improvement for the child-parent psychotherapy group across time, and compared with control subjects, on the Child Behavior Checklist, reduced exposure to community violence and fewer traumatic stress disorder diagnoses, immediately postintervention and at the 6-month follow-up,[44] and benefited even the highest-risk children (those with four or more traumatic or stressful life events).[45] These findings, and those of an efficacy trial comparing child-only with child-mother therapy in a nonrandomized controlled trial,[46] provide promising evidence that these forms of mother-child therapy in families where children are exposed to IPV warrant further evaluation.

Project Support, an intervention for conduct problems in IPV-exposed children recruited from women's shelters,[47] showed greater reductions in conduct problems for children in the intervention group, which involved teaching mothers child-management skills and providing them with instrumental and emotional support. Mothers in the intervention group also showed improvements, compared with control subjects, in parenting behaviors and psychiatric symptoms.

A community-based trauma-focused cognitive-behavior therapy intervention for children with IPV-related PTSD symptoms found that trauma-focused cognitive-behavior therapy improves children's IPV-related PTSD and anxiety symptoms, compared with usual community treatment.[48] Components of the intervention consisted of enhanced combined child-parent sessions, including such strategies as psychoeducation, relaxation skills, cognitive coping skills, and safety enhancement. These sessions also emphasized developing and sharing a narrative about the child's IPV experiences during joint child-parent sessions.

In summary, there is emerging trial-level evidence that various forms of mother-child and child-focused therapies for children exposed to IPV can improve children's behavioral and mental health outcomes.

SYSTEMS ISSUES

IPV is complex and meeting the needs of children requires involvement of health care providers, child protection workers, advocates, and judicial representatives. It is not uncommon for advocates for the child and the nonoffending parent to have difficulties in determining appropriate approaches to ensure everyone's safety. For example, mandatory reporting may raise concern that involvement of child protection authorities could increase violence from the abusive partner. Over the past decade, child protection agencies have developed protocols and procedures that take into account the potential risk to children and the nonoffending partner of such investigations, and sometimes have a special team with expertise assisting families.[26,49] It is important that clinicians communicate to child protection workers their knowledge of and concerns about any risk to the child and other family members regarding violence in the home, and potential for escalation in violence (if known) related to the involvement of child protection.[50] For example, a clinician working with children is often best-situated to work closely with child protection professionals in assessing older children independently regarding their safety and level of support. It is also important for clinicians to encourage parents who are experiencing IPV to consider the effects of such exposure on their parenting and assist them in accessing appropriate resources, such as referrals to advocacy services.

As outlined in a recent clinical statement from the American Academy of Pediatrics about responding to psychological maltreatment of children, clinicians working with children at risk of or exposed to IPV need to ensure there is close collaboration among health care and child protection professionals.[31] A management plan needs to be formulated that ensures close follow-up; where a child's exposure to IPV is ongoing, the clinician needs to advocate on behalf of the child to ensure those needs are prioritized. If the clinician becomes aware that a nonoffending parent has been unable to protect the child from exposure to IPV, it is important that this be reported to the child protection agency.

FUTURE DIRECTIONS

There is no doubt that IPV exposure continues to be a major public health problem for women globally, but it is encouraging that children's experiences of IPV are now being recognized as a type of child maltreatment associated with similar types of impairment as other types of abuse and neglect.[2] It is essential that future efforts focus on evaluation of existing interventions, including the extent to which programs are applicable to other settings, including those with diverse populations, and in low- and middle-income countries.

The concept of "safety planning" has typically focused on women's plans for themselves and their children, without sufficient consideration that some of the strategies that may seem reasonable to women do not apply to children or could be harmful.[51] For example, teaching children to "go to a safe room with a locked door" during times when violence is occurring in the home differs notably from messages that children are given about other types of violence, such as "tell a trusted adult."[51] Safety planning within the context of IPV has generally encompassed such considerations as safe

---

Box 1
Child safety principles and practical strategies

- School-based prevention efforts should not focus exclusively on sexual abuse and should emphasize that any violence in the home is unacceptable; this also destigmatizes the secrecy about family violence.

- Broaden the concept of safety so that it is not just a focus on physical safety, but on emotional, spiritual, and cultural safety.

- Provide information based on the age and developmental stage of the child.

- Frame messages to children within the context of general safety; calling for help; seeking a place of safety outside the home if there is danger inside the home; telling a trusted adult.

- Emphasize the need for adults, not children, to take responsibility for any violence.

- Anticipate possible harms, including increasing self-blame, reinforcing acceptance of violence, and the misapplication of advice in a range of dangerous situations (eg, going to a locked room during a fire).

- Anticipate that exposure to IPV occurs even when parents are not cohabiting (eg, following separation, during visitation).

From MacMillan HL, Wathen CN, Varcoe CM. Intimate partner violence in the family: Considerations for children's safety. Child Abuse Negl 2013;37:1190; with permission.

storage of contact information and resources, and strategies for informing others, such as neighbors, about the need to contact authorities.[52] The evidence for the effectiveness of such safety planning is unknown. Furthermore, the extent to which such plans assist in keeping children safe is unclear.[51] One of the recommendations for future work is development and evaluation of approaches to ensuring children's safety when exposed to IPV. In the absence of evidence about specific approaches to ensuring children's safety when in such settings as homes where there is risk of IPV, **Box 1** outlines some basic principles and practical strategies that it is hoped can guide health care providers in their consideration of children's needs.

SUMMARY

Knowledge about IPV and an understanding of the impairment associated with such exposure is essential for all health professionals working with children. It is clear from what is known about the epidemiology of children's experiences of IPV, that this is associated with significant impairment, including emotional, behavioral, cognitive, and physical health problems. There is an increasing evidence base about interventions aimed at responding to children who have experienced IPV, but the extent to which such interventions are generalizable to other settings beyond the original trials requires replication studies. Emerging evidence on specific forms of mother-child, and child-focused, therapies in families where IPV is present offers hope that referrals from the clinic can improve the health and well-being of these children.

REFERENCES

1. Centers for Disease Control and Prevention. Available at: http://www.cdc.gov/ViolencePrevention/intimatepartnerviolence/index.html. Accessed September 12, 2013.
2. Gilbert R, Widom CS, Browne K, et al. Burden and consequences of child maltreatment in high-income countries. Lancet 2009;373(9657):68–81.
3. Centers for Disease Control and Prevention. Fact sheet: understanding teen dating violence. Available at: http://www.cdc.gov/violenceprevention/pdf/teendatingviolence2012-a.pdf. Accessed September 12, 2013.
4. Finkelhor D, Turner HA, Shattuck A, et al. Violence, crime, and abuse exposure in a national sample of children and youth: an update. JAMA Pediatr 2013;167(7):614–21.
5. Carlson BE. Children exposed to intimate partner violence: research findings and implications for intervention. Trauma Violence Abuse 2000;1:321–40.
6. Feder G, MacMillan HL. Intimate partner violence. In: Goldman L, Schafer AI, editors. Goldman's Cecil medicine. 24th edition. Philadelphia, PA: Elsevier Publishers; 2012. p. 1571–4.
7. Stöckl H, Devries K, Rotstein A, et al. The global prevalence of intimate partner homicide: a systematic review. Lancet 2013;382(9895):859–65.
8. World Health Organization. WHO multi-country study on women's health and domestic violence against women: summary report of initial results on prevalence, health outcomes and women's responses. Geneva (Switzerland): WHO; 2005.
9. World Health Organization/London School of Hygiene and Tropical Medicine. Preventing intimate partner and sexual violence against women: taking acting and generating evidence. Geneva (Switzerland): World Health Organization; 2010.

10. Dahlberg LL, Krug EG. Violence – a global public health problem. In: Krug EG, Dahlberg LL, Mercy JA, et al, editors. World report on violence and health. Geneva (Switzerland): World Health Organization; 2002. p. 3–21.

11. Hamby S, Finkelhor D, Turner H, et al. The overlap of witnessing partner violence with child maltreatment and other victimizations in a nationally representative survey of youth. Child Abuse Negl 2010;34(10):734–41.

12. Levendosky AA, Bogat GA, Martinez-Torteya C. PTSD symptoms in young children exposed to intimate partner violence. Violence Against Women 2013;19(2): 187–201.

13. Gilbert R, Kemp A, Thoburn J, et al. Recognising and responding to child maltreatment. Lancet 2009;373(9658):167–80.

14. Graham-Bermann SA, Castor LE, Miller LE, et al. The impact of intimate partner violence and additional traumatic events on trauma symptoms and PTSD in preschool-aged children. J Trauma Stress 2012;25(4):393–400.

15. Wolfe DA, Crooks CV, Lee V, et al. The effects of children's exposure to domestic violence: a meta-analysis and critique. Clin Child Fam Psychol Rev 2003;6(3): 171–87.

16. Kitzmann KM, Gaylord NK, Holt AR, et al. Child witnesses to domestic violence: a meta-analytic review. J Consult Clin Psychol 2003;71(2):339–52.

17. Evans SE, Davies C, DiLillo D. Exposure to domestic violence: a meta-analysis of child and adolescent outcomes. Aggress Violent Behav 2008;13(2):131–40.

18. Chan YC, Yeung JW. Children living with violence within the family and its sequel: a meta-analysis from 1995–2006. Aggress Violent Behav 2009;14(5): 313–22.

19. Bourget D, Grace J, Whitehurst L. A review of maternal and paternal filicide. J Am Acad Psychiatry Law 2007;35(1):74–82.

20. Jaffe PG, Campbell M, Hamilton LH, et al. Children in danger of domestic homicide. Child Abuse Negl 2012;36(1):71–4.

21. Schwartz JP, Hage SM, Bush I, et al. Unhealthy parenting and potential mediators as contributing factors to future intimate violence: a review of the literature. Trauma Violence Abuse 2006;7(3):206–21.

22. Ehrensaft MK, Cohen P, Brown J, et al. Intergenerational transmission of partner violence: a 20-year prospective study. J Consult Clin Psychol 2003;71:741–53.

23. American Psychiatric Association. Diagnostic and statistical manual of mental disorders. 5th edition. Arlington (VA): American Psychiatric Association; 2013. Available at: dsm.psychiatryonline.org. Accessed June 1, 2013.

24. Scheeringa MS, Myers L, Putnam FW, et al. Diagnosing PTSD in early childhood: an empirical assessment of four approaches. J Trauma Stress 2012;25(4): 359–67.

25. Nemeroff CB, Weinberger D, Rutter M, et al. DSM-5: a collection of psychiatrist views on the changes, controversies and future directions. BMC Med 2013;11:202.

26. Wathen CN, MacMillan HL. Children's exposure to intimate partner violence: impacts and intervnentions. Paediatr Child Health 2013;18(8):419–22.

27. Moyer VA, U.S. Preventive Services Task Force. Primary care interventions to prevent child maltreatment: US Preventive Services Task Force recommendation statement. Ann Intern Med 2013;159(4):289–95.

28. World Health Organization. Responding to intimate partner violence and sexual violence against women: WHO clinical and policy guidelines. Available at: http://apps.who.int/iris.bitstream/10665/852401/1/9789241548595_eng.pdf. Accessed July 10, 2013.

29. MacMillan HL, Wathen CN, Jamieson E, et al, McMaster Violence Against Women Research Group. Screening for intimate partner violence in health care settings: a randomized trial. JAMA 2009;302(5):493–501.
30. Klevens J, Kee R, Trick W, et al. Effect of screening for partner violence on women's quality of life: a randomized controlled trial. JAMA 2012;308(7):681–9.
31. Hibbard R, Barlow J, MacMillan H, Committee on Child Abuse and Neglect, American Academy of Child and Adolescent Psychiatry, Child Maltreatment and Violence Committee. Psychological maltreatment. Pediatrics 2012;130(2):372–8.
32. MacMillan HL, Fleming JE, Jamieson E. Psychiatric assessment of children and adolescents. In: Goldbloom RB, editor. Pediatric clinical skills. 4th edition. New York: Churchill Livingstone; 2011. p. 206–14.
33. Feder GS, Hutson M, Ramsay J, et al. Women exposed to intimate partner violence: expectations and experiences when they encounter health care professionals: a meta-analysis of qualitative studies. Arch Intern Med 2006;166(1):22–37.
34. Feder G, Wathen CN, MacMillan HL. An evidence-based response to intimate partner violence: WHO guidelines. JAMA 2013;310(5):479–80.
35. Thackeray JD, Hibbard R, Dowd MD, Committee on Child Abuse and Neglect, Committee on Injury, Violence, and Poison Prevention. Intimate partner violence: the role of the pediatrician. Pediatrics 2010;125(5):1094–100.
36. Fellmeth GL, Heffernan C, Nurse J, et al. Educational and skills-based interventions for preventing relationship and dating violence in adolescents and young adults. Cochrane Database Syst Rev 2013;(6):CD004534.
37. Nelson HD, Bougatsos C, Blazina I. Screening women for intimate partner violence: a systematic review to update the 2004 U.S. Preventive Services Task Force Recommendation. Ann Intern Med 2012;156:796–808.
38. Taft A, O'Doherty L, Hegarty K, et al. Screening women for intimate partner violence in healthcare settings. Cochrane Database Syst Rev 2013;(4):CD007007.
39. Ramsay J, Carter Y, Davidson L, et al. Advocacy interventions to reduce or eliminate violence and promote the physical and psychosocial well-being of women who experience intimate partner abuse. Cochrane Database Syst Rev 2009;(3):CD005043.
40. Jahanfar S, Janssen PA, Howard LM, et al. Interventions for preventing or reducing domestic violence against pregnant women. Cochrane Database Syst Rev 2013;(2):CD009414.
41. Wathen CN, MacMillan HL. Interventions for violence against women: scientific review. JAMA 2003;289(5):589–600.
42. MacMillan HL, Wathen CN, Barlow J, et al. Interventions to prevent child maltreatment and associated impairment. Lancet 2009;373(9659):250–66.
43. Lieberman AF, Van Horn P, Ippen CG. Toward evidence-based treatment: child-parent psychotherapy with preschoolers exposed to marital violence. J Am Acad Child Adolesc Psychiatry 2005;44(12):1241–8.
44. Lieberman AF, Ghosh Ippen C, VAN Horn P. Child-parent psychotherapy: 6-month follow-up of a randomized controlled trial. J Am Acad Child Adolesc Psychiatry 2006;45(8):913–8.
45. Ghosh Ippen C, Harris WW, Van Horn P, et al. Traumatic and stressful events in early childhood: can treatment help those at highest risk? Child Abuse Negl 2011;35(7):504–13.

46. Graham-Bermann SA, Lynch S, Banyard V, et al. Community-based intervention for children exposed to intimate partner violence: an efficacy trial. J Consult Clin Psychol 2007;75(2):199–209.
47. Jouriles EN, McDonald R, Rosenfield D, et al. Reducing conduct problems among children exposed to intimate partner violence: a randomized clinical trial examining effects of Project Support. J Consult Clin Psychol 2009;77(4):705–17.
48. Cohen JA, Mannarino AP, Iyengar S. Community treatment of posttraumatic stress disorder for children exposed to intimate partner violence: a randomized controlled trial. Arch Pediatr Adolesc Med 2011;165(1):16–21.
49. Cross TP, Mathews B, Tonmyr L, et al. Child welfare policy and practice on children's exposure to domestic violence. Child Abuse Negl 2012;36(3):210–6.
50. Hegarty K, Taft A, Feder G. Violence between partners: working with the whole family. BMJ 2008;337:a839.
51. MacMillan HL, Wathen CN, Varcoe CM. Intimate partner violence in the family: considerations for children's safety. Child Abuse Negl 2013;37(12):1186–91.
52. Taft A, Shakespeare J. Managing the whole family when women are abused by intimate partners: challenges for health professionals. In: Roberts G, Hegarty K, Feder G, editors. Intimate partner abuse and health professionals: new approaches to domestic violence. Edinburgh (United Kingdom): Churchill Livingstone; 2006. p. 145–62.

Child Physical Abuse and Neglect

Samantha Schilling, MD[a],*, Cindy W. Christian, MD[b,c]

KEYWORDS

- Child maltreatment • Mandatory reporting • Child welfare • Child Protective Service

KEY POINTS

- Child maltreatment is common.
- Child physical abuse and neglect are 2 forms of child maltreatment.
- The maltreatment of children is a public health problem.
- There are possible lifelong consequences of child maltreatment to health and well-being.
- Additional resources are needed for the treatment and prevention of child maltreatment.
- Identifying suspected maltreatment and reporting concerns to child welfare can be one of the most challenging and important responsibilities of the pediatric health care provider.

INTRODUCTION

Since the early 1960s, public recognition of child abuse and neglect has improved considerably. The US Government enacted the Child Abuse Prevention and Treatment Act in 1974, which defines maltreatment of a child as "any recent act or failure to act on the part of a parent or caretaker, which results in death, serious physical or emotional harm, sexual abuse or exploitation, or an act or failure to act which presents an imminent risk of serious harm."[1] Decades of research and clinical experience reveal that child abuse and neglect is a public health problem with lifelong health consequences for survivors.[2] Much has been learned about the factors that contribute to the abuse of a child and about characteristics that may prove protective. Despite the progress made, the problem remains widespread and serious. Programs to prevent and intervene in child maltreatment remain fragmented, and a more comprehensive and collaborative approach to public policy concerning child safety and health is needed. The topics of child physical abuse and neglect are discussed in this article. Murray discusses child sexual abuse elsewhere in this issue, and the impact of intimate partner violence on children is discussed in the article by MacMillan.

---

[a] Child Abuse Pediatrics, The Children's Hospital of Philadelphia, 34th Street and Civic Center Boulevard, Philadelphia, PA 19104, USA; [b] Child Abuse and Neglect Prevention, The Children's Hospital of Philadelphia, 34th Street and Civic Center Boulevard, Philadelphia, PA 19104, USA; [c] Pediatrics, The Perelman School of Medicine, The University of Pennsylvania, Philadelphia, PA, USA
* Corresponding author.
E-mail address: Schillings@email.chop.edu

Child Adolesc Psychiatric Clin N Am 23 (2014) 309–319
http://dx.doi.org/10.1016/j.chc.2014.01.001
1056-4993/14/$ – see front matter © 2014 Elsevier Inc. All rights reserved.

childpsych.theclinics.com

EPIDEMIOLOGY

Each year in the United States, Child Protective Service (CPS) agencies receive more than 3 million reports of suspected child maltreatment and investigate more than 2 million of these reports; more than 650,000 children are substantiated by child welfare as maltreatment victims.[3] Most maltreated children are victims of neglect (78.5%), 17.6% are victims of physical abuse, and 9.1% are victims of sexual abuse. More than 1500 child deaths are attributed annually to child abuse or neglect.[3] However, these numbers reflect official investigations and represent only a portion of the children who suffer from maltreatment. For example, data from the Adverse Childhood Experiences studies indicate that 27% of adult women and 30% of adult men are estimated to have been physically abused during childhood, suggesting very high rates of undocumented child maltreatment.[4]

Recent child welfare statistics suggest that the incidence of child abuse and neglect is decreasing. However, child welfare data represent only those cases investigated and confirmed by state child welfare agencies, and thus are influenced by changes in reporting practices, investigation and legal standards, and administrative or statistical procedures.[5] By contrast, researchers examining hospitalization rates for physical abuse have shown either no significant recent changes or recent modest increases in hospitalizations for physical abuse.[6,7]

RISK FACTORS

Child abuse and neglect result from a complex interaction of child, caregiver, and environmental factors. Although child physical abuse and neglect affect children of all ages, ethnicities, and sociodemographic backgrounds, particular factors increase maltreatment vulnerability, and specific situations more commonly trigger maltreatment. Most often multiple factors coexist and are interrelated, increasing the risk for maltreatment of the child.[8]

Child characteristics that predispose a child to maltreatment include those that make a child more difficult to care for, or are in contrast to parental expectations. Examples include children with special health care needs, chronic illnesses, or physical or developmental disabilities.[9] Physical aggression, resistance to parental direction, and antisocial behaviors also more commonly characterize maltreated children.[10] These children exhibit poor emotional regulation, distractibility, negative affect, and a resistance to following directions.[11] A child born prematurely may present special needs, and early and at times prolonged separation may contribute to an increased vulnerability to maltreatment.[12] Although adolescents are more likely than younger children to suffer physical abuse and neglect, because of their smaller size and less mature developmental capacity, infants and toddlers are particularly vulnerable to severe and fatal maltreatment.[13]

Factors that decrease a parent's ability to cope with stress and, therefore, increase the potential for maltreatment include low self-esteem, poor impulse control, and substance abuse.[14] Other parental characteristics associated with child maltreatment include young age, low educational achievement, and mental illness.[15] In addition, parents who were themselves victims of child maltreatment are more likely to have children who are abused and neglected.[16] Parents who maltreat their children are more likely to have unrealistic developmental expectations for child behavior and to have a negative perception of normal behavior. In addition, parents with punitive parenting styles are more likely to maltreat their children.[16]

High-stress situations can increase the potential for child abuse and neglect. Circumstances that occur during the course of normal child development, including colic, nighttime awakenings, and toilet training, are potential triggers for maltreatment.[8] In particular, crying is a common trigger for abusive head trauma.[17] Infant crying generally peaks between 2 and 4 months, and the incidence of abusive head trauma parallels this crying trajectory.[18] Accidents surrounding toilet training are another potential trigger. Immersion burns may be inflicted in response to encopresis or enuresis when a caregiver believes that children should be able to control these bodily functions.[19] The average age of children who have been intentionally burned is 32 months, by which time abusive parents may have expected mastery of bodily functions.[8]

The absence of a robust family social support system places the child at increased risk for maltreatment.[20] Poverty and unemployment are also associated with maltreatment.[20] Young children who live in households with unrelated adults are at exceptionally high risk for physical abuse.[21] Children living in homes with intimate partner violence are at increased risk of being physically abused, in addition to suffering the negative emotional, behavioral, and cognitive consequences from exposure to this family violence.[22,23]

Finally, all of these child, parent, and environmental factors may interact to increase the child's vulnerability to maltreatment. Even if no single factor would be sufficient to overwhelm the caregiver, the combination of stresses may precipitate an abusive crisis.[8]

DEFINITIONS

Federal and state laws define child abuse and neglect. Each state determines the process for investigating abuse, protecting children, and holding perpetrators accountable for their actions or inactions. The Federal Child Abuse Prevention and Treatment Act provides minimum standards to states for defining maltreatment; however, states have the responsibility for specifically defining child abuse for their constituents.[1] State laws vary widely, and defining terms used by states such as "risk of harm," "substantial harm," "substantial risk," and "reasonable discipline" may not be further clarified in legislation, leading to inconsistent interpretations. Some state statutes require "serious bodily injury" or "severe pain" to define abuse, and such subjectivity may hinder consistent and appropriate reporting practices.

Physical Abuse

Although injury to any organ system can occur from physical abuse, some injuries are more common. Bruises, the most common injury resulting from physical abuse, are universal in active children, and are therefore nonspecific. Bruises suggestive of abuse include those that are patterned, such as slap marks or marks caused by a looped extension cord. Bruises in healthy children tend to be distributed over bony prominences; bruises isolated to the torso, ears, or neck should raise concern.[24] Bruises in nonambulatory infants are unusual, and are highly concerning for physical abuse.[25] Approximately 10% of children hospitalized with burns are victims of abuse.[26] Inflicted burns can be the result of contact with hot objects and from immersion injuries. In contrast to accidental scald injuries, these burns have clear demarcation, uniformity of burn depth, and a characteristic pattern.[26] Unexplained fractures, fractures in nonambulatory infants, and the presence of multiple fractures raise suspicion for physical abuse.[27] Certain fracture types also have a high specificity for abuse, such as rib fractures and classic metaphyseal lesions seen in infants. Intentional blunt trauma to the abdomen can result in solid organ and hollow viscus injury. Abusive head trauma is the leading cause of mortality and morbidity from physical abuse.[3] Common findings include subdural hemorrhages, cerebral edema, hypoxic-ischemic injury, and retinal hemorrhages.

Neglect

Neglect occurs when a child's basic needs are not adequately met. Basic needs include food, clothing, stable housing, supervision, protection, health care, education, love, and nurturance. The degree to which children's needs are met falls within a spectrum ranging from ideal to completely inadequate. Extreme situations are easily identified, but most cases are complex and lack precise clarity. Child neglect is a heterogeneous phenomenon varying in type, severity, and chronicity. Both actual and potential harm are of concern. In addition, although much neglect is recognized by an ongoing pattern of poor care, when serious risks are involved single, momentary lapses in care may also constitute neglect.

CLINICAL OUTCOMES

Adverse childhood experiences, including physical abuse and neglect, alter the architecture and function of the developing brain, and influence the neuroendocrine stress response and immune system function.[28] These physiologic disruptions can persist far into adulthood, and lead to lifelong poor physical and mental health.[28] Indeed, more than 80 scientific articles have been published elucidating the multitude of poor health outcomes experienced by adults who were maltreated as children.[4] Childhood maltreatment and family dysfunction produce poor adult health, indirectly via the adoption of high-risk behaviors and maladaptive coping mechanisms, and directly via biological injury. The lifelong consequences are profound, and as diverse as cardiovascular disease,[29] liver cancer,[30] asthma,[31] chronic obstructive pulmonary disease,[32] autoimmune disease,[33] poor dental health,[34] and depression.[35] Furthermore, there is a cumulative effect of traumatic childhood exposures: the more maltreatment, family dysfunction, and social isolation a child experiences, the higher the risk for poor health in adulthood.[36]

Maltreated children also exhibit high rates of physical, developmental, and mental health deficits during childhood. Victims of physical abuse and neglect are more likely to develop a variety of behavioral problems including conduct disorders, aggressive behaviors, poor academic performance, and decreased cognitive functioning.[10,37,38] Other health problems that afflict these vulnerable children include growth failure, obesity, lead poisoning, untreated vision and dental problems, infectious and atopic dermatitis, asthma, infectious diseases, and a range of chronic medical diseases.[39]

THERAPEUTIC STRATEGIES

Prevention and treatment of child maltreatment are complex and challenging. Many of the approaches developed by child welfare agencies, health care providers, therapists, and others have not been rigorously tested, and many families suffer from chronic dysfunction and a multitude of challenges that require broad approaches to management. In addition to addressing the consequences of poverty, substance abuse, mental health, and other common problems encountered by families involved with child welfare, at the core the relationship between parents and children requires intervention. Some strategies in this regard have shown promise.

According to a national panel of child maltreatment experts, Abuse Focused Cognitive Behavioral Therapy (AF-CBT) and Parent-Child Interaction Therapy (PCIT) are the 2 best-practice intervention protocols for the treatment of physical abuse.[40] Both are dyadic interventions designed to alter specific patterns of interaction found in parent-child relationships. AF-CBT represents an approach to working with abused children and their offending caregivers based on learning theory and behavioral principles that target child, parent, and family characteristics related to the maltreatment.[41] The approach is designed to promote the expression of appropriate/prosocial behavior and to discourage the use of coercive, aggressive, or violent behavior. PCIT is a highly specified, step-by-step, live-coached behavioral parent training model. Immediate prompts are provided to a parent by a therapist while the parent interacts with their child. Over the course of 14 to 20 weeks, parents are coached to develop specific positive relationship skills, which then results in child compliance to parent commands.[42,43]

HEALTH CARE PROVIDER MANDATES FOR REPORTING

In every state, health care providers are mandated by law to identify and report all cases of suspected child abuse and neglect. It is the responsibility of CPS to investigate reports of suspected abuse to ensure the ongoing safety of the child. Law enforcement investigates crimes such as serious physical abuse or neglect for possible criminal charges against a perpetrator. Much of the abuse that is recognized by health care providers does not get reported to CPS for investigation.[44] In part this is because clinicians may incorrectly believe that making a report requires certainty in their diagnosis of child abuse, rather than having a reasonable suspicion for maltreatment as the law requires. In addition, many clinicians believe that reporting to CPS is not an effective intervention, and distrust the ability of the child welfare system to protect children.[45]

Health care provider cooperation with CPS investigations is critical to effective decision making by investigators. Health Insurance Portability and Accountability Act (HIPAA) rules allow disclosure of protected health information to CPS without authorization by a legal guardian when the clinician has made a mandatory report, but state laws differ regarding the release of health information during and after investigations are complete.[46] Because CPS and law enforcement investigators do not have a medical background, the clinician's interpretation of the child's injuries in simple language that allows for a meaningful conversation with the investigators is critical for proper investigation, decision making, and protection of the child.[47]

CHALLENGES
Early Identification

Identifying and ensuring the health and safety of abused and neglected children is challenging. Although neglect is the most widespread form of child maltreatment and causes significant morbidity and mortality, the focus of public and professional attention is largely on physical and sexual abuse. Furthermore, neglect is difficult to define. For instance, although a health care provider might view repeated nonadherence to medications as neglect, unless harm has resulted from this inaction, this might not meet a state's CPS criteria for neglect.

Similarly, diagnosing physical abuse can be difficult. Witnesses to the abuse are uncommon, perpetrators infrequently disclose the abuse, child victims are often preverbal, too severely injured, or too frightened to disclose, and injuries can be nonspecific. Although the diagnosis of abuse can be challenging, there is abundant evidence that physicians often miss opportunities for early identification and intervention.[44,45] Previous sentinel injuries are minor injuries such as bruises or intraoral injuries that are noted before a diagnosis of child abuse. Such injuries are often identified by physicians, but are incorrectly attributed to accidental trauma or not reported to CPS for investigation despite physician suspicion for abuse.[44,48] Being cognizant of these sentinel injuries and recognizing and reporting suspected abuse and neglect can save the life of a child, and can protect the child from a lifetime of the physical and mental health sequelae of ongoing maltreatment.

Addressing Mental Health Needs of Maltreated Children

Between 50% and 80% of maltreated children have mental health problems.[49,50] Despite the need for mental health services by abused and neglected children, barriers exist to the delivery and use of services, and not all maltreated children who need treatment receive it or receive it in a timely fashion. Systemic barriers to the delivery of mental health services to maltreated children include lack of funding and accountability, few Medicaid providers, lack of cooperation among providers, waiting lists, and lack of appropriate services.[51] For instance, despite the demonstrated efficacy of AF-CBT and PCIT in treating physical abuse, there is little evidence that they are widely offered to abused children and their families.[40]

By contrast, studies have revealed that youth in foster care covered by Medicaid insurance receive psychotropic medications 3 times more often than Medicaid-insured youth not in foster care.[52] Furthermore, polypharmacy is highly prevalent, with more than 40% of the youth receiving 3 or more psychotropic drugs.[52] In response to these issues, the federal Fostering Connection to Success and Increasing Adoptions Act of 2008 and the Child and Family Services Improvement and Innovation Act require that states develop protocols for the appropriate use and monitoring of psychotropic medications for children in foster care.[53] These mandates have forced states to address these issues by improving behavioral health systems, developing preauthorization criteria for the use of psychotropic medications, identifying criteria for mandatory case reviews, and developing case-consultation systems for primary care providers.

Interdisciplinary Collaboration

The commitment to maltreated children includes a commitment to working outside of the health care community. Physicians need to collaborate with child welfare, judicial, and education colleagues to advocate for the health and well-being of these vulnerable children. In practice, coordination with other professionals to provide immediate and long-term treatment for maltreatment victims can be challenging. The collaborative process can be hindered by the lack of supportive agency–level structures and policies, inadequate resources, poor communication, differences in confidentiality policies, and a lack of knowledge of health providers about child welfare and legal systems (and vice versa). Intersystem collaboration is paramount to achieving the shared goal of ensuring the health and safety of children.

IMPORTANT TOOLS FOR PRACTICE

Ultimately, health care providers need to remain vigilant to the possibility of child maltreatment, be aware of their professional mandates, and be willing to advocate on behalf of these vulnerable patients. The extensive differential diagnosis of physical abuse depends on the type of injury, and requires careful, objective assessments of all children with suspected maltreatment. However, for children who present with pathognomonic injuries to multiple organ systems, an exhaustive search for medical diagnoses is unwarranted. All children younger than 24 months who present with suspicious injuries should undergo a skeletal survey looking for occult or healing fractures. Brain imaging may be indicated to screen for occult head trauma, particularly in young infants with multiple fractures, facial injuries, or rib fractures.

Reports should be made when there is reasonable cause to suspect abuse. In all states, the law provides some type of immunity for good-faith reporting. However, failing to report may result in malpractice suits, criminal offenses, licensing penalties, and, most importantly, continued harm to the child. Mandated reporters must become familiar with their state-specific reporting procedures and laws. Some states require both verbal and written reports. Most states specify the types of information that should be included in a report of suspected abuse or neglect, such as the name and address of the child, the child's parents, the child's age, conditions in the child's home environment, the nature and extent of the child's injuries, and information about other children in the same environment. Information on state-specific laws about mandated reporting can be found at http://www.childwelfare.gov.

Optimal care for a maltreated child depends on the clinician's working knowledge of community resources that can provide safety, advocacy, treatment, and support. Health care providers are ideally positioned to help families enhance their ability to protect children and to address factors that put them at increased risk for maltreatment. Families trust and rely on their provider's guidance and referral to resources that prioritize the health and welfare of families; thus it is paramount that the provider becomes knowledgable about such local resources.

FUTURE DIRECTIONS

Future approaches to the prevention of child maltreatment and the protection of children require meaningful collaboration between child welfare, judicial, education, health, and mental health professionals and systems. There have been recent calls for more rigorous legislative requirements for the reporting of child abuse.[54] Both federal and state legislation can improve laws to protect children and mandate improved interdisciplinary work. For example, identifying HIPAA exceptions that allow for information sharing across systems when children are placed in foster care would reduce real and perceived barriers to the information sharing that is needed to address the health needs of children in care. Health care providers require training on the effects of child maltreatment and toxic stress, assessment tools for primary care providers are needed to identify families and children in need of intervention and support, effective behavioral and treatment strategies need to be identified and adopted broadly, and the behavioral and mental health systems in the country require expansion to meet the needs of the population.

Reducing rates of maltreatment, supporting families, and improving pediatric and adult health outcomes for maltreatment victims requires community-wide strategies and a multisystem public health approach. Future policies and practices must address the overutilization of psychotropic medications in this vulnerable population, and ensure that maltreated children and their families have access to mental health treatments that have been studied and shown to be effective. Equally important is prioritizing permanency and stability for children in foster care, as 1 in 3 of these children fail to achieve a long-lasting placement.[55] Finally, the prevalence of child maltreatment may decline further when policy makers, health care providers, and applicable systems refine, promote, and implement effective prevention strategies that augment current treatments.

SUMMARY

Few problems have as profound an impact on the health and well-being of children as child abuse and neglect. Experiencing child maltreatment increases the risk of developing behaviors in adolescence and adulthood that predict adult morbidity and early mortality. The child welfare, foster, and health care systems have struggled to collaborate to address the health needs of children who have been maltreated. Although recognizing maltreatment and advocating for the safety of a child is a great challenge, intervening on behalf of a vulnerable child has the potential to greatly improve the child's future health outcomes and life trajectory.

REFERENCES

1. CAPTA, The CAPTA Reauthorization Act of 2010, Public Law 111-320, (42 U.S.C. 5106a). Available at: http://www.acf.hhs.gov/programs/cb/laws_policies/cblaws/capta/capta2010.pdf. Accessed November 10, 2013.
2. Middlebrooks JS, Audage NC. The effects of childhood stress on health across the lifespan. Atlanta (GA): Centers for Disease Control and Prevention, National Center for Injury Prevention and Control; 2008.
3. U.S. Department of Health and Human Services, Administration for Children and Families, Administration on Children, Youth and Families, Children's Bureau. 2012. Child maltreatment 2011. Available at: http://www.acf.hhs.gov/programs/cb/research-data-technology/statistics-research/child-maltreatment. Accessed November 10, 2013.
4. Adverse Childhood Experiences (ACE) Study. Prevalence of individual childhood experiences. Atlanta, GA: Centers for Disease Control and Prevention; 2013. Available at: www.cdc.gov/ace/prevalence.htm. Accessed November 10, 2013.
5. Jones L, Finkelhor D. Updated trends in child maltreatment. Crimes Against Children Research Center. 2007. Available at: www.unh.edu/ccrc/pdf/Updated%20Trends%20in%20Child%20Maltreatment%202007.pdf. Accessed November 10, 2013.
6. Leventhal JM, Gaither JR. Incidence of serious injuries due to physical abuse in the United States: 1997 to 2009. Pediatrics 2012;130:e847–52.
7. Farst K, Ambadwar PB, King AJ, et al. Trends in hospitalization rates and severity of injuries from abuse in young children, 1997-2009. Pediatrics 2013; 131:e1796–802.
8. Flaherty EG, Stirling J, The Committee of Child Abuse and Neglect. The pediatrician's role in child maltreatment prevention. Pediatrics 2010;126:833–41.
9. Hibbard RA, Desch L, The Committee on Child Abuse and Neglect and the Council on Children with Disabilities. Maltreatment of children with disabilities. Pediatrics 2007;119:1018–25.
10. Kolko DJ. Characteristics of child victims of physical violence: research findings and clinical implications. J Interpers Violence 1992;7:244–76.
11. Shields A, Cicchetti D. Reactive aggression among maltreated children: the contributions of attention and emotion dysregulation. J Clin Child Psychol 1998;27:381–95.
12. Wu SS, Ma C, Carter RL, et al. Risk factors for infant maltreatment: a population-based study. Child Abuse Negl 2004;28:1253–64.
13. Finkelhor D, Ormrod R, Turner H, et al. The victimization of children and youth: a comprehensive, national survey. Child Maltreat 2005;10:5–25.
14. Kelleher K, Chaffin M, Hollenberg J, et al. Alcohol and drug disorders among physically abusive and neglectful parents in a community-based sample. Am J Public Health 1994;84:1586–90.
15. Sidebotham P, Heron J. Child maltreatment in the "children of the nineties": a cohort study of risk factors. Child Abuse Negl 2006;30:497–522.
16. Oates RK, Davis AA, Ryan MG. Predictive factors for child abuse. Aust Paediatr J 1980;16:239–43.

17. Brewster AL, Nelson JP, Hymel KP, et al. Victim, perpetrator, family, and incident characteristics of 32 infant maltreatment deaths in the United States Air Force. Child Abuse Negl 1998;22:91–101.
18. Barr RG, Trent RB, Cross J. Age-related incidence curve of hospitalized shaken baby syndrome cases: convergent evidence for crying as a trigger to shaking. Child Abuse Negl 2006;30:7–16.
19. Daria S, Sugar N, Feldman KW, et al. Into hot water head first: distribution of intentional and unintentional immersion burns. Pediatr Emerg Care 2004;20: 302–10.
20. Kotch JB, Browne DC, Dufort V, et al. Predicting child maltreatment in the first 4 years of life from characteristics assessed in the neonatal period. Child Abuse Negl 1999;23:305–19.
21. Schnitzer PG, Ewigman BG. Child deaths resulting from inflicted injuries: household risk factors and perpetrator characteristics. Pediatrics 2005;116: e687–93.
22. Christian CW, Scribano P, Seidl T, et al. Pediatric injury resulting from family violence. Pediatrics 1997;99:e8.
23. Holt S, Buckley H, Whelan S. The impact of exposure to domestic violence on children and young people: a review of the literature. Child Abuse Negl 2008; 32:797–810.
24. Pierce MC, Kaczor K, Aldridge S, et al. Bruising characteristics discriminating physical child abuse from accidental trauma. Pediatrics 2010;125:67–74.
25. Sugar NF, Taylor JA, Feldman KW. Bruises in infants and toddlers: those who don't cruise rarely bruise. Arch Pediatr Adolesc Med 1999;153:399–403.
26. Purdue GF, Hunt JL, Prescott PR. Child abuse by burning—an index of suspicion. J Trauma 1988;28:221–4.
27. Leventhal JM, Thomas SA, Rosenfield NS, et al. Fractures in young children: distinguishing child abuse from unintentional injuries. Am J Dis Child 1993;147: 87–92.
28. Shonkoff JP, Garner AS. The lifelong effects of early childhood adversity and toxic stress. Pediatrics 2012;129:e232–46.
29. Dong M, Giles WH, Felitti VJ, et al. Insights into causal pathways for ischemic heart disease: adverse childhood experiences study. Circulation 2004;110: 1761–6.
30. Dong M, Dube SR, Felitti VJ, et al. Adverse childhood experiences and self-reported liver disease: new insights into the causal pathway. Arch Intern Med 2003;163:1949–56.
31. Haczku A, Panettieri RA. Social stress and asthma: the role of corticosteroid insensitivity. J Allergy Clin Immunol 2010;125:550–8.
32. Anda RF, Brown DW, Dube SR, et al. Adverse childhood experiences and chronic obstructive pulmonary disease in adults. Am J Prev Med 2008;34: 396–403.
33. Dube SR, Fairweather D, Pearson WS, et al. Cumulative childhood stress and autoimmune diseases in adults. Psychosom Med 2009;71:243–50.
34. Poulton R, Caspi A, Milne BJ, et al. Association between children's experience of socioeconomic disadvantage and adult health: a life-course study. Lancet 2002; 360:1640–5.
35. Edwards VJ, Holden GW, Felitti VJ, et al. Relationship between multiple forms of childhood maltreatment and adult mental health in community respondents: results from the adverse childhood experiences study. Am J Psychiatry 2003;160: 1453–60.

36. Felitti VJ, Anda RF, Nordenberg D, et al. Relationship of childhood abuse and household dysfunction to many of the leading causes of death in adults: the adverse childhood experiences (ACE) study. Am J Prev Med 1998;14: 245–58.

37. Hildyard KL, Wolfe DA. Child neglect: developmental issues and outcomes. Child Abuse Negl 2002;26:679–95.

38. Perez CM, Widom CS. Childhood victimization and long-term intellectual and academic outcomes. Child Abuse Negl 1994;18:617–33.

39. Steele JS, Buchi KF. Medical and mental health of children entering the Utah foster care system. Pediatrics 2008;122:e703–9.

40. Closing the quality chasm in child abuse treatment: identifying and disseminating best practices. Chadwick Center for Children and Families and National Call to Action. 2004. Available at: http://www.chadwickcenter.org/Documents/Kaufman%20Report/ChildHosp-NCTAbrochure.pdf. Accessed November 10, 2013.

41. Kolko DJ, Swenson CC. Assessing and treating physically abused children and their families: a cognitive behavioral approach. Thousand Oaks (CA): Sage Publications; 2002.

42. Timmer SG, Urquiza AJ, Zebell NM, et al. Parent-child interaction therapy: application to maltreating parent-child dyads. Child Abuse Negl 2005;29:825–42.

43. Chaffin M, Silovsky JF, Funderburk B, et al. Parent-child interaction therapy with physically abusive parents: efficacy for reducing future abuse reports. J Consult Clin Psychol 2004;72:500–10.

44. Sheets LK, Leach ME, Koszewski IJ, et al. Sentinel injuries in infants evaluated for child physical abuse. Pediatrics 2013;131:701–7.

45. Jones R, Flaherty EG, Binns HJ, et al. Clinicians' description of factors influencing their reporting of suspected child abuse: report of the child abuse reporting experience study research group. Pediatrics 2008;122:259–66.

46. The Committee on Child Abuse and Neglect. Child abuse, confidentiality, and the Health Insurance Portability and Accountability Act. Pediatrics 2010;125:197–201.

47. Kellogg ND, The Committee on Child Abuse and Neglect. Evaluation of suspected child physical abuse. Pediatrics 2007;119:1232–41.

48. Flaherty EG, Sege RD, Griffith J, et al. From suspicion of physical child abuse to reporting: primary care clinician decision-making. Pediatrics 2008;122:611–9.

49. Leslie LK, Jeanne GN, Lee M, et al. The physical, developmental, and mental health needs of young children in child welfare by initial placement type. J Dev Behav Pediatr 2005;26:177–85.

50. McMillen JC, Zima BT, Scott LD, et al. Prevalence of psychiatric disorders among older youths in the foster care system. J Am Acad Child Adolesc Psychiatry 2005;44:88–95.

51. Staudt MM. Mental health services utilization by maltreated children: research findings and recommendations. Child Maltreat 2003;8:195–203.

52. Zito JM, Safer DJ, Sai D, et al. Psychotropic medication patterns among youth in foster care. Pediatrics 2008;121:e157–63.

53. U.S. Department of Health and Human Services, Administration for Children and Families, Administration on Children, Youth and Families, Children's Bureau. 2012. Effective use of psychotropic medication for children in foster care. Available at: http://www.nrcpfc.org/fostering_connections/download/IM%20Oversight%20of%20Psychotropics%20Medication%20for%20Children%20in%20Foster%20Care-Title%20IV-B%20Health%20Care%20Oversight%20%20Coordination%20Plan.pdf. Accessed November 20, 2013.

54. Task Force on Child Protection Joint State Government Commission. General Assembly of the Commonwealth of Pennsylvania. Child protection in Pennsylvania: proposed recommendations. 2012. Available at: http://jsg.legis.state.pa.us/resources/documents/ftp/publications/2012-285-Child%20Protection%20Report%20FINAL%20PDF%2011.27.12.pdf. Accessed November 20, 2013.
55. Rubin DM, O'Reilly AL, Luan X, et al. The impact of placement stability on behavioral well-being for children in foster care. Pediatrics 2007;119:336–44.

Child Sexual Abuse

Laura K. Murray, PhD[a],*, Amanda Nguyen, MA[a],
Judith A. Cohen, MD[b]

KEYWORDS

- Child sexual abuse • Prevalence • Treatment

KEY POINTS

- Child sexual abuse (CSA) is truly a global problem, often defying myths and stereotypes, and does not appear to be decreasing over time.
- There are many different definitions of CSA, adding to the challenges of measurement, assessment, and treatment.
- Globalization and modern technology may increase the risk of abuse and exploitation, but may also offer opportunities to strengthen our responses, particularly in areas with lower resources.
- Several therapies have been shown to be efficacious in treating the psychological sequelae of CSA.
- The results of treatment studies are encouraging, as many include youth from high-stress homes and foster care systems, and those who have experienced polyvictimization.
- Results suggest that a wide range of symptoms are decreased, including individual symptoms of posttraumatic stress disorder, depression, anxiety, and behavioral problems, as well as family and relationship problems.
- At present, there is a shift from developing new treatments toward moving effective treatments from the laboratory to real practice settings with wider-scale dissemination and implementation.
- Future research must examine the barriers and facilitators within efforts at dissemination and implementation, and evaluate various strategies to improve reach and uptake.

Sexual abuse toward children and adolescents is a stark reality worldwide. A common misperception about child sexual abuse (CSA) is that it is a rare event perpetrated against girls by male strangers in poor, inner-city areas. To the contrary, CSA is a much too common occurrence that results in harm to millions of children, boys and

The authors have no conflict of interest.
[a] Department of Mental Health, Johns Hopkins University School of Public Health, 624 North Broadway, 8th Floor, Baltimore, MD 21205, USA; [b] Center for Traumatic Stress in Children and Adolescents, Allegheny General Hospital, Drexel University College of Medicine, 4 Allegheny Center, 8th Floor, Pittsburgh, PA 15212, USA
* Corresponding author.
E-mail address: lamurray@jhsph.edu

Child Adolesc Psychiatric Clin N Am 23 (2014) 321–337
http://dx.doi.org/10.1016/j.chc.2014.01.003
1056-4993/14/$ – see front matter © 2014 Elsevier Inc. All rights reserved.

Acronyms	
CBITS	Cognitive-Behavioral Intervention for Trauma in School
CBT	Congnitive behavioral therapy
CDC	Centers for Disease Control and Prevention
CPS	Child Protective Services
CSA	Child sexual abuse
D&I	Dissemination and Implementation
EBT	Evidence-based treatments
EMDR	Eye movement desensitization and reprocessing
FIAM	Fostering Individualized Assistance Program
RCTs	Randomized controlled trials
UNICEF	United Nations Children's Fund
WHO	World Health Organization

girls alike, in large and small communities, and across a range of cultures and socio-economic backgrounds. These acts are perpetrated by many types of offenders, including men and women, strangers, trusted friends or family, and people of all sexual orientations, socioeconomic classes, and cultural backgrounds.[1]

PHENOMENOLOGY AND DEFINITIONS

CSA encompasses many types of sexually abusive acts toward children, including sexual assault, rape, incest, and the commercial sexual exploitation of children. Although there are some differences among these, the unifying term of "child sexual abuse" is used throughout this article to describe commonalities across these experiences. There are many definitions of CSA in use, each of which may have subtle differences in coverage or terminology that influence surveillance and reporting efforts, and potentially lead to different policy, service, or legal implications. According to the US Centers for Disease Control and Prevention (CDC), child sexual abuse is "any completed or attempted (noncompleted) **sexual act**, **sexual contact** with, or exploitation (ie, **noncontact** sexual interaction) of a child by a caregiver."[2] The CDC provides specific definitions for each of the boldface terms, distinguishing sexual acts as those involving penetration, abusive sexual contact as intentional touching with no penetration, and noncontact sexual abuse such as exposing a child to sexual activity, taking sexual photographs or videos of a child, sexual harassment, prostitution, or trafficking.[2] The World Health Organization (WHO) defines CSA as:

> The involvement of a child in sexual activity that he or she does not fully comprehend, is unable to give informed consent to, or for which the child is not developmentally prepared and cannot give consent, or that violate the laws or social taboos of society. Child sexual abuse is evidenced by this activity between a child and an adult or another child who by age or development is in a relationship of responsibility, trust or power, the activity being intended to gratify or satisfy the needs of the other person. This may include but is not limited to: the inducement or coercion of a child to engage in any unlawful sexual activity; the exploitative use of child in prostitution or other unlawful sexual practices; the exploitative use of children in pornographic performances and materials.[3]

Of note, these definitions include as CSA acts that both do and do not involve physical touching or physical force, including completed sex acts, attempted sex acts, abusive sexual touching, and noncontact assaults such as harassment, threats, forced exposure to pornography, and taking unwanted sexual images, such as filming or photography. In some instances, the recipient may not be aware of their own victimization, or that violence has been perpetrated against them. This breadth of scope reflects the recognition that imposing sexual intent of any sort on someone against his or her will is an inherently violent act, regardless of the use of physical force or resulting contact or injury. These definitions also raise the important consideration of consent, and identify categories of people who are unable to consent or resist because of age, disability, state of consciousness or intoxication, or fear of harm to self or others.

Because a legal age of majority is required for consent, all sexual acts between an adult and underage child (even with child assent) are, by definition, CSA. The United Nations Children's Fund (UNICEF) endorses the Council of Europe's definition of child sex abuse, which includes activities involving a child under the legal age as provided by national law, as well as sexual activities with children that involve coercion, abuse of a position of trust or influence, or exploitation of a vulnerable or dependent child.[4] Additional acts of CSA toward children involve the sexual exploitation of children through prostitution or abusive images; profiting from or any role in the facilitation, observation, or exploitation of a child's involvement in sexual performances; causing a child to witness sex abuse or sex acts; and child solicitation.[4]

EPIDEMIOLOGY

Accurate measurement of the prevalence of childhood CSA is made difficult by several methodological issues. Definitions of CSA typically vary across studies, such as in terms of the age used to define childhood, whether an age difference is specified, or if peer abuse is included, as well as the types of acts considered as sexual abuse (eg, both contact and noncontact). Decisions of sample selection (eg, convenience or probability sampling), survey methods (face-to-face interviews or self-administered questionnaires), and number and detail of screening questions also all influence the resulting prevalence estimates.[5]

Most prevalence surveys rely on adult retrospective reporting and may be subject to recall bias, while objective informant observations are likely to underreport because of the large proportion of CSA that goes unseen. The WHO 2002 *World Report on Violence and Health* suggests that cases reported to authorities may reflect a more physically violent subset with injuries requiring treatment, as these cases are less easily hidden. It likens the magnitude of CSA or sexual violence to an iceberg, in which only the smallest portion is reported to authorities, a larger yet still incomplete portion is reported on surveys, and an unquantifiable amount remains unreported because of shame, fear, or other factors.[6] Feelings of guilt and shame, such as perceptions of responsibility for the abuse, lack of honor, and loss of self-worth, influence disclosure.[7–9] Other studies have also found inverse associations between disclosure and the severity of abuse, with children more likely to disclose noncontact abuse than contact abuse.[10]

With these considerations in mind, several studies have been undertaken to document the prevalence of CSA in countries around the world. The 2006 *World Report on Violence against Children*[11–14] provided estimates that in 2002 approximately 150 million girls and 73 million boys were subject to contact CSA worldwide, including 1.2 million trafficked children and 1.8 million exploited through prostitution or pornography.

In the United States, a population-based sample of face-to-face interviews with more than 34,000 adults found that 10% of respondents reported experiencing contact CSA before age 18 years, 25% of whom were men.[15] A nationally representative study using telephone-based interviews with 4549 children and their caregivers reported that 6.1% of children had been victims of CSA (contact and noncontact) in the past year and 9.8% in their lifetime; when looking only at adolescents aged 14 to 17 years, these numbers escalated to 16.3% and 27.3%, respectively.[16]

Two recent meta-analyses of global prevalence studies produced strikingly similar estimates. The first analysis included 65 articles involving 37 male and 63 female samples across 22 countries, totaling more than 10,000 individuals. Definitions of CSA in the studies varied, with an upper age limit ranging from 12 to 17 years and approximately two-thirds of the studies including noncontact CSA. The investigators reported a combined mean prevalence of CSA in 7.9% of males and 19.7% of females, with the highest rates occurring in Africa and the lowest in Europe.[17]

The second analysis included data from 331 studies representing nearly 10 million individuals.[18] In this analysis, the total combined prevalence was 11.8%, with 7.6% of males and 18% of females reporting experiences of CSA. In this analysis, Asia reported the lowest combined prevalence for both boys and girls, while Africa had the highest prevalence for boys and Australia the highest prevalence for girls. This analysis also compared informant with self-report studies, and found that informant studies produced a much more conservative estimate of 0.4%, compared with 12.7% when assessed via self-report.

RISK FACTORS

Childhood sexual abuse often occurs alongside other forms of abuse or neglect, and in family environments in which there may be low family support and/or high stress, such as high poverty, low parental education, absent or single parenting, parental substance abuse, domestic violence, or low caregiver warmth.[15,19] Children who are impulsive, emotionally needy, and who have learning or physical disabilities, mental health problems, or substance use may be at increased risk.[19,20] The risk of CSA also appears to increase in adolescence.[16,20]

Out-of-home youth may be particularly at risk for CSA, initially as a condition that leads to their out-of-home status and later as a consequence of situations such as violent street life.[21–23] These youth may be exploited and forced to trade sex for survival needs such as food, shelter, money, or drugs.[24] In many countries, children in conflict with the law may be at risk of abuse by authorities both on the street and in detention; when detained, they may also be inappropriately housed with adults and made vulnerable to CSA and exploitation.[25]

Children living in conflict and postconflict environments are also at increased risk for CSA, attributable to the breakdown of normal protective structures or the use of CSA as an act of war.[26–28] Some of the children at particular risk in these settings are unaccompanied children who have been separated from their families and may lack adequate protection; children in detention; child soldiers; adolescents; children with disabilities; working children; adolescent mothers, who may lack support or resources; and children born of rape, who may be cast aside by their communities.[29]

FACTORS INFLUENCING DISCLOSURE

Experiences of childhood CSA often go undisclosed and unrecognized. A review of the literature[10] reveals the many factors that inhibit disclosure. In addition to being developmentally vulnerable, children are often manipulated to feel guilty or responsible for the abuse. These children may fear the disclosure will not be believed, or that it will negatively affect their own well-being and that of their families. Moreover, they may be concerned about consequences for the perpetrator, as often the perpetrators are familiar figures who develop complex, confusing, and ambivalent relationships with the child.

A study by Kogan[30] involving a subset of 263 adolescent girls from a nationally representative sample in the United States showed that younger children were not likely to disclose CSA immediately, whereas children aged 7 to 13 years were most likely to tell an adult within a month, and older adolescents were more likely to tell their peers. Kogan hypothesized that adolescents may be more aware of the potential negative reactions of family members; this may be a particular concern when the perpetrator is known to the family, as a close or familial relationship with the perpetrator decreased the likelihood of disclosure. In this sample, girls who feared for their lives or experienced penetration were more likely to tell an adult, suggesting that seeking protection or requiring medical treatment likely influences disclosure.

Priebea and Svedinb[31] sought to explore variables influencing disclosure in a population-based sample of 4339 high school seniors of both sexes in Sweden. In the total sample, 65% of the girls and 23% of the boys reported experiencing CSA. The investigators suggested that the high prevalence may be due to better recall of youth in comparison with adults, as well as a definition that included peer abuse. Of those who had experienced CSA, most youth (81% of girls and 69% of boys) reported disclosing the abuse to someone; however, approximately 40% of the youth talked about their experience only to a same-aged peer, whereas only 8.3% had spoken to a professional, and even fewer (6.8%) said their experience had been reported to social services or police. Contrary to the previous findings, in this study youth who had experienced greater severity of abuse were more likely to feel they could not talk to anyone about the abuse, and they were less likely to talk to a parent or family member. Factors associated with lower disclosure for girls included experiencing contact versus noncontact abuse, single versus multiple instances of abuse, a known abuser rather than a stranger, and perceiving their parents as noncaring. For boys, lower disclosure was associated with attending a vocational program rather than a traditional high school, living with both parents, and perceptions of parents as overprotective or not caring.

Other factors, such as culture and gender, may also influence willingness to report experiences of CSA. Fontes and Plummer[32] presented a thoughtful analysis of the many ways that decisions to disclose CSA are influenced by the social and cultural context, noting that although no one value is exclusive to a particular culture, issues and values may weigh differently in different cultures and influence the ability to disclose. The investigators provided several examples of potential barriers to disclosure, including of the roles of modesty; taboos and shame; sexual scripts that normalize CSA (eg, it is normal for men to want sex, so abuse is a girl's fault for tempting a man); the emphasis on virginity and honor; girls' reports of CSA being discounted as fabricated because of their lower status within a community; fear that disclosure would lead to obligations to avenge lost honor through further violence; respect for elders and filial piety; the influence of religious beliefs and teachings; and structural factors such as language barriers and immigration status.

With respect to gender, Romano and De Luca[33] summarized research suggesting several reasons why boys may be less likely than girls to report these experiences. These investigators described how female sexual abuse is more widely recognized and screened for, leading to higher reporting; along this same line of thought, boys may be more reluctant to seek support owing to gender norms reinforcing self-reliance, which in turn leads to a continued underestimation of the problem of male CSA. Boys may also experience more confusion about the abuse; they may mistakenly believe that admitting CSA by male perpetrators would mean that they are homosexual; and they may be confused as to whether sexual acts with an older person are abusive because of their visible physiologic responses, emotional grooming by the abuser, and some societal views that sexual exploration with someone not much older than them is a neutral or even a positive experience, rather than potentially traumatic experience.

COURSE AND OUTCOMES

The heterogeneity of definitions of child sexual abuse is also reflected in the widely varied reactions, ranging from severe psychological impact to no evidence of negative psychological sequelae.[34] For those who are affected, the mental health effects of childhood sexual abuse are varied.[35] Child survivors of sexual abuse are at increased risk for anxiety, inappropriate sexual behavior and preoccupations, anger, guilt, shame, depression, posttraumatic stress disorder (PTSD), and other emotional and behavioral problems throughout their life span.[36–40] Research shows that survivors of child sexual abuse are more likely to experience social and/or health problems in adulthood, such as alcohol problems, use of illicit drugs, suicide attempts, and marriage/family problems.[41] Numerous studies show that CSA survivors are vulnerable to later sexual revictimization in both adolescence and adulthood.[42,43] Finally, CSA has a clear correlation with high-risk sexual behaviors (eg, multiple sexual partners) and may have a connection with later abuse on others.[44–46] The effects of CSA are often compounded by other types of co-occurring abuse and dysfunction, producing a cumulative effect on risk factors for negative health outcomes, including adult diseases such as heart, lung, and liver disease, and cancer.[47] Although much of this literature focuses on the outcomes for girls, a meta-analysis of the impact of childhood CSA on boys shows similar outcomes.[46] Although the design limitations in CSA research often preclude causal inference, twin studies have demonstrated that the association between CSA and such adverse health outcomes is independent of other risk factors in the home environment.[48]

Although survivors of CSA are at risk of poor health outcomes, these outcomes are not fixed. Factors supporting healthier outcomes include self-esteem and social support from family and peers, as well as family expressiveness and cohesion, whereas family conflict negatively affects resilience. In fact, some literature suggests that social support and family characteristics may be more influential than particular risk factors or characteristics of the experienced abuse in determining resilience.[49–51]

SYSTEMS INVOLVEMENT

There are numerous systems involved after a child experiences sexual abuse, which may include Child Protective Services (CPS), police, legal teams, medical teams, other child protection agencies, foster care and child welfare agencies, and/or residential treatment facilities. CPS is generally responsible for the investigation of and intervention in cases of suspected sexual abuse whereby the offender is in a caretaking role for the child. Law enforcement agencies are usually responsible for the investigation of cases involving offenders in non-caretaking roles. However, CPS are often involved in situations where the perpetrator is not the caregiver, but the child's caretaker fails to protect the child. On receiving a report, CPS conduct an investigation, within a specified time frame (typically within 24 or 48 hours or up to 5 days) to determine whether abuse has occurred. The child usually participates in an interview conducted either by CPS alone or CPS in conjunction with law enforcement. The length and number of interview sessions may vary depending on the case, age of the child, and who is interviewing (eg, the skill and years of experience of the interviewer). A child who has been sexually abused also usually receives a medical examination, ideally by a professional who specializes in CSA evaluations.[52] In the case of recent abuse or concern of injury, it is important that this examination be conducted as soon as possible, and in accordance with established forensic practice. Caregivers and family members are also interviewed. These results are provided to CPS, law enforcement, and often a legal team. There are 2 or 3 courts that are potentially involved in a sexual abuse case: the Juvenile Court, responsible for child protection; the Criminal Court, responsible for offender prosecution; and/or the Family Court.

CPS ultimately determine whether the abuse is likely to recur in the future and whether the child's safety can be ensured in the home (the first choice). If CPS determine that the child is not safe within his or her own home, they may suggest removal of the child and placement with a relative or a foster family, or in some cases a residential treatment facility if there is more severe symptomatology. Efforts may also include removing the offender from the home.

Many of these agencies are involved in specific tasks, many of which are short term. However, sexual abuse is usually not a short-term problem, and requires different interventions at different times. Thus, the coordination of multiple services is important to ensure the long-term protection and healing of the child. Some communities have set up multidisciplinary teams and links between agencies[53,54] that serve to coordinate care. In other communities, services are poorly integrated. How child protection systems and legal institutions need to respond is discussed in the WHO World Violence Report,[6] with key recommendations highlighting the need for better assessment and monitoring, better response systems, policy development, better data, documentation of effective responses, and improved training and education for professionals. There are additional guidelines for best practices in investigating allegations of CSA that highlight agencies and processes commonly used, such as medical providers, forensic interviewing, and psychosocial evaluations.[55] Online resources and research publications discuss the challenges of responding to and evaluating CSA cases, such as nondisclosure of abuse by family members or the child, difficult decisions of whether to remove a child from a home, and again the complicated process of coordinating the multiple agencies involved.

THERAPEUTIC STRATEGIES

Treatment of a child and familial system after sexual abuse is multifaceted and generally requires a biopsychosocial approach. Depending on the presence and extent of physical injury, medical professionals may be involved in ongoing treatment. Children and their caretakers (family or foster caretakers) are usually assigned a case manager. The role of a case manager is to link the child and family to necessary services, and continue to assess need. Case managers often help the family connect with medical and mental health services, as well as any legal or court appointments. This article focuses on the mental and behavioral health of the family and child after sexual abuse.

There is a growing evidence base of effective psychotherapeutic treatments for sexually abused children and their families. Unfortunately, it is common for sexually abused children to have other types of traumatic experiences; for example, being removed from their home, witnessing domestic violence, and experiencing multiple instances of sexual abuse, physical abuse, and/or neglect.[37,47,56] Most of the treatment studies conducted have included populations with multiple traumatic experiences and/or a particular diagnosis common after trauma (eg, PTSD).[37] A recent Cochrane review examined the effectiveness of psychological therapies in treating children and adolescents who have been diagnosed with PTSD.[57] Fourteen randomized controlled trials (RCTs) were included, totaling 758 participants who had experienced sexual abuse, civil violence, natural disaster, domestic violence, and motor vehicle accidents. The therapies used in these 14 studies were: (1) cognitive-behavioral therapy (CBT); (2) exposure-based; (3) psychodynamic; (4) narrative; (5) supportive counseling; and (6) eye-movement desensitization and reprocessing (EMDR). Most compared a psychological therapy group with a control group, showing significant improvement across symptoms of PTSD, depression, and anxiety. Of therapies assessed, CBT was shown to have the greatest efficacy, with significant improvement and lower PTSD symptoms documented for up to a year following treatment. Depression scores were also lower with CBT treatment, and no adverse effects were identified. For narrative therapy and EMDR, this review reported no statistically significant difference in PTSD or depression symptom scores in comparison with controls. A review by Silverman and colleagues[58] also evaluated RCTs of psychosocial treatments for children exposed to traumatic events.[59,60] Results showed that trauma-focused cognitive-behavioral therapy (TF-CBT) was the only treatment that met criteria for a "well-established treatment, based on Chambless and colleagues'[60] categories of evidence." School-based group CBT[61,62] was determined to be "probably efficacious," and 7 other treatments (resilient peer treatment, family therapy, client-centered therapy, cognitive-processing therapy, child-parent psychotherapy, CBT for PTSD, and EMDR) were classified as "possibly efficacious."

TF-CBT is one of the most rigorously evaluated treatments for CSA.[63] TF-CBT is a hybrid model that integrates elements of exposure-based, cognitive-behavioral, affective, humanistic, attachment, family, and empowerment therapies into a treatment designed to address the unique needs of children with problems related to traumatic life experiences such as sexual abuse. This treatment was developed to ideally include both the child (aged 3–18 years) and a supportive caregiver, in weekly parallel sessions. Eight components are delivered and practiced over a period of approximately 12 to 16 weeks. The components of TF-CBT include: (1) psychoeducation; (2) relaxation; (3) affective modulation; (4) cognitive processing; (5) trauma narrative (gradual exposure) and cognitive restructuring of the trauma; (6) in vivo desensitization; (7) conjoint parent/child session; and (8) enhancing safety skills. Although the treatment is designed with specific components, each with a set of goals, TF-CBT is highly flexible in meeting the individual presentation of symptoms and the needs of different children and families.

Multiple RCTs have demonstrated TF-CBT to be a highly effective treatment for the sequelae of child trauma exposure, including depression, anxiety, and PTSD symptoms.[64,65] Many of these RCTs had clear inclusion criteria of a sexual abuse experience,[64,66–71] although many of the children had experienced multiple traumas. Follow-up studies demonstrated sustained benefit at 6 months, 1 year, and 2 years after treatment.[68,72,73] Recent RCTs, quasi-experimental trials, and open trials included children exposed to multiple traumatic events.[74–76] There is also a growing body of literature on the implementation of TF-CBT for youth with ongoing traumas.[77–79] TF-CBT has been adapted and used effectively with a variety of populations including Latino youth,[80] Native American youth,[81] and orphans and vulnerable children in Zambia.[82,83] Research suggests broad applicability and acceptability among ethnically diverse therapists, children, and parents.[84,85]

CHALLENGES
Dissemination and Implementation

Research shows that despite high rates of CSA and known negative sequelae, many children who have experienced sexual abuse either do not receive treatment or receive treatment that has not proved to be effective.[86,87] The wide-scale dissemination and implementation (D&I) of evidence-based treatments (EBT) is an area of high interest, and is also wrought with many challenges.[88] For example, effective D&I usually requires ongoing, multilevel strategies across numerous partnerships (eg, trainers, providers, organizations, policy-makers) that can be expensive and time-consuming. Some studies have sought to identify specific barriers to D&I of EBT to guide the use of specific strategies. Barriers may include clinician attitudes toward EBT, contextual or institutional factors (eg, organizational culture and climate, leadership), client attitudes, and population characteristics.[89] Another barrier to D&I of EBT is the cost of training and ongoing supervision, especially with attrition. Research has begun to lay out various strategies that can be helpful with D&I.[90] For example, training accompanied by regular supervision and/or consultation has been found to be effective with community mental health professionals trained in manualized treatments.[91–93]

Although the D&I of effective treatments for CSA is a challenge, some notable progress has been made. For example, the National Child Traumatic Stress Network[94] was established by the US Congress in 2000 with the mission of raising the standard of care and increasing access to effective treatment for children who have experienced traumas such as CSA. More recently, increasing numbers of state-wide initiatives to implement treatments for sexual abuse, such as TF-CBT, are showing positive results and are overcoming some common D&I challenges.[95–97]

These initiatives demonstrate different strategies used for D&I, and discuss important successes and lessons to help in future endeavors. One reoccurring challenge is gaining buy-in from therapists to complete the entire training process. Strategies used to aid in this include more careful identification of practitioners most likely to complete and use an EBT, offering additional consultation call and advanced training opportunities for clinicians, and varying call times to help with difficult schedules. Most groups found it important to match the national certification in TF-CBT with state requirements as another incentive. Strategies used to disseminate and effectively implement EBT have included a combination of assessing organizational readiness, live training sessions, and ongoing consultations. Another key strategy that has seen success across many states is the use of learning collaboratives, an approach using groups within an organization to study and adapt implementation practices to capitalize on shared learning and collaboration. It is clear that different strategies and approaches are needed for varying contexts and settings, and ideally EBT should be provided during graduate school to truly produce a readily trained workforce of mental health professionals proficient in evidence-based trauma treatments.

Intrafamilial Sexual Abuse

CSA committed by someone within the family is often cited as a particular challenge. In these cases, it is usually more common that a child needs to be removed from the home for some time, along with any siblings. These family systems often undergo stress during investigations. There is some research suggesting that children abused by someone within the family represent a distinctly different group from those abused outside the family. Distinct features may include an increased guilt about and/or reluctance to disclose abuse[98,99] and a higher likelihood of recantation.[100] There may be coercion from caregivers to recant and/or change a disclosure, and often there is significant financial stress introduced into family systems when the breadwinner is forced out. There is also some evidence to suggest that children who have experienced intrafamilial abuse show less improvement following therapy[101] and may be more subject to the cumulative impact of polyvictimization,[37] owing to exposure to both sexual and emotional abuse. However, most treatment studies do not distinguish between those abused within the family or by someone outside the family, creating challenges in truly teasing out the differences.

Cultural Considerations in CSA Populations

Some publications discuss concern about the cross-cultural sensitivity and applicability of EBT.[102,103] Culturally competent treatment has been emphasized in several published guidelines.[104–106] Some challenges to better understanding the cross-cultural effectiveness include low minority recruitment in clinical trials, uncommon examination of culture as a moderator of treatment, limited descriptions of culturally modified changes to treatment, and cultural validity of treatment outcome measures. Nevertheless, a recent review found that some trauma-focused treatments were probably efficacious for ethnic minorities.[84] The three treatments include: (1) TF-CBT; (2) the Fostering Individualized Assistance Program (FIAM),[107] which is an individualized case management intervention; and (3) cognitive-behavioral intervention for trauma in school (CBITS).[62] Although challenges remain and more studies are needed, Huey and Polo[84] recommended using an existing EBT for ethnic minorities rather than unstudied treatments.

Fewer evaluations of child and adolescent EBT for sexually abused populations have been conducted globally. A recent, small-scale RCT assessed group-based TF-CBT with war-affected, sexually exploited girls in the Democratic Republic of Congo.[108] Compared with a wait-list control condition, TF-CBT participants had significantly greater reductions in traumatic stress symptoms and other psychosocial difficulties. Researchers noted a mean decrease of 22.5 symptoms from pretest to posttest in the treatment group, compared with a mean increase of 2.6 symptoms in the control group ($P<.001$). An open trial of TF-CBT in Zambia demonstrated the feasibility of integrating TF-CBT into existing human immunodeficiency virus (HIV) care systems (eg, hospices, HIV-centered clinics), with promising clinical outcomes.[82] Of particular interest may be the specific modifications across cultures made to TF-CBT, which were conceptualized as alterations in technique rather than changes in core components or goals of the treatment.[83] There is also growing evidence from research in global mental health as a whole that with careful adaptation to local context, EBTs developed in high-income settings can be feasibly, acceptably, and effectively delivered in low-resource settings with different cultural backgrounds.[109]

SUMMARY

CSA is truly a global problem, often defying myths and stereotypes, and it does not appear to be decreasing over time. There are many different definitions of CSA, adding to the challenges of measurement, assessment, and treatment. Globalization and modern technology may increase the risk of abuse and exploitation, but may also offer opportunities to strengthen our responses, particularly in areas of lower resources. It is clear that CSA is associated with the risk of negative psychosocial and health outcomes, but processes of resilience have also identified several protective factors (eg, family support, parent-child relationships, social support) that could be strengthened through prevention and early intervention efforts.

Several therapies have been shown to be efficacious in treating the psychological sequelae of CSA.[58] The results of treatment studies are encouraging, as many include youth from high-stress homes and foster care systems, and those who have experienced polyvictimization. Results suggest that a wide range of symptoms are decreased, including individual symptoms of PTSD, depression, anxiety, and behavioral problems, as well as family and relationship problems. At present, there is a shift from developing new treatments toward moving effective treatments from the laboratory to real practice settings with wider-scale D&I. This agenda raises its own set of challenges regarding flexibility and fidelity: the delicate balance of staying true to an evidence-based model and assuring that it meets the needs of diverse populations and settings.[110] Future research must examine the barriers and facilitators within D&I efforts, and evaluate various strategies to improve reach and uptake.

REFERENCES

1. Cromer LD, Goldsmith RE. Child sexual abuse myths: attitudes, beliefs, and individual differences. J Child Sex Abuse 2010;19:618–47.
2. Leeb RT, Paulozzi L, Melanson C, et al. Child maltreatment surveillance: uniform definitions for public health and recommended data elements, version 1.0. Atlanta (GA): Centers for Disease Control and Prevention, National Center for Injury Prevention and Control; 2008. Available at: http://www.cdc.gov/violenceprevention/pdf/cm_surveillance-a.pdf.
3. World Health Organization. Report of the consultation on child abuse prevention (WHO/HSC/PVI/99.1). Geneva (Switzerland): World Health Organization; 1999. Available at: http://www.who.int/mip2001/files/2017/childabuse.pdf.
4. UNICEF. Definitions of select child protection terms. 2010. Available at: http://www.unicef.org/protection/57929_58022.html#core. Accessed November 6, 2013.
5. Goldman JD, Padayachi UK. Some methodological problems in estimating incidence and prevalence in child sexual abuse. J Sex Res 2000;37(4):305–14.
6. Krug EG, Dahlberg LL, Mercy JA, et al, editors. Sexual violence: world report on violence and health. Geneva (Switzerland): World Health Organization; 2002. Available at: http://whqlibdoc.who.int/publications/2002/9241545615_eng.pdf.
7. Schönbucher V, Maier T, Mohler-Kuo M, et al. Disclosure of child sexual abuse by adolescents: a qualitative in-depth study. J Interpers Violence 2012;27(17): 3486–513. http://dx.doi.org/10.1177/0886260512445380.
8. Goodman-Brown TB, Edelstein RS, Goodman GS, et al. Why children tell: a model of children's disclosure of sexual abuse. Child Abuse Negl 2003;27(5): 525–40.
9. Fontes LA. Sin vergüenza: addressing shame with Latino victims of child sexual abuse and their families. J Child Sex Abuse 2007;16:61–82.
10. Paine ML, Hansen DJ. Factors influencing children to self-disclose sexual abuse. Clin Psychol Rev 2002;22:271–95.
11. Pinheiro PS. World report on violence against children: United Nations Secretary-General's study on violence against children. Geneva (Switzerland): ATAR Roto Presse SA; 2006. Available at: http://www.unicef.org/violencestudy/reports.html.
12. World Health Organization. Global estimates of health consequences due to violence against children. Background paper to the UN secretary-general's study on violence against children. Geneva (Switzerland): World Health Organization; 2006.
13. Andrews G, Corry J, Slade T, et al. Child sexual abuse. In: Ezzati M, Lopez AD, Rodgers A, et al, editors. Comparative quantification of health risks: global and regional burden of disease attributable to selected major risk factors, vol. 2. Geneva (Switzerland): World Health Organization; 2004. p. 1851–940. Available at: http://www.who.int/publications/cra/chapters/volume1/0000i-xxiv.pdf.
14. International Labour Organization. A future without child labour. Global Report. Geneva (Switzerland): International Labour Organization; 2002.

15. Perez-Fuentes G, Olfson M, Villegas L, et al. Prevalence and correlates of child sexual abuse: a national study. Compr Psychiatry 2013;54(1):16–27.
16. Finkelhor D, Turner H, Ormrod R, et al. Violence, abuse, and crime exposure in a national sample of children and youth. Pediatrics 2009;124(5):1411–23.
17. Pereda N, Guilera G, Forns M, et al. The prevalence of child sexual abuse in community and student samples: a meta-analysis. Clin Psychol Rev 2009; 29(4):328–38.
18. Stoltenborgh M, van Ijzendoorn MH, Euser EM, et al. A global perspective on child sexual abuse: metal-analysis of prevalence around the world. Child Maltreat 2011;16(2):79–101.
19. Butler AC. Child sexual assault: risk factors for girls. Child Abuse Negl 2013; 37(9):643–52. http://dx.doi.org/10.1016/j.chiabu.2013.06.009.
20. Davies EA, Jones AC. Risk factors in child sexual abuse. J Forensic Psychiatr 2013;20(3):146–50.
21. Tyler KA, Hoyt DR, Whitbeck LB, et al. The impact of childhood sexual abuse on later sexual victimization among runaway youth. J Res Adolesc 2001;11(2): 151–76.
22. Stewart AJ, Steiman M, Cauce AM, et al. Victimization and posttraumatic stress disorder among homeless adolescents. J Am Acad Child Adolesc Psychiatry 2004;43(3):325–31.
23. Rew L, Taylor-Seehafer M, Fitzgerald ML. Sexual abuse, alcohol and other drug use, and suicidal behaviors in homeless adolescents. Issues Compr Pediatr Nurs 2001;24(4):225–40.
24. Tyler KA, Johnson KA. Trading sex: voluntary or coerced? The experiences of homeless youth. J Sex Res 2006;43(3):208–16.
25. Wernham M. An outside chance: street children and juvenile justice, an international perspective. London: Consortium of Street Children; 2004. Available at: http://www.crin.org/resources/infoDetail.asp?ID=4382.
26. Wood EJ. Variation in sexual violence during war. Polit Soc 2006;34:307–41.
27. Ward J, Marsh M. Sexual violence against women and girls in war and its aftermath: realities, responses, and required resources. A briefing paper prepared for symposium on sexual violence in conflict and beyond. Brussels, June 21–23, 2006. Available at: https://unfpa.org/emergencies/symposium06/docs/finalbrusselsbriefingpaper.pdf.
28. Carpenter RC. Recognizing gender-based violence against civilian men and boys in conflict situations. Secur Dialog 2006;37:83–103.
29. UNHCR. Sexual and gender-based violence against refugees, returnees and internally displaced persons. 2003. Available at: http://www.rhrc.org/resources/gbv/gl_sgbv03.pdf. Accessed November 6, 2013.
30. Kogan SM. Disclosing unwanted sexual experiences: results from a national sample of adolescent women. Child Abuse Negl 2004;28(2):147–65.
31. Priebea G, Svedinb CG. Child sexual abuse is largely hidden from the adult society: an epidemiological study of adolescents' disclosures. Child Abuse Negl 2008;32:1095–108.
32. Fontes LA, Plummer C. Cultural issues in disclosures of child sexual abuse. J Child Sex Abuse 2010;19:491–518.
33. Romano E, De Luca RV. Male sexual abuse: a review of effects, abuse characteristics, and links with later psychological functioning. Aggress Violent Beh 2001;6(1):55–78.
34. Kendall-Tackett KA, Williams LM, Finkelhor D. Impact of sexual abuse on children: a review and synthesis of the literature. Psychol Bull 1993;113:164–80.

35. Maniglio R. The impact of child sexual abuse on health: a systematic review of reviews. Clin Psychol Rev 2009;29(7):647–57. http://dx.doi.org/10.1016/j.cpr.2009.08.003.

36. Cutajar MC, Mullen PE, Ogloff JR, et al. Psychopathology in a large cohort of sexually abused children followed up to 43 years. Child Abuse Negl 2010; 34(11):813–22. http://dx.doi.org/10.1016/j.chiabu.2010.04.004.

37. Finkelhor D, Ormrod RK, Turner HA. Poly-victimization: a neglected component in child victimization. Child Abuse Negl 2007;31:7–26.

38. Lalor K, McElvaney R. Child sexual abuse, links to later sexual exploitation/high-risk sexual behavior, and prevention/treatment programs. Trauma Violence Abuse 2010;11(4):159–77. http://dx.doi.org/10.1177/1524838010378299.

39. Mills R, Scott J, Alati R, et al. Child maltreatment and adolescent mental health problems in a large birth cohort. Child Abuse Negl 2013;37(5):292–302.

40. Nanni V, Uher R, Danese A. Childhood maltreatment predicts unfavorable course of the illness and treatment outcome and depression: a meta-analysis. Am J Psychiatry 2012;163(2):141–51.

41. Dube S, Anda R, Whitfield C, et al. Long term consequences of childhood sexual abuse by gender of victim. Am J Prev Med 2005;28:430–8.

42. Classen C, Palesh O, Aggarwal R. Sexual revictimization: a review of the literature. Trauma Violence Abuse 2005;6:103–29.

43. Humphrey JA, White JW. Women's vulnerability to sexual assault from adolescence to young adulthood. J Adolesc Health 2000;27:419–24.

44. Fergusson D, Horwood J, Lynskey M. Childhood sexual abuse, adolescent sexual behaviours and sexual revictimization. Child Abuse Negl 1997;21:789–803.

45. Noll J, Trickett P, Putnam F. A prospective investigation of the impact of childhood sexual abuse on the development of sexuality. J Consult Clin Psychol 2003;71:575–86.

46. Homma Y, Wang N, Sawyc E, et al. The relationship between sexual abuse and risky sexual behavior among adolescent boys: a meta-analysis. J Adolesc Health 2012;51(1):18–24.

47. Felitti VJ, Anda RF, Nordenberg D, et al. Relationship of childhood abuse and household dysfunction to many of the leading causes of death in adults: the adverse childhood experiences (ace) study. Am J Prev Med 1998;14:245–58.

48. Nelson EC, Heath AC, Madden PA, et al. Association between self-reported child sexual abuse and adverse psychosocial outcomes: results from a twin study. Arch Gen Psychiatry 2002;59(2):139–45. http://dx.doi.org/10.1001/archpsyc.59.2.139.

49. Jonzon E, Lindblad F. Risk factors and protective factors in relation to subjective health among adult female victims of child sexual abuse. Child Abuse Negl 2006;30:127–43.

50. McClure F, Chavez D, Agars M, et al. Resilience in sexually abused women: risk and protective factors. J Fam Psychol 2008;23(2):81–8.

51. Fassler IR, Amodeo M, Griffin ML, et al. Predicting long-term outcomes for women sexually abused in childhood: contribution of abuse severity versus family environment. Child Abuse Negl 2005;29:269–84.

52. Sheela L, Lahoti MD, McClan N, et al. Evaluating the child for sexual abuse. Am Fam Physician 2001;63(5):883–93.

53. Wolf M. Putting standards into practice: a guide to implementing NCA standards for children's advocacy centers. Washington, DC: National Children's Alliance; 2000.

54. Jackson SL. A USA national survey of program services provided by child advocacy centers. Child Abuse Negl 2004;28(4):411–21.
55. American Professional Society on the Abuse of Children. Available at: http://www.apsac.org/. Accessed November 5, 2013.
56. Saunders BE. Understanding children exposed to violence: toward an integration of overlapping fields. J Interpers Violence 2003;18(4):356–76.
57. Gillies D, Taylor F, Gray C, et al. Psychological therapies for the treatment of post-traumatic stress disorder in children and adolescents. Cochrane Database Syst Rev 2012;(12):CD006726. http://dx.doi.org/10.1002/14651858.CD006726.pub2.
58. Silverman WK, Ortiz CD, Viswesvaran C, et al. Evidence-based psychosocial treatments for children and adolescents exposed to traumatic events. J Clin Child Adolesc Psychol 2008;37(1):156–83. http://dx.doi.org/10.1080/15374410701818293.
59. Chambless DL, Hollon SD. Special section: empirically supported psychological therapies. J Consult Clin Psychol 1998;66(1):7–18.
60. Chambless DL, Sanderson WC, Shoham V, et al. An update on empirically validated therapies. Clin Psychol Psychother 1996;49:5–18.
61. Kataoka SH, Stein BD, Jaycox LH, et al. A school-based mental health program for traumatized Latino immigrant children. J Am Acad Child Adolesc Psychiatry 2003;42:311–8.
62. Stein BD, Jaycox LH, Kataoka SH, et al. A mental health intervention for school children exposed to violence. J Am Med Assoc 2003;290:603–11.
63. Cohen JA, Mannarino AP, Deblinger E. Treating trauma and traumatic grief in children and adolescents. New York: Guilford Press; 2006.
64. Cohen JA, Deblinger E, Mannarino AP, et al. A multi-site, randomized controlled trial for sexually abused children with PTSD symptoms. J Am Acad Child Adolesc Psychiatry 2004;43:393–402.
65. Dorsey S, Briggs-King EC, Woods BA. Cognitive-behavioral treatment for post-traumatic stress disorder in children and adolescents. Child Adolesc Psychiatr Clin N Am 2011;20(2):255–69. http://dx.doi.org/10.1016/j.chc.2011.01.006.
66. Cohen JA, Mannarino AP. A treatment outcome study for sexually abused preschool children: initial findings. J Am Acad Child Adolesc Psychiatry 1996;35:42–50.
67. Cohen JA, Mannarino AP. A treatment study for sexually abused preschool children: outcome during a one-year follow-up. J Am Acad Child Adolesc Psychiatry 1997;36:1228–35.
68. Cohen JA, Mannarino AP. Interventions for sexually abused children: initial treatment outcome findings. Child Maltreat 1998;3:17–26.
69. Deblinger E, Lippmann J, Steer R. Sexually abused children suffering posttraumatic stress symptoms: initial treatment outcome findings. Child Maltreat 1996;1:310–21.
70. Deblinger E, Stauffer LB, Steer RA. Comparative efficacies of supportive and cognitive behavioral group therapies for young children who have been sexually abused and their nonoffending mothers. Child Maltreat 2001;6:332–43.
71. King N, Tonge BJ, Mullen P, et al. Treating sexually abused children with post-traumatic stress symptoms: a randomized clinical trial. J Am Acad Child Adolesc Psychiatry 2000;59(11):1347–55.
72. Deblinger E, Mannarino AP, Cohen JA, et al. A follow-up study of a multisite, randomized, controlled trial for children with sexual abuse-related PTSD symptoms. J Am Acad Child Adolesc Psychiatry 2006;45(12):1474–84.

73. Deblinger E, Steer RA, Lippmann J. Two-year follow-up study of cognitive behavioral therapy for sexually abused children suffering post-traumatic stress symptoms. Child Abuse Negl 1999;23:1371–8.

74. CATS Consortium. Implementing CBT for traumatized children and adolescents after September 11: lessons learned from the Child and Adolescent Trauma Treatments and Services (CATS) project. J Clin Child Adolesc Psychol 2007; 36(4):581–92. http://dx.doi.org/10.1080/15374410701662725.

75. Cohen JA, Mannarino AP, Iyengar S. Community treatment of PTSD for children exposed to intimate partner violence: a randomized controlled trial. Arch Pediatr Adolesc Med 2011;165(1):16–21. http://dx.doi.org/10.1001/archpediatrics. 2010.247.

76. Jaycox LH, Cohen JA, Mannarino AP, et al. Children's mental health care following Hurricane Katrina: a field trial of trauma-focused psychotherapies. J Trauma Stress 2010;23(2):223–31. http://dx.doi.org/10.1002/jts.20518.

77. Murray LK, Cohen JA, Mannarino AP. Trauma-focused cognitive behavioral therapy for youth who experience continuous traumatic exposure. Peace Confl 2013;19(2):180–95. http://dx.doi.org/10.1037/a0032533.

78. Cohen JA, Mannarino AP, Kliethermes M, et al. Trauma-focused CBT for youth with complex trauma. Child Abuse Negl 2012;36(6):528–41. http://dx.doi.org/ 10.1016/j.chiabu.2012.03.007.

79. Cohen JA, Mannarino AP, Murray LK. Trauma-focused CBT for youth who experience ongoing traumas. Child Abuse Negl 2011;25(8):637–46. http://dx.doi.org/ 10.1016/j.chiabu.2011.05.002.

80. de Arellano MA, Danielson CK. Culturally-modified trauma-focused therapy for treatment of Hispanic child trauma victims. Paper presented at the Annual San Diego Conference on Child and Family Maltreatment. San Diego, January 2006.

81. BigFoot DS, Schmidt S. Honoring children-mending the circle: cultural adaptation of trauma-focused cognitive-behavioral therapy children. J Clin Psychol 2010;66(8):847–56. http://dx.doi.org/10.1002/jclp.20707.

82. Murray LK, Familiar I, Skavenski S, et al. An evaluation of trauma-focused cognitive behavioral therapy for children in Zambia. Child Abuse Negl 2013;12. http:// dx.doi.org/10.1016/j.chiabu.2013.04.017.

83. Murray LK, Dorsey S, Skavenski SA, et al. Identification, modification, and implementation of an evidence-based psychotherapy for children in a low-income country: the use of TF-CBT in Zambia. Int J Ment Health Syst 2013;7(1):24.

84. Huey SJ, Polo AJ. Evidence-based psychosocial treatments for ethnic minority youth. J Clin Child Adolesc Psychol 2008;37(1):262–301. http://dx.doi.org/10. 1080/15374410701820174.

85. Murray LK, Skavenski S, Michalopoulos L, et al. Counselor and client perspectives of trauma-focused cognitive behavioral therapy for children in Zambia: A qualitative study. J Clin Child Adolesc Psychol 2014 Jan 8. [Epub ahead of print].

86. Burns B, Phillips S, Wagner H, et al. Mental health need and access to mental health services by youths involved with child welfare: a national survey. J Am Acad Child Adolesc Psychiatry 2004;43:960–70.

87. Kolko D, Cohen J, Mannarino A, et al. Community treatment of child sexual abuse: a survey of practitioners in the National Child Traumatic Stress Network. Adm Policy Ment Health 2009;36:37–49.

88. Fixsen DL, Naoom SF, Blase KA, et al. Implementation research: a synthesis of the literature (FMHI Publication No. 231). Tampa (FL): University of South

Florida, Louis de la Parte Florida Mental Health Institute, The National Implementation Research Network; 2005.

89. Cook JM, Biyanova T, Coyne JC. Barriers to adoption of new treatments: an internet study of practicing community psychotherapists. Adm Policy Ment Health 2009;36:83–90. http://dx.doi.org/10.1007/s10488-008-0198-3.

90. Powell BJ, McMillen JC, Proctor EK, et al. A compilation of strategies for implementing clinical innovations in health and mental health. Med Care Res Rev 2012;69(2):123–57. http://dx.doi.org/10.1177/1077558711430690.

91. Herschell AD, Kolko DJ, Baumann BL, et al. The role of therapist training in the implementation of psychosocial treatments: a review and critique with recommendations. Clin Psychol Rev 2010;30:448–66. http://dx.doi.org/10.1016/j.cpr. 2010.02.005.

92. Beidas RS, Edmunds JE, Marcus SC, et al. Training and consultation to promote implementation of an empirically supported treatment: a randomized trial. Psychiatr Serv 2012;63(7):660–5. http://dx.doi.org/10.1176/appi.ps.201100401.

93. Beidas R, Glickman A, Nadeem E, editors. Special issue: going beyond training and hoping: evidence-based supervision, consultation, and ongoing support strategies in schools and community settings. Adm Policy Ment Health 2013:40(6).

94. The National Child Traumatic Stress Network. Available at: www.nctsn.org. Accessed November 7, 2013.

95. Sigel BA, Kramer TL, Conners-Burrow NA, et al. Statewide dissemination of trauma-focused cognitive-behavioral therapy (TF-CBT). Child Youth Serv Rev 2013;35:1023–9.

96. Cohen JA, Mannarino AP. Disseminating and implementing trauma-focused CBT in community settings. Trauma Violence Abuse 2008;9:214–26.

97. Allen B, Johnson JC. Utilization and implementation of trauma-focused cognitive behavioral therapy for the treatment of maltreated children. Child Maltreat 2012; 17(1):80–5. http://dx.doi.org/10.1177/1077559511418220.

98. DiPietro EK, Runyan DK, Fredrickson DD. Predictors of disclosure during medical evaluation for suspected sexual abuse. J Child Sex Abuse 1997;1:133–42.

99. Hershkowitz I, Horowitz D, Lamb ME. Trends in children's disclosure of abuse in Israel: a national study. Child Abuse Negl 2005;29:1203–14.

100. Malloy LC, Lyon TD, Quas J. Filial dependency and recantation of child sexual abuse allegations. J Am Acad Child Adolesc Psychiatry 2007;46:162–70.

101. Hetzel-Riggin MD, Brausch AM, Montgomery BS. A meta-analytic investigation of therapy modality outcomes for sexually abused children and adolescents: an exploratory study. Child Abuse Negl 2007;31:125–41.

102. Gray-Little B, Kaplan D. Race and ethnicity in psychotherapy research. In: Snyder CR, Ingram RE, editors. Handbook of psychological change: psychotherapy processes & practices for the 21st century. Hoboken (NJ): Wiley; 2000. p. 591–613.

103. Miranda J, Azocar F, Organista KC, et al. Recruiting and retaining low-income Latinos in psychotherapy research. J Consult Clin Psychol 1996;64:868–74.

104. American Psychological Association. Guidelines on multicultural education, training, research, practice, and organizational change for psychologists. Washington, DC: APA; 2002. Available at: http://www.apa.org/pi/oema/resources/policy/multicultural-guidelines.aspx.

105. Bernal G, Bonilla J, Bellido C. Ecological validity and cultural sensitivity for outcome research: issues for cultural adaptation and development of psychosocial treatments with Hispanics. J Abnorm Child Psychol 1995;23:67–82.

106. De Arellano MA, Danielson CK. Assessment of trauma history and trauma-related problems in ethnic minority child populations: an informed approach. Cognit Behav Pract 2008;15(1):53–66.

107. Clark HB, Prange ME, Lee B, et al. An individualized wraparound process for children in foster care with emotional-behavioral disturbances: follow-up findings and implications from a controlled study. In: Epstein MH, Kutash K, Duchnowski A, editors. Outcomes for children and youth with emotional and behavioral disorders and their children: programs and evaluation best practices. Austin (TX): Pro-Ed; 1998. p. 513–42.

108. O'Callaghan P, McMullen J, Shannon C, et al. A randomized controlled trial of trauma-focused cognitive behavioral therapy for sexually exploited, war-affected Congolese girls. J Am Acad Child Adolesc Psychiatry 2013;52(4): 359–69. http://dx.doi.org/10.1016/j.jaac.2013.01.013.

109. Patel V, Chowdhary N, Rahman A. Improving access to psychological treatments: lessons from developing countries. Behav Res Ther 2011;49(9):523–8. http://dx.doi.org/10.1016/j.brat.2011.06.012.

110. Kendall PC, Beidas RS. Smoothing the trail for dissemination of evidence-based practices for youth: flexibility within fidelity. Prof Psychol Res Pr 2007;38:13–20.

Complex Trauma

Matthew Kliethermes, PhD*, Megan Schacht, PhD,
Kate Drewry, MSW, LCSW

KEYWORDS

- Complex trauma • Children and adolescents • Interpersonal trauma
- Childhood victimization

KEY POINTS

- Complex trauma exposure involves chronic/multiple traumas during developmentally vulnerable time periods.
- Exposure to complex trauma is a common occurrence for children and adolescents.
- Complex trauma exposure disrupts early attachment relationships and brain development.
- Complex trauma outcomes involve significant difficulties with emotional, behavioral, somatic, and cognitive dysregulation.

Acronyms	
ADHD	Attention deficit/hyperactivity disorder
BTT	Betrayal trauma theory
DTD	Developmental trauma disorder
HPA	Hypothalamic-pituitary-adrenal
PTSD	Post-traumatic stress disorder

INTRODUCTION

The construct of complex trauma has evolved significantly in the past 25 years. Part of the challenge with the development of this concept is that the term complex trauma has been used to refer to both the traumatic event and the unique sequelae of symptoms associated with this type of trauma. One of the earliest attempts to delineate the concept of complex trauma was attempted by Terr[1] who differentiated type I and type II traumas. According to this model, type I traumas tend to be single events resulting in symptoms more closely aligned with posttraumatic stress disorder (PTSD), whereas

Disclosure: The authors have no industry disclosures to report.
Children's Advocacy Services of Greater St Louis, Department of Psychology, University of Missouri–St Louis, Weinman Building, 1 University Boulevard, St Louis, MO 63121, USA
* Corresponding author.
E-mail address: kliethermesm@umsl.edu

Child Adolesc Psychiatric Clin N Am 23 (2014) 339–361
http://dx.doi.org/10.1016/j.chc.2013.12.009   childpsych.theclinics.com
1056-4993/14/$ – see front matter © 2014 Elsevier Inc. All rights reserved.

type II traumas tend to be repeated, long-standing events that may present with a range of symptoms including denial, dissociation, rage, self-destructive behavior, and unremitting sadness.

The definition of complex traumatic experiences has evolved into one that refers to severe events that tend to be chronic and undermine a child's personality development and fundamental trust in relationships.[2] Building from this characterization, a complex traumatic event has been further defined as a traumatic event that is repetitive and occurs over an extended period of time, undermines primary caregiving relationships, and occurs at sensitive times with regard to brain development. Complex trauma events vary widely and include physical abuse, sexual abuse, emotional abuse, neglect, witnessing domestic violence, exposure to community violence, and medical trauma. The lack of consensus on a definition of complex trauma has posed challenges for researchers because definitions can have varying emphasis placed on the number of traumatic events, the types of traumatic events, the developmental periods in which they occur, or the resulting symptom profile.[3]

The term complex trauma is also used to refer to the unique pattern of symptoms associated with this type of experience. Research has struggled to identify the sequelae of complex trauma; however, it has consistently identified that the impact of complex trauma is distinctive compared with more acute traumas.[2,4–6] Domains of impairment associated with complex trauma exposure may include deficits in relationships and attachment, emotional and behavioral dysregulation, cognitive/attentional deficits, and biological changes that may affect physical health. Further, symptoms such as dissociation, changes to self-perception, and overall shifts in beliefs about the world are frequently seen among youth who have experienced complex trauma.[7]

Delineating the construct of complex trauma both from the perspective of defining the traumatic event as well as its resulting sequelae is important to further research efforts and to avoid unnecessary pathologizing of traumatized children. Even more importantly, fully understanding the impact of complex trauma on children will best facilitate clinicians' ability to enhance protective factors and develop treatment interventions to help children recover.

Complex Trauma Prevalence

Given the dual definitions of complex trauma, the prevalence of complex trauma can be thought of in 2 ways. First, it can refer to the frequency of exposure to complex traumatic experiences. Second, it can refer to the frequency of complex trauma outcomes in response to such exposure.

Prevalence of complex traumatic events

Exposure to repetitive or multiple forms of victimization is common in childhood. Finkelhor and colleagues[4] found that 22% of a nationally representative sample of 2030 children aged 2 to 17 years had experienced 4 or more different forms of victimization in the past year. Victimization was broadly defined to include exposure to violent and property crime (eg, assault, theft), child welfare violations (eg, child abuse), warfare/civil disturbances, and bullying. The same researchers[8] conducted a screening of lifetime exposure to victimization in a nationally representative sample of 4053 youth aged 2 to 17 years. Almost 66% of the sample had been exposed to more than 1 form of victimization, 30% had been exposed to 5 or more types of victimization, and 10% had experienced 11 or more.

Polyvictimization can also start at a young age. For example, in the Turner and colleagues[8] study, 40% of polyvictims were younger than 13 years of age. A study of

213 children aged 2 to 4 years found that 64.3% had a history of trauma exposure, and that 34.7% of those exposed to trauma had experienced 2 or more traumas.[9] A portion of this sample included children referred to sites providing mental health or developmental delay services, whereas the remainder were nonreferred children recruited from the same communities. As discussed later, prevalence of complex trauma exposure is even higher among at-risk populations such as youth in foster care[10] and those who are justice involved.[11]

Prevalence of complex trauma outcomes

Given the ongoing debate regarding the validity of complex trauma as a separate diagnostic entity in adults[12] and children[13] it is challenging to specify the prevalence of complex trauma outcomes. However, research does support a dose-response relationship with exposure to more trauma types resulting in increased symptom breadth and complexity for children[14–16] and adults.[14,17,18]

Furthermore, evidence is beginning to emerge regarding the prevalence of developmental trauma disorder (DTD),[6] a proposed syndrome designed to describe outcomes associated with complex trauma exposure. Stolbach and colleagues[19] found that, among youth who met criteria for complex trauma exposure, 31% met the proposed criteria for DTD. This finding suggests that a sizable percentage of youth presenting for trauma-focused services are showing clinically significant complex trauma outcomes. Further, a study of 330 former Ugandan child soldiers with severe histories of chronic trauma exposure found that slightly more than 78% met the proposed criteria for DTD.[20] Overall, these findings suggest that outcomes conceptualized as complex trauma are common following exposure to chronic, interpersonal trauma.

Causes of Complex Trauma Exposure

The causes of complex trauma can also be considered in the context of exposure and outcomes. With regard to exposure, multiple individual and environmental characteristics have been identified as precipitants for repeated victimization. For example, Finkelhor and colleagues[21] identified 4 primary precipitants for polyvictimization: (1) living in a dangerous community; (2) living in a dangerous family environment; (3) living in a nondangerous but chaotic family environment; and (4) having emotional problems that result in increased risky behavior, interpersonal antagonism, and risk of victimization. Further, being a polyvictim seems to be a risk factor for future polyvictimization.[22]

Causes of Complex Trauma Outcomes

Complex trauma outcomes (discussed later) could be conceptualized as a developmental disorder triggered by exposure to complex trauma. It is theorized that complex trauma outcomes are influenced by the developmental period during which trauma exposure occurs, but that they also disrupt subsequent development.[7] Therefore, complex trauma outcomes consist of common traumatic stress reactions (eg, PTSD, depression, insecure attachment, dissociation) and developmental disruptions caused by contextual factors related to complex trauma exposure (eg, impaired caregiving, multiple placements) and traumatic stress reactions (eg, chronic hyperarousal disrupting development of emotion regulation). Further, impairment seems to be more chronic and severe when trauma exposure has an earlier onset,[23,24] increased duration,[23,25] consists of multiple types of trauma,[26] and is interpersonal in nature,[27] which are all part of the definition of complex trauma exposure. So, how does complex trauma exposure result in these outcomes? Possible causal factors include disrupted brain development and disorganized attachment.

Complex trauma and disrupted brain development

First, considerable research indicates that trauma exposure can result in structural and functional changes in brain development.[28] The areas of the brain most affected by trauma exposure are the structures that make up the stress response system. For example, neurobiological findings following trauma exposure include neuroendocrine dysregulation; reduction in hippocampal, amygdala, and prefrontal cortex volume; and decrease in corpus callosum size.[29,30] These structural changes are thought to be the causal underpinnings of common posttraumatic symptoms such as hyperarousal, reexperiencing, emotional and behavioral dysregulation, dissociation, numbing, attention difficulties, and executive function deficits.[31,32]

These changes have been conceptualized as an alternate developmental pathway designed to be an adaptation to a high-stress environment.[31] Biologic systems shift from a focus on learning to a focus on survival.[33] Brain organization and activation become focused on structures that promote rapid, autonomic responses to avoid harm and regulate arousal (eg, brainstem, midbrain, amygdala) rather than structures involved in complex learning and long-term adaptation (eg, medial and dorsolateral prefrontal cortex). This survival-focused brain can defend against immediate harm, but does so at the expense of systems that prevent exhaustion, injury, and illness and promote self-regulation and learning.[34] These alterations in brain structure and function result in a combination of affective, somatic, behavioral, and interpersonal impairments perhaps best conceptualized as a dysregulation syndrome.[35] The alterations also likely explain the variety of developmental deficits identified in children exposed to trauma, including speech-language disorders,[36] executive functioning deficits,[37] working memory,[38] and overall cognitive ability.[39]

It remains difficult to distinguish how the brain changes related to complex trauma differ from those seen in research specific to PTSD. For example, changes in brain function and structure have been detected less than a month after trauma exposure,[40,41] suggesting that extended activation of the human stress response may not be a causal necessity. In contrast, research has suggested that earlier onset and longer duration of trauma exposure are associated with more significant structural changes in the brain.[23,25] It also seems possible that the structural changes are more closely related to the presence and severity of PTSD rather than characteristics of trauma exposure.[30,42] However, this relationship is also unclear because other researchers have shown changes in the brain structure of trauma-exposed individuals regardless of diagnostic status.[30,43] In addition, there seems to be some validity to the idea that trauma exposure affects brain development differentially depending on what region of the brain is developing most actively when the trauma occurs. Andersen and colleagues[44] showed that adult hippocampal volume was most related to sexual abuse occurring between 3 and 5 years of age and between 11 and 13 years of age, corpus callosum area was most related to sexual abuse between ages 9 and 10 years, and frontal cortex volume was most related to sexual abuse during ages 14 to 16 years. Based on these findings, it seems reasonable to suspect that the changes in brain structure seen after trauma exposure occur on a continuum influenced by a variety of factors (eg, genetic predisposition; onset, severity, and duration of trauma exposure; severity and duration of traumatic stress reactions; disrupted attachment; and developmental status), many of which are defining aspects of complex trauma. However, further research is needed to clarify the relationship between complex trauma and changes in brain function and structure.

Complex trauma and disrupted attachment

A second critical causal factor related to complex trauma outcomes is caregiver-child attachment. By definition, complex trauma is thought to occur in caregiving or relational contexts,[2] and attachment has been implicated in the expression of complex trauma outcomes. The first year of life largely revolves around development of a secure attachment relationship between infant and caregiver allowing for emotional communication and coregulation.[45] Schore[46] states that secure attachment promotes brain development, development of social bonds, and development of brain structures critical for the regulation of stress (ie, hypothalamic-pituitary-adrenal axis). This contention seems to be supported because researchers have shown increased cortisol reactivity in insecurely attached children[47,48] and differences in gray matter volume in the right temporal pole and left lateral orbitofrontal cortex in adults who showed attachment-related anxiety.[49]

Disorganized attachment is associated with a variety of negative outcomes including externalizing disorders, aggression, and oppositional defiant disorder.[50] It is thought that youth with a disorganized attachment style lack an organized strategy for coping with stress and instead show behavioral disorganization or disorientation when confronted by stress.[51] Further, disorganized youth are typically unable to use the attachment relationship to modulate distress. This inability seems to continue throughout childhood because these youth are more likely to have social skill deficits, including inconsistent or overly rigid interpersonal behavior.[52]

In the context of complex trauma the attachment relationship is commonly disrupted and disorganized. The caregiver overstimulates the child through traumatic behavior and/or understimulates the child through neglect. Further, the caregiver does not repair this misattunement, fails to protect the child from stressors, and fails to help the child regulate arousal.[46] Brain structures associated with self-regulation subsequently remain underdeveloped resulting in a chronic state of dysregulation characterized by both hyperarousal and hypoarousal.[53] This combination of attachment disruption and maltreatment is thought to lead to more chronic and severe symptoms, beyond the effects of maltreatment alone.[54–56] In this context, complex trauma outcome causes could be construed as the interaction between traumatic stress responses and disorganized attachment. Pearlman and Courtois[57] note that research from trauma/dissociation and attachment/development supports the idea that most chronically abused individuals show an insecure disorganized and dissociative attachment style. Thus the distress and dysregulation associated with trauma exposure occurs in the context of inability to regulate oneself through attachment. Further, given that trauma exposure likely occurred in the context of an attachment relationship, interpersonal interactions may further trigger trauma-related distress. This distress could contribute to the chronic dysregulation associated with complex trauma. Some research supports this possibility because unresolved attachment in adults has been associated with several symptoms reminiscent of complex trauma, including dissociation, inconsistent sense of self, and relationship problems.[58]

PHENOMENOLOGY

Numerous studies have attempted to describe the sequelae of complex trauma and, although there is some convergence among this literature, there is not yet a clear symptom profile.[7,13,14,59] As mentioned previously, youth with multiple traumatic exposures typically fare worse than those with a single traumatic exposure and the highest level of symptom distress is associated with exposure to multiple interpersonal traumas.[60] Further, an increase in the number of different types of traumas experienced is associated with an increase in symptom complexity.[14]

Several attempts have been made to identify symptom clusters that can accurately capture the sequelae of complex trauma exposure. What these attempts have identified is that the Diagnostic and Statistical Manual of Mental Disorders (DSM), Fourth Edition, Text Revision (DSM-IV-TR) criteria for PTSD do not seem to accurately and comprehensively capture the sequelae of complex trauma.[14,22] Additional symptom clusters associated with complex trauma exposure include affect regulation, consciousness, self-perception, perception of the perpetrator, relations with others, systems of meaning, alterations in attention and consciousness, somatization, and disturbances in self-regulatory capacities.[12,14,61] Given the recent evolution of the PTSD diagnosis with the DSM-5 it will be interesting to see how research evolves in this area. It seems that the DSM-5 PTSD criteria may be able to more comprehensively include youth with complex trauma within the diagnosis. Nonetheless, given that extensive literature has shown that the experience of complex trauma results in a significantly different symptom profile than acute trauma, it will continue to be important to understand the sequelae of complex trauma in order to develop useful case conceptualizations.

Dysregulation of Affect and Behavior

Perhaps the most readily apparent symptom clusters of complex trauma are those associated with affective and behavioral dysregulation. In general, anxiety, depression, and anger/aggression are frequently comorbid with posttraumatic stress and the experience of complex trauma.[62] Severe, ongoing trauma has the potential to affect children by overloading their ability to cope with emotions, altering their ability to access and identify emotions, impairing their ability to tolerate emotional expression; and impairing their ability to regulate their impulses.[7,13,63] These youth subsequently tend to present with rapidly vacillating moods with extreme responses seemingly triggered by minor stressors or by nothing.

Dysregulation of behavior may present as either undercontrolled or overcontrolled behavioral patterns. The function of overcontrolled behavior is to manage overwhelming affect and feelings of helplessness by attempting to rigidly regulate what behavior patterns and routines children may have under their control. In contrast, undercontrolled behavior is often a reflection of deficits in impulse control, planning, and executive functioning.[7] These adaptations to the overwhelming stress of complex trauma are children's best attempts to cope with their experiences, but ultimately tend to put them more at risk for further traumatization. Their deficits in both emotional and behavioral regulation leave them without the skills necessary to navigate social situations and also result in behavioral reactions that may put them at further risk (eg, aggression, self-injurious behaviors).[64]

Disturbances of Attention/Consciousness, Cognition, and Information Processing

Disturbances of attention and consciousness may present in a variety of ways: dissociation, inattention, a lack of sustained curiosity, difficulty planning and anticipating, and so forth.[7,13] One way to conceptualize these reactions is as overdevelopment of avoidance responses.[65] Avoidance is a common trauma response and often generalized beyond the initial trauma stimulus (eg, anxiety related to bathrooms or nighttime). However, with complex trauma the avoidance becomes even more extreme and generalizes to symptoms such as dissociation, memory loss, and impaired executive functioning.

Difficulties with attention and arousal have created much debate over the comorbidity of attention deficit/hyperactivity disorder (ADHD) in children who have experienced complex trauma. Although ADHD and complex trauma seem to be distinct syndromes, their overlapping symptoms make them difficult to differentiate in children exposed to complex trauma. Although complex trauma has not been found to be a risk factor for ADHD,[66] additional research is needed to determine how to distinguish between ADHD and cognitive regulatory deficits related to complex trauma/dissociation.

In addition to inattention, dissociative symptoms may present as memory loss, depersonalization, derealization, disengagement, and numbing. It is unclear to what extent dissociation helps differentiate complex trauma symptoms, but research suggests that dissociation plays a unique role in overall sequelae of complex trauma.[67] For example, one study identified that dissociation uniquely contributes to relationship difficulties, likely because of the impaired interpersonal skills that evolve when dissociative symptoms become more prevalent.[68]

Interpersonal Difficulties

Complex trauma has the potential to cause a variety of interpersonal difficulties, in large part through its influence on a child's attachment and internal representation of themselves in relation to others.[55] This condition may manifest as difficulties with trust, low interpersonal effectiveness, revictimization, victimizing others, and poor boundaries.[69,70] Because most complex trauma experiences threaten the primary attachment relationship (eg, domestic violence, sexual abuse, neglect), it is logical that a resulting symptom cluster would be disruptions to a child's ability to develop high-quality, adaptive interpersonal skills. Children with complex trauma histories often do not experience safety within their relationships and are not able to use their primary caregiving relationships as a secure base on which to develop internal working models of themselves and others. In addition, secondary traumatic stressors that these children often continue to confront (eg, disruptions in foster placements, transitions in family composition) may further impede their ability to develop interpersonal skills and quality attachment relationships and also present additional risk factors to overcome. A study of 347 children in long-term foster and kinship care consistently identified significant social and interpersonal difficulties.[71]

Distortions in Attributions

Disruptions in attachment and the ability to regulate emotions and impulses is often linked to the evolution of distortions related to sense of self and expectations of others and the world.[72] Complex trauma often occurs within the context of formative caregiving relationships that shape children's beliefs about themselves and the world around them. The abuse can involve the creation of distorted attributions (eg, being told that they are damaged), but the children may also develop distorted attributions as a way of coping with the trauma, their environment, and resulting symptoms (eg, believing they deserve the abuse and do not deserve anything better). Overall, these distortions facilitate the development of self-blame, low self-esteem, and poor self-efficacy.[73] These maladaptive beliefs may build a foundation for impaired social interactions and further mental health deficits.[13]

Biology

Complex trauma can interfere with many neurologic and physiologic developmental processes causing biological compromise.[7] The neurobiological impact of trauma can impede the maturation of specific brain structures; neuroendocrine responses; and the coordination of cognition, emotion regulation, and behavior.[74] The biological impact of trauma can decrease children's overall awareness of their bodies. Further, trauma may manifest as somatic symptoms, increased electrical irritability in limbic structures,[75] or may lead to serious long-term health risk behaviors and diseases.[76]

PREDICTING CLINICAL OUTCOMES FOR COMPLEX TRAUMA EXPOSURE

Trying to appreciate how clinical outcomes associated with complex trauma exposure vary across development is like trying to pick the winning number on a roulette wheel. Because of the ever-changing developmental landscape, the frequency of victimization, and the ongoing presence of secondary adversities, there are many possible outcomes.

Exposure to interpersonal violence has been found to place children at greater overall risk for psychosocial impairment and PTSD than exposure to noninterpersonal violence and/or community violence.[77] Therefore, the presence of interpersonal victimization could be a helpful predictor. However, victimization rates have been found to be generally high across the developmental span of childhood. Further, research has shown that some of the commonly held beliefs about exposure to trauma, such as young children being more frequently exposed to domestic violence, are not necessarily as robust as was once thought.[78] In general, boys experience more peer assaults as they proceed through adolescence, sibling assaults peak in middle childhood and decline with age, and sexual victimization of girls increases in later adolescence.[78] These findings suggest that trying to predict clinical outcomes by exposure to interpersonal victimization at a given developmental period may be impractical.

Family system factors may offer more insight into understanding clinical outcomes across the developmental spectrum. Risk factors that influence the development of PTSD in children include externalizing characteristics, family mental health difficulties, family adversity, low intelligence quotient, and chronic environmental stressors.[79] These findings suggest that trying to anticipate clinical outcomes by evaluating the risk and protective factors (both intrinsic and extrinsic) to a child may be a more valid and reliable approach.

Overall, research has indicated that a multifaceted approach is required to understand the link between complex trauma experiences and outcomes.[55,80] This approach includes considering traumatic stressors and their related events as well as the intrinsic/extrinsic factors of the child and their ongoing adjustment. The resulting picture may be intricate and difficult to predict, but also accurately reflects the complexity of both the traumas experienced and the children who live through them.

Family Issues

Offending caregiver dynamics

For many children and adolescents exposed to complex trauma, parents or other primary caregivers are the source of their trauma. Children who experience trauma caused by those responsible for protecting and nurturing them are likely to develop insecure attachment patterns, including disorganized attachment. As many as 90% of maltreated children show an insecure attachment style,[81] with disorganized attachment style being present in half to three-quarters.[82] Similar to complex trauma outcomes, disorganized attachment is associated with emotion regulation difficulties, externalizing problems, and impaired social functioning.[83]

Betrayal trauma theory offers another framework for understanding the impact of caregiver-perpetrated or family-perpetrated trauma on children and adolescents. According to this theory, the violation of trust that occurs when children are victimized by caregivers or others in positions of trust constitutes a threat to their survival.[82] Because a child's awareness of caregiver-inflicted trauma might cause withdrawal from that caregiver, thereby disrupting the attachment relationship that affords safety and protection to the child, it may be psychologically necessary for the child to remain unaware of the betrayal. This so-called betrayal blindness, although enabling the child to preserve a sense of security, may be associated with significant difficulties related to dissociation (the mechanism by which betrayal blindness occurs), cognition, mental health symptoms, and interpersonal functioning.[82] For example, research indicates that experiencing childhood betrayal trauma is associated with later difficulty in recognizing interpersonal betrayals and detecting trustworthiness in people.

Trauma that originates in the family is likely to generate significant secondary adversities for children and adolescents.[81] Caregiver-perpetrated trauma may necessitate placement in foster care or residential facilities, requiring adjustment to new caregivers, homes, neighborhoods, communities, and schools. Separation from family and peers, uncertainty about the future, loss of familiar routines, and the stress of system involvement can exacerbate trauma-related symptoms or create additional psychological distress in children placed outside the home. Other secondary adversities often resulting from intrafamilial trauma include economic problems caused by parental incarceration or estrangement, significant rifts in immediate or extended family relationships, residential instability, and legal system involvement.

Resilience/Coping

The family is a child's first and generally most significant social environment, and as such plays an important role in determining how children and adolescents adapt to complex trauma exposure. The role of the family environment in influencing the outcomes of traumatized children is especially significant given that family variables (eg, caregiver support, parenting practices) are potential targets of intervention, whereas variables specific to the trauma exposure (eg, type and duration of exposure) are often immutable.[84,85] Certain family characteristics and relationship qualities are associated with resilience and adaptive functioning among children who are maltreated or exposed to chronic stress. Other types of family conditions and behaviors seem to contribute to, or exacerbate, trauma symptoms.[86]

Parenting practices can mediate the impact of trauma on children and adolescents. Research suggests that there is great variability in parenting practices among families experiencing child maltreatment and family violence, and aspects of parenting predict differential outcomes for traumatized children.[87,88] Valentino and colleagues[89] found that hostile/coercive parenting was associated with greater PTSD and internalizing symptoms in children exposed to trauma; in the same study, engaged and supportive parenting strongly predicted child-reported adjustment. Graham-Bermann and colleagues[90] found that parenting warmth and effectiveness differentiated children who seemed to be coping adequately following exposure to domestic violence from those with problems in adjustment.

Caregiver support is a primary protective factor in children exposed to trauma, predicting the degree to which children experience and resolve trauma reactions. Research findings consistently show that children who have a supportive caregiver show fewer behavioral and emotional symptoms following trauma.[84,87,91] As noted by Cook and colleagues,[7] supportive caregiving responses following trauma can be conceptualized as involving 3 factors: (1) believing and validating the child's experience, (2) tolerating the child's affect, and (3) the caregivers' regulation of their own emotional response. In contrast, when caregivers deny children's experiences, the children's recovery is impeded because they cannot integrate the traumatic experiences or develop positive coping strategies.[7]

Research on trauma and attachment provides additional support to the salience of the parent-child relationship in the aftermath of trauma. Attachment theory posits that children are biologically driven to seek proximity to a caregiver, especially in situations perceived as frightening or dangerous.[92] Through a secure attachment with the caregiver, children learn to regulate their emotions and make sense of what is happening in the environment. Secure attachment can mitigate the impact of overwhelming stressors and support recovery and healing following exposure to trauma.[93]

Systemic Issues

Implications for children in care

Children and adolescents in the child welfare system have high rates of trauma exposure, including complex trauma exposure. A recent study of foster children referred for treatment found that 70.4% of the sample reported at least 2 forms of recurrent interpersonal trauma perpetuated by caregivers (ie, sexual abuse, physical abuse, emotional abuse, neglect, or domestic violence); 11.7% reported having experienced all 5 trauma types.[10] Among children involved with the child welfare system, children with complex trauma histories experience more mental health symptoms, including symptoms of traumatic stress, compared with children with other types of trauma.[10,94]

Findings related to the prevalence of complex trauma exposure among children in the child welfare system and the adverse mental health outcomes associated with such exposure have important practice implications. First, child welfare professionals need increased awareness of the nature of complex trauma exposure and its relationship to adverse mental health outcomes. When workers better understand how children are affected by complex trauma experiences, they will be better able to determine treatment priorities and address service gaps.[10] In addition, frontline workers should be trained to complete trauma screening on all children who enter the child welfare system, ideally using a standardized assessment tool that has been empirically validated.[10] Identifying children with trauma histories, including complex trauma histories, helps ensure that they are linked with appropriate treatment providers. In addition, foster parents, residential care workers, and other frontline providers should receive specialized training related to meeting the needs of children with complex trauma histories. For example, foster parents should learn how to identify trauma triggers and support children's development of self-regulation capacities. The National Child Traumatic Stress Network has developed the Resource Parent Curriculum for this purpose; see the Network's Web site (www.nctsn.org) for more information.

Juvenile justice

The correlation between trauma exposure and involvement in the juvenile justice system has been well documented. Approximately 90% of youth in juvenile justice facilities report having experienced at least one potentially traumatic event.[64,95] Because of definitional issues, estimates of complex trauma among justice-involved youth are more difficult to determine. However, Ford and colleagues[96] report that a hierarchical cluster analysis of a large representative sample of youth in detention settings yielded an estimated prevalence of 35% with complex trauma histories. Another study[11] found that more than half (62.14%) of their justice-involved sample had experienced trauma in the first 5 years of life and 90% experienced multiple trauma types over their lifetimes. In addition, arrest and juvenile justice confinement experiences can be traumatic for some youth, compounding their already complex trauma histories, increasing their risk for additional trauma, and/or triggering memories of prior traumatic experiences.[97]

The disruption of self-regulation capacities that stems from complex trauma poses challenges in milieu management and treatment in juvenile justice settings.[96] Many youth with complex trauma histories are unlikely to have the self-regulation skills necessary to participate in the educational and recreational milieu activities or respond positively to motivational or crisis prevention interventions offered in these settings.[96] A complex trauma perspective favors milieu interventions that build skills in self-regulation rather than assuming that youth already possess them.[96]

The Sanctuary Model is an example of an intervention that can be used to address the needs of youth with complex trauma histories in the juvenile justice system. Developed by Dr Sandra Bloom[98] and her colleagues in the 1980s, the Sanctuary Model recognizes the treatment environment as a core modality for healing the wounds of psychological trauma, and intervenes at the level of organizational culture to create new, developmentally grounded, trauma-informed routines for the children being served, their families, staff members, and the organization as a whole.[98] This model is currently being implemented as a systematic organizational change process for more than 250 human service delivery systems including juvenile programs[98] and has been associated with significant decreases in negative interactions between youth and staff in juvenile detention centers.[99]

Clinical Assessment of Complex Trauma

Effective assessment of complex trauma exposure and outcomes in children and adolescents requires the integration of knowledge from a variety of areas, including trauma, child development, neurodevelopment, attachment, family systems, and child welfare. Furthermore, this knowledge must be exercised while developing a therapeutic alliance with a youth (and often caregivers) who presents with self-regulation and interpersonal deficits, and frequent safety concerns. This process is clinically and personally challenging.

Complex trauma assessment should be embedded in the typical assessment process at the initiation of services. It is critical to establish a genuine working alliance with the youth and caregiver(s). This alliance relies on a careful balance between identifying vulnerabilities (the standard goal of most assessments) while accommodating those vulnerabilities (eg, titrating the assessment process to avoid the youth decompensating) and validating youths' strengths and accomplishments.[63] However, as long as sensitive issues (eg, trauma history) are discussed in a noncoercive, collaborative fashion, screening does not seem to cause increased deterioration or crises.[64] The building of a working alliance is likely to be tested by the presence of safety risks or unreported abuse. It is important to respond immediately and calmly to such disclosures to enhance the youth's actual or perceived safety and control.[63] This enhancement can often be accomplished through transparency, providing a clear rationale for the clinician's actions and trying to make events as predictable and controllable as possible for the youth (eg, clearly explaining the investigatory process to a youth when having to make a hotline report).

Developing a detailed trauma history is a crucial aspect of assessing youth exposed to complex trauma.[63,100] Formal screening instruments may be helpful in this process. Such instruments include the Traumatic Experiences Screening Instrument[101] and the UCLA Posttraumatic Stress Disorder Reaction Index.[102] However, even when directly evaluated, it is common for traumatic experiences to go undisclosed during initial assessment. Additional disclosures may occur more organically over time as the youth develops increased trust with the service provider.[100] Thus assessment of complex trauma is often an ongoing process that occurs throughout the course of treatment.

Although developing a detailed trauma history is important, focusing only on past events is not sufficient.[63] It is equally important to identify current or potential events that may be retraumatizing (eg, facing a perpetrator while testifying at court) or result in the youth reenacting prior traumatic experiences (eg, a sexually abused youth engaging in sexualized behavior). These triggers and reenactments can profoundly affect the youth's daily functioning and often present as observable behavior patterns (eg, youths becoming belligerent every time their employers give feedback regarding their work performance).

The assessment of complex trauma involves more than identifying past traumas and future triggers. It is also necessary to assess relevant areas of current functioning. As mentioned previously, youth exposed to complex trauma typically present with dysregulation associated with affect, behavior, attention/consciousness, cognition, interpersonal functioning, attributions toward self and others, and biological functioning. Related to these deficits, Ford and colleagues[63] recommend that assessment should identify problems and strengths affecting a youth's ability to:

1. Identify/prepare for triggers/reenactments and develop coping skills to prevent harm to self or others
2. Develop or restore emotion regulation (ie, ability to access emotions [especially trauma-related emotions such as shame and betrayal], capacity to tolerate emotional expression)
3. Acquire or regain the capacity to accurately monitor bodily sensations and arousal
4. Develop or restore cognitive and behavioral self-regulation to reduce the occurrence/severity of maladaptive behaviors (eg, substance abuse, self-harm, sexualized behaviors)
5. Experience safety and attunement in family, peer, and therapeutic relationships and subsequently develop secure inner models of relationships
6. Develop a personal identity of resiliency and self-determination

These areas can be assessed many ways, but because of complex biographic histories and symptom presentations, it is unlikely that the assessment process can be accomplished through any single measure or technique.[65] Instead it is recommended to use a variety of approaches with multiple informants.[103] For example, the assessment process for youth exposed to complex trauma could include the following:

1. Biopsychosocial interviews conducted with the youth, caregiver(s), and other relevant familial (eg, grandparent) or professional (eg, caseworker, teacher) entities
2. Semistructured interview for child and adolescent psychiatric disorders (eg, Kiddie Schedule for Affective Disorders and Schizophrenia[104])
3. Behavioral observations of youth in multiple settings (eg, home, school, community)
4. Wide range of youth-report measures (eg, Youth Self Report,[105] Multiphasic Personality Inventory-A[106])
5. Wide range of adult-report measures (eg, Behavior Assessment System for Children,[107] Child Behavior Checklist,[105] Teacher Report Form[105])
6. Trauma-specific youth-report assessment measures (eg, Trauma Symptom Checklist for Children[108])
7. Trauma-specific adult-report assessment measures (eg, Trauma Symptom Checklist for Young Children,[109] Child Sexual Behavior Inventory[110])

The Challenge of Diagnosing Youth Exposed to Complex Trauma

As discussed earlier, evaluating youth exposed to complex trauma is challenging. However, this is intensified by the lack of a psychiatric diagnosis that fully accounts for the symptom presentation of youth exposed to complex trauma.[13] Using DSM-IV-TR criteria, PTSD has not been the most common diagnosis for traumatized youth, and comorbid diagnoses are common.[111]

Therefore it has been argued that PTSD criteria, particularly before DSM-5, do not fully describe the symptom presentation of many traumatized youth. A wide variety of diagnoses (eg, ADHD, oppositional defiant disorder, and bipolar disorder) tends to be used to capture the range of presented difficulties. This variety of diagnoses results in a confusing diagnostic picture that obscures causal factors and may result in effective trauma-focused treatments being underused and under-reimbursed for this population.[13]

One attempt to address this situation has been the revision of PTSD criteria for DSM-5.[112] The DSM-5 PTSD criteria included a new symptom domain based on negative alterations in cognitions or mood (eg, persistent negative beliefs about oneself, others, or the world; persistent negative emotional states), expanded the hyperarousal domain to include reckless or destructive behavior (eg, reckless driving, excessive substance use), and added a PTSD subtype characterized by dissociation. DSM-5 PTSD criteria seem to capture outcomes of complex trauma more fully than previous iterations. The new criteria seem to better describe the impaired self-regulation across multiple domains (ie, affect, physiology, cognition, behavior, motivation, relationships, and self-identity).[113]

Another effort to better capture the sequelae of complex trauma has been the formulation of DTD. DTD is an attempt to organize the self-regulation deficits derived from clinical observation and research focused on complex trauma and distinguish it as a separate diagnosis that includes symptoms of PTSD but also extends beyond PTSD criteria.[63] DTD symptom clusters include PTSD symptoms as well as affective/physiologic dysregulation, attentional/behavioral dysregulation, and self/relational dysregulation.[63] Although DTD was not included in DSM-5, it is undergoing validation in an international field trial,[63] which may result in its inclusion in future iterations of the DSM.

Debate regarding the validity and usefulness of DTD will likely be a hallmark of the field for the near future. For example, Schmid and colleagues[114] summarize arguments for and against formalized DTD criteria. Arguments in support of DTD suggest that DTD will (1) allow more specific diagnosis, (2) sensitize professionals and the public to the impact of chronic trauma, (3) highlight the developmental course of mental disorders, (4) stimulate research on complex trauma, (5) help explain the high rate of comorbidity among traumatized youth, (6) promote development and refinement of effective treatments, and (7) decrease social and legal stigmatization of traumatized youth. Arguments against the formalization of DTD criteria include (1) the presence of overlap with other diagnoses (eg, borderline personality disorder); (2) lack of clarity regarding the cause of DTD; (3) not all severely traumatized children develop any disorder, much less DTD; (4) the possibility that emotional dysregulation may precede complex trauma rather than be caused by it; (5) lack of age/developmentally sensitive criteria; (6) DTD may result in true comorbid diagnoses going untreated; and (7) increased pressure to identify past trauma experiences resulting in disrupted therapeutic relationships or false trauma memories.

In conclusion, the diagnosis of complex trauma outcomes is a contentious topic and will likely remain so for the foreseeable future. The heart of this debate is whether or not complex trauma outcomes represent a distinct disorder from PTSD or are better conceptualized as simply a more severe form of PTSD. However, the current knowledge base regarding this question is insufficient to make that distinction,[12,114] highlighting the need for further investigation.

Treatment of Youth Exposed to Complex Trauma

Treating youth exposed to complex trauma can be a complicated, overwhelming process. The needs of these youth are typically intense, varied, and rapidly changing, particularly early in treatment. It can be argued that no gold standard treatment exists for this population; however, substantial progress has been made in identifying effective treatment approaches.

The general consensus among experts is that a phase-based approach is most effective.[5,115,116] In this approach, treatment occurs sequentially, with later phases building on previous phases. For example, early in treatment, youth may be taught skills to alleviate current emotional dysregulation but also to provide the tools needed for subsequent trauma processing. Although treatment is generally sequential, phases may not always proceed in a linear fashion, and previous phases may be revisited as needed, allowing the therapist to sensitively respond to the chaos and changing needs of the population.[117]

Several models of phase-based treatment of complex trauma have been developed. Ford and colleagues[115] describe one approach, consisting of 3 phases: (1) engagement, safety, and stabilization; (2) recalling traumatic memories; and (3) enhancing daily living. In phase 1, the therapist works to form a therapeutic alliance and increase the youth's sense of safety. This phase is often a significant and lengthy portion of treatment in light of characteristic difficulties with dysregulation, attachment, and environmental instability. When these difficulties have become manageable, the second phase of treatment begins. This phase focuses on trauma-related content and processing traumatic memories. This phase occurs at a safe, manageable pace through graduated exposure and ongoing use of the self-regulation skills learned in phase 1. When symptoms of posttraumatic stress (eg, intrusive memories, arousal to trauma cues, maladaptive trauma-related beliefs) have been addressed, the therapist and client move to phase 3, focusing on developing a healthy lifestyle that is not ruled by trauma triggers or reenactments.

Multiple evidence-based treatment models have been adapted or created to adhere to a phase-based approach and have shown effectiveness. Effective treatment models tend to have similar characteristics that include (1) prioritization of safety and stability, (2) heavy emphasis on relationships, (3) interventions that balance immediate needs and long-term goals, (4) focus on strengths and resiliency, (5) consistent development of self-regulation skill in multiple domains (eg, emotion, information processing, awareness, somatic, relational), (6) mastery of traumatic memories, and (7) prevention of and preparation for losses and crises.[118]

The following list (in alphabetical order) provides some examples of evidence-based treatment models that have been developed or adapted for youth exposed to complex trauma. This list should not be considered exhaustive and, because of length constraints, does not provide a detailed description of each model.

Attachment, self-regulation, and competency

Components-based intervention framework for youth exposed to complex trauma and their surrounding systems of care.[119,120]

Child-parent psychotherapy

Psychodynamic, caregiver-child dyadic model for preschoolers.[121]

Dialectical behavior therapy
Flexible, principle-driven, manualized treatment model that integrates cognitive-behavioral principles with mindfulness practice to enhance self-regulation.[122,123]

Eye movement desensitization and reprocessing
Trauma-focused treatment model that emphasizes information processing systems and the resolution of physiologically stored memories.[124,125]

Integrative treatment of complex trauma
Multicomponent therapy for children and adolescents that integrates complex trauma, attachment theory, the self-trauma model, and aspects of trauma-focused cognitive behavior therapy.[126]

Parent-child interaction therapy
Manualized parent-training program based on social learning and attachment theories for children aged 2 to 7 years with externalizing behavior problems.[127]

Real-life heroes
Integrated trauma and resiliency–centered treatment model for latency-aged youth with history of exposure to complex trauma.[128]

Seeking safety
Structured psychoeducational model for co-occurring PTSD and substance abuse.[129]

Structured psychotherapy for adolescents responding to chronic stress
Group intervention for adolescents integrating aspects of trauma-focused treatment and dialectical behavior therapy.[130]

Trauma affect regulation: guide for education and therapy
Brief group or individual program for youth with complex trauma histories and their families.[131]

Trauma-focused cognitive behavior therapy
Phase-oriented individual treatment model for traumatized youth and nonoffending caregivers.[103,132]

Trauma systems therapy
Systemic-based intervention focused equally on dysregulation in youth exposed to complex trauma and factors in the social environment that trigger and maintain dysregulation.[133]

SUMMARY

It is difficult to overstate the current and future importance of complex trauma to child and adolescent mental health and to society. As described in this article, large numbers of children and adolescents are exposed to chronic trauma and polyvictimization during highly vulnerable developmental periods. This exposure disrupts early attachment relationships and takes a severe toll on the developing brain, resulting in complex and severe symptom presentations resulting from impaired self-regulation. The subsequent needs of these youth place high demands on the resources of systems with which they interact, including biologic and adoptive families, education, child welfare, medical, and juvenile justice. Because of the diversity and severity of complex trauma outcomes, the provision of mental health services to this population is replete with challenges. However, gifted researchers and clinicians are increasingly devoting resources to address the needs of this population. The fruits of this labor can be seen in the development of a comprehensive conceptual framework and multiple, promising evidence-based treatment models. Challenges remain for youth exposed to complex trauma and the professionals who work with them, but the knowledge and tools that have developed over the last 25 years give cause for optimism.

REFERENCES

1. Terr L. Childhood traumas. Am J Psychiatry 1991;148:10–20.
2. Ford JD, Courtois CA. Defining and understanding complex trauma and complex traumatic stress disorders. In: Courtois CA, Ford JD, editors. Treating complex traumatic stress disorders: an evidence-based guide. New York: The Guilford Press; 2009. p. 13–30.
3. Weathers F, Keane T. The Criterion A problem revisited: controversies and challenges in defining and measuring psychological trauma. J Trauma Stress 2007; 20:107–21.
4. Finkelhor D, Ormrod RK, Turner HA. Poly-victimization: a neglected component in child victimization. Child Abuse Negl 2007;31:7–26.
5. Cook A, Spinazzola J, Ford J, et al. Complex trauma in children and adolescents. Psychiatr Ann 2005;35(5):390–8.
6. van der Kolk BA. Developmental trauma disorder. Psychiatr Ann 2005;35(5): 401–8.
7. Cook A, Blaustein M, Spinazzola J, et al, editors. Complex trauma in children and adolescents. National Child Traumatic Stress Network; 2003. Available at: http://www.nctsnet.org/nctsn_assets/pdfs/edu_materials/ComplexTrauma_All. pdf. Accessed October 28, 2013.
8. Turner HA, Finkelhor D, Ormrod R. Poly-victimization in a national sample of children and youth. Am J Prev Med 2010;38:323–30.
9. Grasso DJ, Ford JD, Briggs-Gowan MJ. Early life trauma exposure and stress sensitivity in young children. J Pediatr Psychol 2012;38(1):94–103.
10. Greeson JK, Briggs EC, Kisiel CL, et al. Complex trauma and mental health in children and adolescents placed in foster care: findings from the National Child Traumatic Stress Network. Child Welfare 2011;90:91–108.
11. Dierkhising CB, Ko SJ, Woods-Jaeger B, et al. Trauma histories among justice-involved youth: findings from the National Child Traumatic Stress Network. Eur J Psychotraumatol 2013;4:1–12.
12. Resick PA, Bovin MJ, Calloway AL, et al. A critical evaluation of the complex PTSD literature: implications for DSM-5. J Trauma Stress 2012;25(3):241–51.
13. D'Andrea W, Ford J, Stolbach B, et al. Understanding interpersonal trauma in children: why we need a developmentally appropriate trauma diagnosis. Am J Orthop 2012;82(2):187–200.
14. Cloitre M, Stolbach BC, Herman JL, et al. A developmental approach to complex PTSD: childhood and adult cumulative trauma as predictors of symptom complexity. J Trauma Stress 2009;22(5):399–408.
15. Ford JD, Elhai JD, Connor DF, et al. Poly-victimization and risk of posttraumatic, depressive, and substance use disorders and involvement in delinquency in a national sample of adolescents. J Adolesc Health 2010;46(6):545–52.
16. Ford JD, Wasser T, Connor DF. Identifying and determining the symptom severity associated with polyvictimization among psychiatrically impaired children in the outpatient setting. Child Maltreat 2011;16(3):216–26.
17. Anda RF, Brown DW, Felitti VJ, et al. Adverse childhood experiences and prescribed psychotropic medications in adults. Am J Prev Med 2007;32(5):389–94.

18. Briere J, Kaltman S, Green BL. Accumulated childhood trauma and symptom complexity. J Trauma Stress 2008;21(2):223–6.

19. Stolbach BC, Minshew R, Rompala V, et al. Complex trauma exposure and symptoms in urban traumatized children: a preliminary test of proposed criteria for developmental trauma disorder. J Trauma Stress 2013;26(4):483–91.

20. Klasen F, Gehrke J, Metzner F, et al. Complex trauma symptoms in former Ugandan child soldiers. J Aggress Maltreat Trauma 2013;22(7):698–713.

21. Finkelhor D, Ormrod R, Turner H, et al. Pathways to poly-victimization. Child Maltreat 2009;14(4):316–29.

22. Finkelhor D, Ormrod RK, Turner HA. Re-victimization patterns in a national longitudinal sample of children and youth. Child Abuse Negl 2007;31(5): 479–502.

23. De Bellis MD, Keshavan MS, Clark DB, et al. Developmental traumatology part II: brain development. Biol Psychiatry 1999;45:1271–84.

24. Ogle CM, Rubin DC, Siegler IC. The impact of the developmental timing of trauma exposure on PTSD symptoms and psychosocial functioning among older adults. Dev Psychol 2013;49(11):2191–200.

25. Cohen JA, Perel JM, De Bellis MD, et al. Treating traumatized children: clinical implications of the psychobiology of posttraumatic stress disorder. Trauma Violence Abuse 2002;3(2):91–108.

26. Teicher MH, Samson JA, Polcari A, et al. Sticks, stones, and hurtful words: relative effects of various forms of childhood maltreatment. Am J Psychiatry 2006; 163(6):993–1000.

27. Ehring T, Quack D. Emotion regulation difficulties in trauma survivors: the role of trauma type and PTSD symptom severity. Behav Ther 2010;41(4):587–98.

28. Gabowtiz D, Zucker M, Cook A. Neuropsychological assessment in clinical evaluation of children and adolescents with complex trauma. J Child Adolesc Trauma 2008;1:163–78.

29. Wilson DR, Hansen DJ, Li M. The traumatic stress response in child maltreatment and resultant neuropsychological effects. Aggress Violent Behav 2011; 16:87–97.

30. Karl A, Schaefer M, Malta LS, et al. A meta-analysis of structural brain abnormalities in PTSD. Neurosci Biobehav Rev 2006;30(7):1004–31.

31. Teicher MH, Andersen SL, Polcari A, et al. The neurobiological consequences of early stress and childhood maltreatment. Neurosci Biobehav Rev 2003;27(1–2): 33–44.

32. Watts-English T, Fortson BL, Gibler N, et al. The psychobiology of maltreatment in childhood. J Soc Issues 2006;62(4):717–36.

33. Ford JD. Neurobiological and developmental research: clinical implications. In: Courtois CA, Ford JD, editors. Treating complex traumatic stress disorders: an evidence-based guide. New York: The Guilford Press; 2009. p. 31–58.

34. Ford JD, Blaustein ME, Habib M, et al. Developmental trauma therapy models. In: Ford JD, Courtois CA, editors. Treating complex traumatic stress disorders in child and adolescents: scientific foundations and therapeutic models. New York: The Guilford Press; 2013. p. 261–76.

35. Althoff RR, Ayer LA, Rettew DC, et al. Assessment of dysregulated children using the Child Behavior Checklist: a receiver operating characteristic curve analysis. Psychol Assess 2010;22(3):609–17.

36. Kernic MA, Holt VL, Wolf ME, et al. Academic and school health issues among children exposed to maternal intimate partner abuse. Arch Pediatr Adolesc Med 2002;156(6):549–55.

37. Beers SR, De Bellis MD. Neuropsychological function in children with maltreatment-related posttraumatic stress disorder. Am J Psychiatry 2002; 159(3):483–6.
38. Bücker J, Kapczinski F, Post R, et al. Cognitive impairment in school-aged children with early trauma. Compr Psychiatry 2012;53(6):758–64.
39. Pugh RH, Tepper FL, Halpern-Felsher BL, et al. Changes in abused children's social and cognitive skills from intake to discharge in a residential treatment center. Resid Treat Child Youth 1997;14(3):65–83.
40. Lui S, Huang X, Chen L, et al. High-field MRI reveals an acute impact on brain function in survivors of the magnitude 8.0 earthquake in China. Proc Natl Acad Sci U S A 2009;106(36):15412–7.
41. Chen L, Lui S, Wu QZ, et al. Impact of acute stress on human brain microstructure: an MR diffusion study of earthquake survivors. Hum Brain Mapp 2013; 34(2):367–73.
42. Bossini L, Tavanti M, Calossi S, et al. Magnetic resonance imaging volumes of the hippocampus in drug-naïve patients with post-traumatic stress disorder without comorbidity conditions. J Psychiatr Res 2008;42(9):752–62.
43. Bremner JD. Traumatic stress: effects on the brain. Dialogues Clin Neurosci 2006;8(4):445–61.
44. Andersen SL, Tomada A, Vincow ES, et al. Preliminary evidence for sensitive periods in the effect of childhood sexual abuse on regional brain development. J Neuropsychiatry Clin Neurosci 2008;20(3):292–301.
45. Schore AN. Relational trauma, brain development, and dissociation. In: Ford JD, Courtois CA, editors. Treating complex traumatic stress disorders in child and adolescents: scientific foundations and therapeutic models. New York: The Guilford Press; 2013. p. 3–23.
46. Schore AN. Relational trauma and the developing right brain: the neurobiology of broken attachment bonds. In: Baradon T, editor. Relational trauma in infancy. London: Routledge; 2010. p. 19–47.
47. Bernard K, Dozier M. Examining infants' cortisol responses to laboratory tasks among children varying in attachment disorganization: stress reactivity or return to baseline? Dev Psychol 2010;46(6):1771–8.
48. Luijk MP, Velders FP, Tharner A, et al. FKBP5 and resistant attachment predict cortisol reactivity in infants: gene-environment interaction. Psychoneuroendocrinology 2010;35(10):1454–61.
49. Benetti S, McCrory E, Arulanantham S, et al. Attachment style, affective loss and gray matter volume: a voxel-based morphometry study. Hum Brain Mapp 2010; 31(10):1482–9.
50. Lyons-Ruth K, Jacobvitz D. Attachment disorganization: unresolved loss, relational violence, and lapses in behavioral and attentional strategies. In: Cassidy J, Shaver PR, editors. Handbook of attachment: theory, research, and clinical applications. New York: The Guilford Press; 1999. p. 520–54.
51. MacDonald HZ, Beeghly M, Grant-Knight W, et al. Longitudinal association between infant disorganized attachment and childhood posttraumatic stress symptoms. Dev Psychopathol 2008;20(2):493–508.
52. Jacobvitz D, Hazen N. Developmental pathways from infant disorganization to childhood peer relationships. In: Solomon J, George C, editors. Attachment disorganization. New York: The Guilford Press; 1999. p. 127–59.
53. Schore AN. Early relational trauma, disorganized attachment, and the development of a predisposition to violence. In: Siegel D, Solomon M, editors. Healing trauma: attachment, mind, body, and brain. New York: WW Norton; 2003. p. 107–67.

54. Aspelmeier JE, Elliott AN, Smith CH. Childhood sexual abuse, attachment, and trauma symptoms in college females: the moderating role of attachment. Child Abuse Negl 2007;31(5):549–66.
55. Cicchetti D, Toth SL. A developmental psychopathology perspective on child abuse and neglect. J Am Acad Child Adolesc Psychiatry 1995;34(5): 541–65.
56. Ford JD, Connor DF, Hawke J. Complex trauma among psychiatrically impaired children: a cross-sectional, chart-review study. J Clin Psychiatry 2009;70(8): 1155–63.
57. Pearlman LA, Courtois CA. Clinical applications of the attachment framework: relational treatment of complex trauma. J Trauma Stress 2005;18(5):449–59.
58. Bailey HN, Moran G, Pederson DR. Childhood maltreatment, complex trauma symptoms, and unresolved attachment in an at-risk sample of adolescent mothers. Attach Hum Dev 2007;9(2):139–61.
59. Dorahy MJ, Corry M, Shannon M, et al. Complex PTSD, interpersonal trauma and relational consequences: findings from a treatment receiving Northern Irish sample. J Affect Disord 2009;112:71–80.
60. Green BL, Goodman LA, Krupnick JL, et al. Outcome of single versus multiple trauma exposure in a screening sample. J Trauma Stress 2000;13:271–86.
61. Cloitre M, Courtois CA, Charuvastra A, et al. Treatment of complex PTSD: results of the ISTSS Expert Clinician Survey on best practices. J Trauma Stress 2011; 24:615–27.
62. Heim C, Nemeroff CB. The role of childhood trauma in the neurobiology of mood and anxiety disorders: preclinical and clinical studies. Biol Psychiatry 2001;49: 1023–39.
63. Ford JD, Nader K, Fletcher KE. Clinical assessment and diagnosis. In: Ford JD, Courtois CA, editors. Treating complex traumatic stress disorders in child and adolescents: scientific foundations and therapeutic models. New York: The Guilford Press; 2013. p. 116–39.
64. Ford JD, Hartman JK, Hawke J, et al. Traumatic victimization, posttraumatic stress disorder, suicidal ideation, and substance abuse risk among juvenile justice-involved youth. J Child Adolesc Trauma 2008;1:75–92.
65. Briere J, Spinazzola J. Phenomenology and psychological assessment of complex posttraumatic states. J Trauma Stress 2005;18(5):401–12.
66. Ford JD, Connor D. ADHD and posttraumatic stress disorder (PTSD). Current Attention Disorder Reports 2009;1:61–6.
67. Ford JD. Dissociation in complex posttraumatic stress disorder or disorders of extreme stress not otherwise specified (DESNOS). In: Dell PF, O'Neil JA, editors. Dissociation and the dissociative disorders: DSM-V and beyond. New York: Routledge; 2009. p. 471–83.
68. Dorahy MJ, Corry M, Shannon M, et al. Complex trauma and intimate relationships: the impact of shame, guilt and dissociation. J Affect Disord 2013;147: 72–9.
69. Kernhof K, Kaufhold J, Grabhorn R. Object relations and interpersonal problem in sexually abused female patients: an empirical study with the SCORS and the IIP. J Pers Assess 2008;90:44–51.
70. Taylor S, Asmundson GJ, Carleton RN. Simple versus complex PTSD: a cluster analytic investigation. J Anxiety Disord 2006;20:459–72.
71. Tarren-Sweeney M. An investigation of complex attachment- and trauma-related symptomatology among children in foster and kinship care. Child Psychiatry Hum Dev 2013;44(6):727–41.

72. Baldwin MW, Fehr B, Keedian E, et al. An exploration of the relational schemata underlying attachment styles: self-report and lexical decision approaches. Pers Soc Psychol Bull 1993;19:746–54.

73. Burack JA, Flanagan T, Peled T, et al. Social perspective-taking skills in maltreated children and adolescents. Dev Psychol 2006;42:207–17.

74. van der Kolk BA. The neurobiology of childhood trauma and abuse. Child Adolesc Psychiatr Clin N Am 2003;12:293–317.

75. Marsella AJ, Friedman MJ, Gerrity ET, et al, editors. Ethnocultural aspects of posttraumatic stress disorder: Issues research, and clinical applications. Washington, DC: American Psychological Association; 1996.

76. Felitti VJ, Anda RF, Nordenberg D, et al. Relationship of childhood abuse and household dysfunction to many of the leading causes of death in adults: the Adverse Childhood Experiences (ACE) study. Am J Prev Med 1998;14: 245–58.

77. Luthra R, Abramovitz R, Greenberg R, et al. Relationship between type of trauma exposure and posttraumatic stress among urban children and adolescents. J Interpers Violence 2009;24:1919–27.

78. Finkelhor D, Ormrod RK, Turner HA. The developmental epidemiology of childhood victimization. J Interpers Violence 2009;24:711–31.

79. Koenen K, Moffitt TE, Poulton R, et al. Early childhood factors associated with the development of post-traumatic stress disorder: results from a longitudinal birth cohort. Psychol Med 2007;37:181–92.

80. Pynoos RS, Steinberg AM, Wraith R. A developmental model of childhood traumatic stress. In: Cicchetti D, Cohen D, editors. Developmental psychopathology vol. 2: risk, disorder, and adaptation. Oxford (England): John Wiley & Sons; 1995. p. 72–95.

81. van der Kolk BA. Child abuse and victimization. Psychiatr Ann 2005;35(3): 374–8.

82. Kaehler LA, Babcock R, DePrince AP, et al. Betrayal trauma. In: Ford JD, Courtois CA, editors. Treating complex traumatic stress disorders in child and adolescents: scientific foundations and therapeutic models. New York: The Guilford Press; 2013. p. 62–78.

83. Alexander PC. Relational trauma and disorganized attachment. In: Ford JD, Courtois CA, editors. Treating complex traumatic stress disorders in child and adolescents: scientific foundations and therapeutic models. New York: The Guilford Press; 2013. p. 39–61.

84. Deblinger E, Steer RA, Lippmann J. Two-year follow-up study of cognitive behavioral therapy for sexually abused children suffering post-traumatic stress symptoms. Child Abuse Negl 1999;23(12):1371–8.

85. Yancey CT, Hansen DJ. Relationship of personal, familial, and abuse-specific factors with outcome following childhood sexual abuse. Aggress Violent Behav 2010;15(6):410–21.

86. Turner HA, Finkelhor D, Ormrod R. Family context, victimization, and child trauma symptoms: variations in safe, stable, and nurturing relationships during early and middle childhood. Am J Orthop 2012;82(2):209–19.

87. Haskett ME, Nears K, Ward CS, et al. Diversity in adjustment of maltreated children: factors associated with resilient functioning. Clin Psychol Rev 2006;26(6): 796–812.

88. Howell KH. Resilience and psychopathology in children exposed to family violence. Aggress Violent Behav 2011;16(6):562–9.

89. Valentino K, Berkowitz S, Stover CS. Parenting behaviors and posttraumatic symptoms in relation to children's symptomatology following a traumatic event. J Trauma Stress 2010;23(3):403–7.
90. Graham-Bermann SA, Gruber G, Howell KH, et al. Factors discriminating among profiles of resilience and psychopathology in children exposed to intimate partner violence (IPV). Child Abuse Negl 2009;33(9):648–60.
91. Elliott AN, Carnes CN. Reactions of nonoffending parents to the sexual abuse of their child: a review of the literature. Child Maltreat 2001;6(4):314–31.
92. Bowlby J. Attachment and loss. New York: Basic Books; 1980.
93. Blaustein M, Kinniburgh K. Intervention beyond the child: the intertwining nature of attachment and trauma. British Psychological Society 2007;26:48–53. Briefing paper.
94. Kisiel C, Fehrenbach T, Small L, et al. Assessment of complex trauma exposure, responses, and service needs among children and adolescents in child welfare. J Child Adolesc Trauma 2009;2:143–60.
95. Abram KM, Teplin LA, Charles DR, et al. Posttraumatic stress disorder and trauma in youth in detention. Arch Gen Psychiatry 2004;61:403–10.
96. Ford JD, Chapman J, Connor DF, et al. Complex trauma and aggression in secure juvenile justice settings. Crim Justice Behav 2012;39:694–724.
97. National Child Traumatic Stress Network. Trauma-focused interventions for youth in the juvenile justice system. Available at: http://www.nctsn.org/products/trauma-focused-interventions-youth-juvenile-justice-system-2004. Accessed September 24, 2013.
98. Bloom SL. Sanctuary model. In: Ford JD, Courtois CA, editors. Treating complex traumatic stress disorders in child and adolescents: scientific foundations and therapeutic models. New York: The Guilford Press; 2013. p. 277–94.
99. National Juvenile Justice Trainers Association Honors NYS Office of Children and Family Services. New York State Office for Children and Family Services web site. Available at: http://ocfs.ny.gov/main/news/2008/2008_10_07_jjtAward.asp. Accessed September 24, 2013.
100. Courtois CA. Complex trauma, complex reactions: assessment and treatment. Psychother Theor Res Pract Train 2004;41(4):412–25.
101. Ippen CG, Ford J, Racusin R, et al. Traumatic events screening inventory - parent report revised. 2002. Available at: http://www.ptsd.va.gov/professional/pages/assessments/assessment-pdf/TESI-C.pdf. Accessed September 18, 2013.
102. Steinberg AM, Brymer MJ, Decker KB, et al. The University of California at Los Angeles post-traumatic stress disorder reaction index. Curr Psychiatry Rep 2004;6(2):96–100.
103. Kliethermes M, Wamser R. Adolescents with complex trauma. In: Cohen JA, Mannarino AP, Deblinger E, editors. Trauma-focused CBT for children and adolescents: treatment applications. New York: The Guilford Press; 2012. p. 175–96.
104. Kaufman J, Birmaher B, Brent D, et al. Schedule for affective disorders and schizophrenia for school-age children-present and lifetime version (K-SADS-PL): initial reliability and validity data. J Am Acad Child Adolesc Psychiatry 1997;36(7):980–8.
105. Achenbach TM, Rescorla LA. Manual for the ASEBA school-age forms and profiles. Burlington (VT): University of Vermont, Research Center for Children, Youth, & Families; 2001.

106. Butcher JN, Williams CL, Graham JR, et al. Minnesota Multiphasic Personality Inventory-Adolescent Version (MMPI-A): manual for administration, scoring and interpretation. Minneapolis (MN): University of Minnesota Press; 1992.
107. Reynolds CR, Kamphaus RW. Behavior assessment scale for children manual. 2nd edition. New York: Pearson; 2006.
108. Briere J. Trauma symptom checklist for children (TSCC) professional manual. Odessa (FL): Psychological Assessment Resources; 1996.
109. Briere J. Trauma symptom checklist for young children (TSCYC). Odessa (FL): Psychological Assessment Resources; 2005.
110. Friedrich WN. The child sexual behavior inventory professional manual. Odessa (FL): Psychological Assessment Resources; 1998.
111. Copeland WE, Keeler G, Angold A, et al. Traumatic events and posttraumatic stress in childhood. Arch Gen Psychiatry 2007;64(5):577-84.
112. American Psychiatric Association, DSM-5 Task Force. Diagnostic and statistical manual of mental disorders: DSM-5. 5th edition. Arlington (VA): American Psychiatric Publishing; 2013.
113. Ford JD. Hijacked by your brain: how to free yourself when stress takes over. Psychology Today Web site. Available at: http://www.psychologytoday.com/blog/hijacked-your-brain/201306/ptsd-becomes-more-complex-in-the-dsm-5-part-1. Published June 11, 2013. Accessed November 25, 2013.
114. Schmid M, Petermann F, Fegert JM. Developmental trauma disorder: pros and cons of including formal criteria in the psychiatric diagnostic systems. BMC Psychiatry 2013;13:3.
115. Ford JD, Courtois CA, Steele K, et al. Treatment of complex posttraumatic self-dysregulation. J Trauma Stress 2005;18(5):437-47.
116. Herman JL. Complex PTSD: a syndrome in survivors of prolonged and repeated trauma. J Trauma Stress 1992;5:377-91.
117. Courtois CA. Recollections of sexual abuse: treatment principles and guidelines. New York: Norton; 1999.
118. Ford JD, Cloitre M. Best practices in psychotherapy for children and adolescents. In: Courtois CA, Ford JD, editors. Treating complex traumatic stress disorders: an evidence-based guide. New York: The Guilford Press; 2009. p. 59-81.
119. Kinniburgh KJ, Blaustein M, Spinazzola J, et al. Attachment, self-regulation, and competency. Psychiatr Ann 2005;35(5):424-30.
120. Blaustein M, Kinniburgh K. Treating traumatic stress in children and adolescents: how to foster resilience through attachment, self-regulation, and competency. New York: The Guilford Press; 2010.
121. Klatzkin A, Lieberman AF, Van Horn P. Child-parent psychotherapy and historical trauma. In: Ford JD, Courtois CA, editors. Treating complex traumatic stress disorders in child and adolescents: scientific foundations and therapeutic models. New York: The Guilford Press; 2013. p. 295-314.
122. Linehan MM. Cognitive-behavioral treatment of borderline personality disorder. New York: The Guilford Press; 1993.
123. DeRosa RR, Rathus JH. Dialectical behavior therapy with adolescents. In: Ford JD, Courtois CA, editors. Treating complex traumatic stress disorders in child and adolescents: scientific foundations and therapeutic models. New York: The Guilford Press; 2013. p. 225-45.
124. Shapiro F. Eye movement desensitization and reprocessing: basic principles, protocols and procedures. 2nd edition. New York: The Guilford Press; 2001.

125. Wesselmann D, Shapiro F. Eye movement desensitization and reprocessing. In: Ford JD, Courtois CA, editors. Treating complex traumatic stress disorders in child and adolescents: scientific foundations and therapeutic models. New York: The Guilford Press; 2013. p. 203–24.
126. Briere J, Lanktree CB. Treating complex trauma in adolescents and young adults. Los Angeles (CA): Sage; 2011.
127. Urquiza AJ, Timmer S. Parent-child interaction therapy. In: Ford JD, Courtois CA, editors. Treating complex traumatic stress disorders in child and adolescents: scientific foundations and therapeutic models. New York: The Guilford Press; 2013. p. 315–28.
128. Kagan R. Rebuilding attachments with traumatized children: healing from losses, violence, abuse, and neglect. Binghamton (NY): Haworth Press; 2004.
129. Najavits LM, Gallop RJ, Weiss RD. Seeking safety therapy for adolescent girls with PTSD and substance use disorder: a randomized controlled trial. J Behav Health Serv Res 2006;33(4):453–63.
130. DeRosa R, Pelcovitz D. Group treatment for chronically traumatized adolescents: igniting SPARCS of change. In: Brom D, Pat-Horenczyk R, Ford JD, editors. Treating traumatized children: risk, resilience, and recovery. London: Routledge; 2008. p. 225–39.
131. Ford JD, Russo E. Trauma-focused, present-centered, emotional self-regulation approach to integrated treatment for posttraumatic stress and addiction: trauma adaptive recovery group education and therapy (TARGET). Am J Psychother 2006;60(4):335–55.
132. Cohen JA, Mannarino AP, Deblinger E. Treating trauma and traumatic grief in children and adolescents. New York: The Guilford Press; 2006.
133. Saxe GN, Ellis BH, Kaplow JB. Collaborative treatment of traumatized children and teens: the trauma systems therapy approach. New York: The Guildford Press; 2007.

Universal Preventive Interventions for Children in the Context of Disasters and Terrorism

Betty Pfefferbaum, MD, JD[a],*, Vandana Varma, MBBS[a],
Pascal Nitiéma, MD, MPH, MS[a], Elana Newman, PhD[b]

KEYWORDS

- Children and adolescents • Disaster • Disaster interventions
- Disaster mental health services • Preparedness • Screening • Terrorism
- Universal interventions

KEY POINTS

- Universal disaster services are used for children in general populations without consideration of their disaster exposures, experiences, or reactions.
- Universal disaster services include screening and case finding as well as preparedness and postevent preventive interventions.
- Universal services are typically administered in a group format in settings where children naturally congregate, such as schools.

Continued

Disclosures: This work was funded in part by the National Institute of Mental Health, the National Institute of Nursing Research, and the Substance Abuse and Mental Health Services Administration (5 R25 MH070569), which established the Child and Family Disaster Research Training and Education Program at the Terrorism and Disaster Center (TDC) at the University of Oklahoma Health Sciences Center. TDC is a partner in the National Child Traumatic Stress Network and is funded, in part, by the Substance Abuse and Mental Health Services Administration (1 U79 SM57278).
None of the authors of this article have any actual or potential conflicts of interest. Points of view in this document are those of the authors and do not necessarily represent the official position of the National Child Traumatic Stress Network; the National Institute of Mental Health; the National Institute of Nursing Research; the Substance Abuse and Mental Health Services Administration; the Tulsa Institute of Trauma, Abuse, and Neglect; the University of Oklahoma Health Sciences Center; or the University of Tulsa.

[a] Department of Psychiatry and Behavioral Sciences, Terrorism and Disaster Center, College of Medicine, University of Oklahoma Health Sciences Center, 920 Stanton L. Young Boulevard, Oklahoma City, OK 73104, USA; [b] Department of Psychology, Tulsa Institute of Trauma Abuse and Neglect, University of Tulsa, 800 South Tucker Drive, Tulsa, OK 74104, USA
* Corresponding author. Department of Psychiatry and Behavioral Sciences, College of Medicine, University of Oklahoma Health Sciences Center, Oklahoma City, OK.
E-mail address: Betty-Pfefferbaum@ouhsc.edu

Child Adolesc Psychiatric Clin N Am 23 (2014) 363–382
http://dx.doi.org/10.1016/j.chc.2013.12.006
1056-4993/14/$ – see front matter © 2014 Elsevier Inc. All rights reserved.

childpsych.theclinics.com

Continued

- Most universal preventive interventions delivered to children before and after a disaster are multimodal and rely heavily on cognitive behavioral techniques.
- Most universal preventive interventions have demonstrated benefit for at least some of the outcomes measured.
- The field awaits research on several key issues related to the relative efficacy of universal preventive intervention approaches and components, the timing and setting of intervention delivery, and the preparation of providers.

INTRODUCTION

Children are especially vulnerable to the effects of disasters and terrorism, and they constitute an important focus of disaster mental health services. Because disasters threaten children's assumptions that the world is safe and predictable,[1] disaster services may be needed for children who reside in the general community where a disaster strikes as well as for those who are more directly affected by an event through physical presence, the experiences of significant others, damage to property, and/or exposure to secondary adversities. Preventive interventions are classified along a spectrum of risk and need, with universal preventive interventions designed for the general population of children in a disaster community not identified for individual risk. These interventions are contrasted with selected preventive interventions for children who are at an increased risk of developing a mental, emotional, or behavioral disorder based on biologic, psychologic, or social factors and with indicated preventive interventions for children at high risk and identified as being predisposed to, or having minimal detectable signs or symptoms that presage, a disorder.[2] Universal, selected, and indicated services can be linked through a stepped approach with assessment and sequenced interventions based on need.[3]

This article addresses universal preventive interventions administered to general populations of children without consideration of their disaster experiences or emotional states. Thus, these interventions address children with a range of disaster exposures and conditions rather than focusing only on the needs of children who were directly exposed to an event, children whose significant others were directly exposed, or children whose prior experiences or preexisting conditions increase their risk for adverse outcomes. This report describes the organization and structure of services used to meet the needs of children in the general population (practice applications), examines screening and intervention approaches (tools for practice), and suggests future directions for the field.

LITERATURE SEARCH AND REVIEW

A systematic literature search on child disaster and terrorism mental health services and interventions was conducted in July 2013 (**Fig. 1**). Much of the literature described services addressing multiple populations—universal, selected, and indicated—covering a variety of disasters and issues across disaster phases. This literature included empirical studies and descriptive works on disaster services in general (eg, mental health services, crisis intervention, school-based activities) and on specific disasters (see **Fig. 1**).

Forty-seven articles described empirical studies of interventions. In one study that described a 2-phase trial,[4] the 2 stages discussed were analyzed separately. Hence,

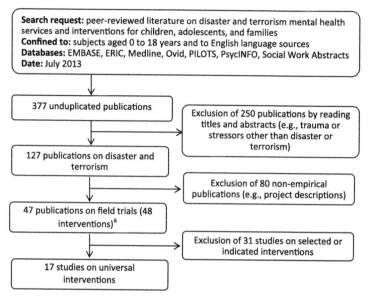

Search request: peer-reviewed literature on disaster and terrorism mental health services and interventions for children, adolescents, and families
Confined to: subjects aged 0 to 18 years and to English language sources
Databases: EMBASE, ERIC, Medline, Ovid, PILOTS, PsycINFO, Social Work Abstracts
Date: July 2013

377 unduplicated publications

Exclusion of 250 publications by reading titles and abstracts (e.g., trauma or stressors other than disaster or terrorism)

127 publications on disaster and terrorism

Exclusion of 80 non-empirical publications (e.g., project descriptions)

47 publications on field trials (48 interventions)[a]

Exclusion of 31 studies on selected or indicated interventions

17 studies on universal interventions

[a]Two stages of one study which described a two-phase trial[4] were analyzed separately, resulting in 48 interventions for review.

Fig. 1. Flow diagram of the literature search and research reviewed.

the final sample of empirical papers for review included 48 intervention studies. These studies were classified as universal, selected, or indicated based on ratings by 2 authors (PN and VV). Universal preventive interventions were defined as those delivered to children regardless of their disaster exposures or experiences or their clinical, emotional, or behavioral status. The inter-rater agreement (weighted kappa) for these ratings was 0.80 (95% confidence interval = 0.64–0.96). Discrepancies were resolved through consensus of the authors. Seventeen studies describing empirical research on universal preventive interventions were selected for analysis (see **Fig. 1**).

Of the 17 empirical studies evaluating universal preventive interventions, 5 addressed preparedness and 12 addressed postdisaster situations. It is noteworthy that many of the studies were well designed, with 14 implementing controlled trials and 7 of those using individual or cluster random assignment (**Table 1**).

PRACTICE APPLICATIONS: ORGANIZATION AND STRUCTURE OF DISASTER MENTAL HEALTH SERVICES

The disaster system of care includes 2 components. The public health component emphasizes wellness and resilience and includes efforts to identify children who need services. The clinical component is designed to treat psychopathology and maladaptive emotional and behavioral reactions to the event and to secondary adversities, including preexisting psychopathology exacerbated by the disaster.[21] Operational in the aftermath of an event, this system of care relies on a network of existing and new clinical, public health, education, faith-based, and community service systems to reach survivors with a range of needs. It may be difficult to implement services depending on the degree of destruction or damage to the community infrastructure and on the chaos and confusion that ensue.

Table 1
Characteristics of studies assessing universal interventions

Study	Disaster/Time Interval Between Event and Intervention	Age and/or Grade	Location/Provider	Type of Intervention	Number of Sessions/Duration of the Intervention	Type of Control	Random Assignment
Preparedness Interventions							
Berger et al,[5] 2007	Terrorism[a]/ongoing	Grades 2-6	School/teacher	Eclectic with CBT	8 Sessions	Waitlist	Yes[b]
Berger et al,[6] 2012	Terrorism[a]/ongoing	11–13 y Grades 7-8	School/teacher	Eclectic with CBT	16 Weekly sessions	Waitlist	Yes[b]
Gelkopf & Berger,[7] 2009	Terrorism[a]/ongoing	Grades 7-8	School/teacher	Eclectic with CBT	12 Sessions	Waitlist	Yes
Ronan & Johnston,[8] 2003	Pre-event preparedness/no disaster	11–13 y	School/teacher	Emergency management hazard education	1 Class period per day over 6 wk for usual education; NS for homework with parents	Usual hazard education	Yes[b]
Wolmer et al,[9] 2011	Pre-event prevention/no disaster	Grades 4-5	School/teacher	Eclectic with CBT	14 Weekly modules	NTC	No
Postdisaster Interventions							
Berger & Gelkopf,[10] 2009	Tsunami/14.5 mo	9-14 y Elementary school	School/teacher	Eclectic with CBT	12 Weekly sessions	Waitlist	Yes[b]
Brown et al,[4] 2006 (classroom)	Terrorist attack/30 mo	8-13 y Grades 3-7	School/mental health professional	Eclectic with CBT	10 Weekly sessions	NA	NA
Goenjian et al,[11] 1997	Earthquake/18 mo	Grades 6-7	School/mental health professional	Eclectic with CBT	4 Group and 2 individual sessions over 3 wk	NTC	No

Study	Disaster/time	Age	Setting/provider	Intervention	Sessions	Control	Well-established
Goenjian et al,[12] 2005	Earthquake/18 mo	15–17 y	School/mental health professional	Eclectic with CBT	4 Group and 2 individual sessions over 3 wk	NTC	No
Hardin et al,[13] 2002	Hurricane/NS	13–18 y	School/mental health professional	Eclectic with CBT	3 Sessions per year for 3 y	Assigned nontreated & nonparticipants	Yes[b]
Ronan & Johnston,[14] 1999	Volcanic eruption/3 mo	7–13 y	School/mental health professional	Eclectic with CBT	1 Session	Exposure	Yes[b]
Sahin et al,[15] 2011	Earthquake/10 mo	NS/NS	School/mental health professional	Psychoeducation	NS	NTC	No
Stewart et al,[16] 1992	Hurricane/NS	13–17 y High school	School/mental health professional	Eclectic with CBT	1 Session	NA	NA
Vijayakumar et al,[17] 2006	Tsunami/12 mo	11–14 y	Community setting/mental health professional and volunteer	Eclectic with CBT	6 Sessions over 6 mo	NTC	No
Wolmer et al,[18] 2003	Earthquake/4.5 mo	Grades 1–5	School/teacher	Eclectic with CBT	8 Twice-weekly sessions	NA	NA
Wolmer et al,[19] 2005	Earthquake/4.5 mo	9–17 y	School/teacher	Eclectic with CBT (follow-up of 2003 study)	8 Twice-weekly sessions	NTC	No
Wolmer et al,[20] 2011	Terrorism[a]/5 mo	8–12 y Grades 3–6	School/teacher	Eclectic with CBT	15 Weekly modules	Waitlist	No

Abbreviations: CBT, cognitive behavioral therapy; NA, not applicable; NS, not specified; NTC, nontreatment control; NWE, not well established treatment.
[a] Study participants had been exposed to repetitive terrorist attacks in the context of armed conflict.
[b] Cluster randomization.

Pre-event and postevent interventions have addressed a variety of natural and human-caused disasters and have been delivered to children and adolescents across ages and in nations around the world (see **Table 1**). The choice of interventions depends on the disaster phase and on the availability of settings and providers as well as on the experiences and needs of the children being served. Each of these is addressed later.

Timing of Intervention Delivery

Universal services are applied across all phases of a disaster. Pre-event services are designed to enhance preparedness and resilience, whereas postevent interventions are used to normalize reactions, reduce trauma and anxiety, and improve coping and recovery. Typically, screening and case finding activities are administered after an event to capture information appropriate to the context and disaster phase. Interventions in the studies examined for this report were delivered before the disaster for preparedness efforts and from several months to more than 2 years after the disaster (see **Table 1**).

Predisaster preparedness interventions have been delivered to universal populations in geographic areas where disasters are likely to recur. Two types of preparedness programs have been tested. One approach provided instructions to children and their parents about disasters and disaster mitigation without directly addressing emotional issues.[8] This approach increased children's hazard knowledge and hazard adjustments and decreased their hazard-related fears. Similar to postdisaster interventions, the second approach, used in the context of terrorism, focused directly on children's emotional health in the context of educational programing about the sociopolitical conflicts that led to the terrorist threat.[5,7] Specifically, 2 classroom interventions delivered to Israeli students attending schools in communities that had suffered repeated terror attacks used psychoeducation, cognitive behavioral techniques, body awareness activities and meditation, and narrative approaches.[5,7] These interventions resulted in improved emotional outcomes, such as posttraumatic stress disorder (PTSD) symptoms, somatic complaints,[5,7] anxiety,[5] depression, and functional problems,[7] for participants.

Several interventions reviewed for this report were efficacious when administered within the first 6 months after the disaster.[14,18–20] In their controlled trial of an intervention delivered 3 months after exposure to volcanic eruptions, Ronan and Johnston[14] found improvement in children's self-reported PTSD symptoms and coping ability with both of the brief interventions tested, a cognitive behavioral intervention and an exposure intervention, with no significant difference between the 2 interventions. Following a massive earthquake in Turkey, Wolmer and colleagues[18] found significant improvement in posttraumatic stress and dissociative symptoms, whereas grief symptoms increased significantly, following an intervention that combined psychoeducation, cognitive behavioral techniques, play activities, and maintaining a personal diary delivered 4 to 5 months after the earthquake. Approximately 3 years after the intervention (3.5 years after the earthquake), the severity of posttraumatic stress, grief, and dissociative symptoms in the intervention and control groups were not significantly different; but the children who participated in the intervention were rated higher in adaptive functioning than the control group.[19]

Evidence suggests that interventions can be beneficial even if delivered many months or even years after a disaster with some evidence of long-term benefit. For example, Brown and colleagues[4] administered their intervention more than 2 years after the September 11 attack with sustained benefit at the 4- to 6-month follow-up. Berger and Gelkopf[10] demonstrated improvement in children's distress symptoms with their intervention administered 14.5 months after the 2004 Indian Ocean tsunami but did not conduct a long-term follow-up assessment to examine the lasting benefit with the intervention. Goenjian and colleagues[11] found that their trauma- and grief-focused psychotherapy intervention, delivered to children 18 months after a massive earthquake in Armenia, resulted in reductions in posttraumatic stress. Moreover, the benefit was evident 5 years after the disaster when, in addition to greater improvement in PTSD symptoms, those who received the intervention showed improvement in depressive symptoms, whereas those who did not experienced worsening of depressive symptoms.[12] Improvement in the PTSD score in the nontreatment group could be attributed to natural recovery, whereas the much greater decrease in those who received the intervention suggests a clinically meaningful effect of the intervention on PTSD symptoms with a large difference in the changes in PTSD scores between both groups (Cohen's d = 0.89). The medium effect size of the difference in changes in depression scores between the 2 groups (Cohen's d = 0.73) also suggests a clinically meaningful effect of the treatment on depression.

It is unclear if either the number of sessions or the duration of an intervention is associated with lasting benefit. As evident in **Table 1**, the number of sessions across interventions ranged from 1 to 16, commonly delivered on a weekly basis. Hardin and colleagues[13] implemented the most prolonged intervention, with 3 sessions per year over a 3-year period. Perhaps most impressive was the sustained benefit with the intervention delivered by Goenjian and colleagues[11,12] in 4 group and 2 individual sessions over 3 weeks.

In general, studies have not considered the importance of timing in their analyses of outcomes and they have not compared the efficacy of interventions delivered during different disaster phases. Moreover, the potential for natural recovery complicates the interpretation of results. Certain trauma-related stress symptoms may recede over time without any therapeutic intervention as observed in 2 nontreatment controls in the reviewed studies.[12,13] Ronan and Johnston[14] considered the possibility of natural recovery and, thus, assessed the effects of time in their comparison of brief exposure and cognitive behavioral interventions in children after a series of volcanic eruptions. The study included 2 phases: the first was a 2-month observational period with no treatment and the second entailed administration of either the exposure or cognitive behavioral intervention. PTSD symptoms and coping scores improved significantly during each of the 2 study phases in both the full sample and the subset of participants with symptomatic PTSD. For participants with symptomatic PTSD in both treatment groups, the decrease in PTSD symptoms during the observational phase was greater than that of the post-treatment period, in contrast to coping scores, which increased more after treatment than in the observational period. The study of a school-based public health intervention delivered to adolescents after Hurricane Hugo also raised the possible influence of natural recovery when, after increased distress in both the intervention and control groups in the first year, there was a steady decrease over the next 2 years for all groups.[13] Hence, some, or all, of an observed treatment effect may reflect natural recovery. It is also possible for symptoms to remain stable or increase when no treatment is administered[11,12] or for recovery of nontreated children to occur at a slower pace relative to those who receive treatment. For example, it took more than 18 months after the baseline assessment to observe a significant decrease in posttraumatic stress symptoms in nontreated students who were exposed to the Armenian earthquake, whereas those who received the intervention had significantly lower posttraumatic stress symptoms 18 months after the baseline assessment.[11,12]

Delivery Sites

Universal disaster services are administered in community settings generally chosen to maximize access. These settings include, for example, schools and preschools, day care programs, primary health care facilities, faith-based institutions, youth centers, volunteer organizations, and even shelters and refugee camps if other sites are unavailable. With respect to the interventions reviewed for this article, all but one, which was administered in a community setting (L. Vijayakumar, written communication, September 2013), were delivered to children in schools. After reviewing 19 trauma intervention studies, including 8 on disaster interventions, Rolfsnes and Idsoe[22] concluded that interventions in schools and by school personnel are beneficial for traumatized children.

Universal preventive interventions, which can be delivered in groups to relatively large numbers of children simultaneously, are especially suited for school settings, which provide access to children who are accustomed to shared experiences. Typically, schooling is one of the first services to be restored after an event. Further, disaster-related problems are likely to emerge in school where children spend many of their waking hours. Schools not only foster development, achievement, and discovery but they also constitute the primary socializing agent for children providing safe environments to acquire and build trusting relationships with adults and peers and to express and process their experiences and emotions. If not damaged or destroyed by the disaster, schools are a source of continuity, stability, and strength to teach safety and preparedness, normalize and monitor reactions, reestablish routines, clarify and process media coverage, restore expectations, teach coping, practice new skills, inspire hope and a focus on the future, and support recovery. Moreover, children derive support from their peers at school.

Services can be delivered in schools without the stigma commonly associated with mental health interventions, and parents and families know and generally trust school personnel and processes. Although parents may not seek services for themselves, they may be receptive to services designed for their children. Thus, schools can be used to reach the broader community through public health activities, such as preparedness, prevention, and universal interventions designed to deliver psychoeducation and social support, assess and monitor affected children, and identify and triage children with problems that warrant more comprehensive evaluation and more intensive professional attention.

Many obstacles complicate the use of schools for delivering disaster services. School administrators must balance the importance of the academic mission with the emotional needs of children, teachers, and staff. Administrators sometimes minimize the effects of a disaster thinking that few children were affected and that those who were can readily be identified.[23] School personnel may be concerned that addressing the disaster will retraumatize children, failing to see the distinction between reexposing children to the actual threat as opposed to memories and information about the threat. Teachers and staff are likely to be stressed by the disaster; thus, addressing their needs must be a priority.[24] The school's response may be hindered if trauma-exposed parents question school policies and the ability of the school to protect their children.[1] Depending on school or school-district policies, active or passive parental consent may be required to conduct screenings and/or deliver services. Parents may be suspicious of services, especially if coupled with research; they may be too busy attending to other primary needs to provide documentation of consent. Moreover, schools may lack certain resources needed to provide services that are typically found in clinical settings, such as sufficient private space to meet with children and families, the availability of licensed mental health professionals, and the capacity and mechanisms to conduct comprehensive assessments and deliver treatment. Furthermore, classroom enrollment may change as a result of displacement, creating challenges in finding children who may need services as well as potential problems integrating displaced children into schools that may lack the resources and preparation to address the needs of these children.[1] Finally, using classroom settings misses children who are denied access to school and/or those who are home schooled.

Providers

The choice of providers to deliver disaster interventions is determined by various factors, including their availability, training, and experience as well as the goals and complexity of the intervention and the venue for intervention delivery. Noting that teachers can administer assessments, reinforce new skills, and provide feedback to students, Wolmer and colleagues[18] prepared teachers as mediators to deliver a classroom-based intervention to children after an earthquake in Turkey. Teachers and school personnel have established relationships with children making them a natural source of support; they are familiar with child development and situational crises, and they are in a position to notice emotional and behavioral changes and changes in functioning. Yet at the same time, they may need additional support and guidance for addressing their own emotional responses. This support can be incorporated into teacher training to enhance their coping as well as their sense of self-efficacy and competence.[25]

As evident in **Table 1**, all of the pre-event preparedness interventions reviewed for this report were delivered by trained teachers, whereas most of the postevent interventions were delivered by mental health professionals. Pre-event situations are not typically designed to address clinical concerns, whereas clinical problems may arise in postevent environments, especially following catastrophic events. For example, Goenjian and colleagues[11] used therapists to deliver both their universal classroom-based group intervention and individual sessions with children after an earthquake in Armenia. Vijayakumar and colleagues[17] used psychologists and volunteers to deliver an intervention to children in a coastal village in India approximately 1 year after the 2004 Indian Ocean tsunami. Many of the children receiving these interventions were severely or moderately affected, though more than 40% were not affected by the disaster. On the other hand, noting the lack of trained mental health professionals, an intervention delivered to Sri Lankan children following the tsunami[10] and one administered to children following an earthquake in Turkey[18,19] were delivered by teachers who were trained and supervised.

Conditions Addressed and Outcomes

Universal services are delivered to children regardless of their disaster exposures, experiences, or reactions. The outcomes studied reflect the focus of the interventions and the characteristics of the children receiving them. **Table 2** presents the outcomes examined in the universal preventive intervention studies reviewed for this report. Appropriately, given their application to children in the general population rather than to selected or indicated populations, most studies did not measure PTSD diagnostic outcomes; the 6 studies that did report PTSD outcomes used cutoff values on rating scales rather than clinical assessment to establish diagnostic outcome.[5–7,9,10,20] Notable pre-event exceptions were terrorism preparedness interventions with Israeli children, many of whom had been exposed to prior terrorist incidents,[5–7,9] another postevent Israeli terrorism intervention study,[20] and an intervention delivered to

Table 2
Outcomes assessed in studies of universal interventions

Study	Event	PTSD Diagnosis or Caseness	PTSS	Anxiety	Depression	Coping	Functioning	Somatic Complaints	Other Outcomes
Preparedness Interventions									
Berger et al,[5] 2007	T	IMP, SUP	IMP, SUP	IMP, SUP	—	—	IMP, SUP	IMP, SUP	—
Berger et al,[6] 2012	T	IMP, SUP	IMP, SUP	IMP, SUP	—	—	IMP, SUP	IMP, SUP	Separation anxiety: IMP, SUP
Gelkopf & Berger,[7] 2009	T	IMP, SUP	IMP, SUP	—	IMP, SUP	—	IMP, SUP	IMP, SUP	—
Ronan & Johnston,[8] 2003	PE	—	—	—	—	NC, NSD	—	—	Hazard adjustments: IMP, SUP; EM knowledge: IMP, SUP; Hazard fears: IMP, NSD
Wolmer et al,[9] 2011	T	SUP	SUP	—	—	—	—	—	Stress/mood: SUP
Postdisaster Interventions									
Berger & Gelkopf,[10] 2009	ND	IMP, SUP	IMP, SUP	—	IMP, SUP	—	IMP, SUP	IMP, SUP	Hope: IMP, SUP
Brown et al,[4] 2006[a] (classroom)	T	—	NC	NC	IMP	—	—	—	Anger: IMP
Goenjian et al,[11] 1997	ND	—	IMP, SUP	—	NC, SUP	—	—	—	—
Goenjian et al,[12] 2005[b]	ND	—	IMP, SUP	—	NC, SUP	—	—	—	—
Hardin et al,[13] 2002	ND	—	—	—	—	—	—	—	Mental distress: IMP, SUP

Study							Outcomes
Ronan & Johnston,[14] 1999	ND	—	—	IMP, NSD	—	IMP, NSD	—
Sahin et al,[15] 2011	ND	IMP, NSD	—	—	—	—	Earthquake knowledge: NSD; Perceived benefit: SUP
Stewart et al,[16] 1992[c]	ND	—	—	—	—	—	Evaluation of intervention
Vijayakumar et al,[17] 2006	ND	NC,NSD	NC,NSD	—	—	NC, NSD	Behavior difficulties: NC, NSD; Affective problems: NC, NSD; Desist smoking: SUP
Wolmer et al,[18] 2003	ND	IMP	—	—	—	—	Grief: WR; Dissociative symptoms: IMP
Wolmer et al,[19] 2005	ND	IMP, NSD	—	—	SUP	—	Grief: IMP, NSD; Dissociative symptoms: IMP, NSD
Wolmer et al,[20] 2011	T	IMP, SUP	—	—	—	—	Stress/mood: IMP; Parent concern: NC; Teacher satisfaction with classroom atmosphere: IMP

Types of intervention and controls are presented in **Table 1**.

Abbreviations: EM, emergency management; IMP, pre-event to postevent improvement in the intervention group; NC, no significant change in outcome after the intervention; ND, natural disaster; NSD, no significant difference between intervention and control; PE, pre-event no disaster; PTSS, posttraumatic stress symptom or reaction; SUP, intervention superior to control; T, terrorism; WR, pre-event to postevent worsening of symptoms.

a There was a significant pre/post improvement in total PTSD score for 22 participants identified as having PTSD, but the difference was not significant for the full sample.

b The decrease in mean depression score in the treatment group was not statistically significant.

c A total of 82% of the participants rated the small group component as very good or excellent and 70% rated the large group component as very good or excellent.

Sri Lankan children following the 2004 Indian Ocean tsunami.[10] Most (95.8%) of the Sri Lankan children studied by Berger and Gelkopf[10] after the tsunami were physically present at the disaster, 60.2% knew someone killed, and 27.1% knew someone injured in the disaster, making it appropriate to address PTSD. Not only did the intervention result in a decrease in the number of probable PTSD cases in the intervention group compared with the waitlist control group but no new cases of probable PTSD were observed in the intervention condition, whereas new probable cases emerged in the waitlist control (see **Table 2**).

As evident in **Table 2**, most interventions have demonstrated benefit in at least some of the outcomes measured, including PTSD or posttraumatic stress reactions or symptoms,[5–7,9–12,14,18–20] other anxiety reactions,[5,6] depression,[4,7,10–12] somatic complaints,[5–7,10] anger,[4] dissociative symptoms,[18,19] grief,[19] hope,[10] and functioning.[5–7,10,19] Not all studies examined emotional or behavioral outcomes exclusively. Two investigations studied children's knowledge after interventions that delivered information about disasters.[8,15] Ronan and Johnston[8] found improvement in problem-focused areas, such as hazard knowledge and hazard adjustment and in hazard-related fears, after an emergency management education program, though there was no improvement in the children's perceived emotional coping ability. Sahin and colleagues[15] found no significant difference in earthquake knowledge between children who received a psychoeducation intervention and the no-treatment control condition, though children who received the intervention reported it to be beneficial. Instead of measuring emotional or behavioral outcomes, Stewart and colleagues[16] asked students who participated in their psychoeducational Hurricane Hugo intervention to rate their experience using written questions with 5 response options ranging from poor to excellent. Most students rated the experience favorably.

All but 4 studies[8,13,15,16] assessed posttraumatic stress reactions or symptoms as an outcome, though not all found improvement from preassessment to postassessment[4,17] or superiority of the intervention over the control condition (see **Table 2**).[17,19] For example, Vijayakumar and colleagues[17] attributed their failure to find improvement in PTSD symptoms in children who participated in their intervention to the fact that the largely psychoeducation intervention was not intended to address trauma symptoms. The intervention focused instead on other behaviors, including the expression of positive emotions and resisting peer pressure to smoke, both of which improved.

Although universal preventive interventions are not intended for children who themselves are, or whose loved ones are, directly exposed to a disaster, these children may receive universal interventions intended for general populations of which they are a part. Study results may be skewed when interventions are delivered to universal populations that include large numbers of children with direct exposure or children with disaster-related losses. For example, following their universal teacher-mediated intervention for children after an earthquake in Turkey, Wolmer and colleagues[18] found improvement in posttraumatic stress symptoms, whereas grief symptoms increased perhaps because the resolution of trauma allowed the grief process to begin or because the intervention did not adequately address grief symptoms; there also may have been a reporting bias created by the participants' reluctance to acknowledge symptoms before the intervention and their willingness to do so after the intervention. In their follow-up study, these investigators[19] found a significant decrease in posttraumatic stress, grief, and dissociation over the course of 3 years. But unfortunately, children in both the intervention and control groups still reported moderate (30%–35%) or severe (17%–18%) levels of posttraumatic stress symptoms. There was no significant difference in levels of posttraumatic stress symptoms between the intervention and nontreatment control groups. The investigators attributed these results to a combination of predisaster vulnerability, postdisaster stress, dysfunctional family life, and inadequate support for some children demonstrating the importance of referral for selected and/or indicated interventions for children at an elevated risk for adverse outcomes. Nevertheless, teacher-rated daily functioning in terms of academic performance, social behavior, and general conduct was significantly better in the intervention group compared with controls.

IMPORTANT TOOLS FOR PRACTICE: SCREENING AND INTERVENTION APPROACHES

Various approaches are used in universal services to administer preparedness and postdisaster interventions and to conduct screening and case-finding activities. These universal services are typically delivered to children in groups.

Screening and Case Finding

The goal of screening is to identify children who are at risk for maladaptive outcomes and/or those who may need formal evaluation and possible treatment. Screening is appropriate if large numbers of children were exposed to an event or if the level of exposure among a population is unknown. Screening is typically conducted in venues where children naturally congregate. For example, schools provide a popular and relatively convenient setting for screening.[3,26] The appropriate timing of screening remains in debate, especially given the ubiquitous distress that accompanies disasters[27]; screening must be reasonable in cost in relation to potential benefits,[28] and it should not be conducted in the absence of a mechanism to refer children for the services that the screening results suggest are needed.[29] **Fig. 2** outlines the steps associated with the screening process, including indications for clinical evaluation and appropriate services (see **Fig. 2**).

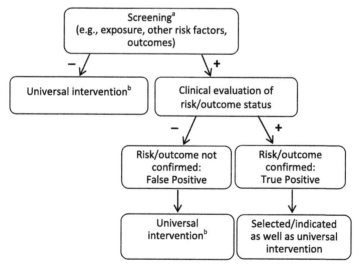

[a]Screening instruments with established high sensitivity and specificity in children similar to the ones being screened (e.g., similar socio-demographic characteristics, culture, trauma, environmental context) should be used.
[b]Children receiving only universal interventions should be reassessed periodically.

Fig. 2. Flow diagram of the screening process.

Screening may set a low threshold to increase sensitivity (the likelihood of testing positive for an individual with the condition), while sacrificing specificity (the likelihood of testing negative for an individual who does not have the condition). False positives occur with children being incorrectly labeled as in need of services, which may subject children to unnecessary evaluation and treatment.[30] False negatives may occur if the instrument fails to detect the condition presented by the respondent (low sensitivity), if children deny problems, or as a result of natural fluctuation in trauma reactions after a disaster.[27]

Children who screen positive for psychiatric risk (most often PTSD or major depression) should be referred for a more comprehensive evaluation (see **Fig. 2**).[31,32] A school-based survey of middle and high school students conducted 7 weeks after the Oklahoma City bombing underscored the importance of individual assessment for those identified as most distressed or symptomatic who may have suffered a preexisting condition, experienced prior trauma, or possessed other risk factors.[33] Although seeking counseling was related to exposure, to initial reactions, and to current posttraumatic stress, worry about safety, and trouble handling demands in general, few students with the highest posttraumatic stress levels sought counseling; there was no relationship between posttraumatic stress and seeking counseling for this group.[33] The findings also support the need for outreach and psychoeducation to inform families about when services may be needed and to link symptomatic children to those services.

For practical administration, screening tools should be brief, uncomplicated, and easy to administer and score; appropriate in content reflecting the context and disaster phase; and acceptable to those being screened.[28,29] Screening instruments should reflect developmental and normative expectations, the language and culture of those being assessed, and the needs of children with special health and mental health problems.[34] In the disaster context, screening tools for children typically query aspects of children's exposure and experiences (eg, disaster-related injuries, losses, life disruptions, adversities, current needs) and their subjective reactions (eg, horror/terror, general distress, posttraumatic stress reactions, anxiety, depression, changes in behavior, impaired functioning). These tools typically do not assess predisaster problems or the numerous individual, family, and social factors that may influence children's reactions.[32]

Several instruments have been used to assess children's reactions to traumatic events and conditions[35] that arise in the postdisaster environment, such as PTSD symptoms, depressive symptoms, other anxiety symptoms, and behavior problems.[36] **Table 3** presents the instruments used to measure selected outcomes in the universal child disaster interventions reviewed for this report. Unfortunately, although studies have been conducted on screening tools in Chinese[37] and Thai[38] samples, the sensitivity and specificity of most instruments for use in screening has not been well established in the context of disasters or terrorism (see **Table 3**).

Intervention Approaches and Components

Universal preventive interventions, administered before and after a disaster, are used for general populations of children whose disaster exposures and experiences may vary greatly. These public health interventions may benefit all children by normalizing disaster reactions, helping children process their experiences, fostering coping and adaptive skill development, enhancing future planning and preparedness, and promoting recovery.

All of the interventions reviewed for this report were administered to children in groups. The benefits of group application include learning from other group members

Table 3
Instruments used to measure the principal outcomes assessed in studies of universal interventions

Outcome	Instrument	Studies
PTSD/PTSS (n = 13)	Post-Traumatic Stress Disorder Reaction Index (PTSD-RI, Steinberg et al,[39] 2004)	Berger et al,[5] 2007 Berger et al,[6] 2012 Berger & Gelkopf,[10] 2009 Gelkopf & Berger,[7] 2009 Goenjian et al,[11] 1997 Goenjian et al,[12] 2005 Ronan & Johnston,[14] 1999 Vijayakumar et al,[17] 2006 Wolmer et al,[18] 2003 Wolmer et al,[19] 2005 Wolmer et al,[20] 2011 Wolmer et al,[9] 2011
	Child PTSD Symptom Scale (CPSS, Foa et al,[40] 2001)	Brown et al,[4] 2006
Anxiety (n = 4)	Screen for Child Anxiety-Related Emotional Disorders (SCARED, Birmaher et al,[41] 1997)	Berger et al,[5] 2007 Berger et al,[6] 2012
	Multidimensional Anxiety Scale for Children (MASC, March et al,[42] 1997)	Brown et al,[4] 2006
	Youth Self-Rating scale (YSR, Achenbach,[43] 1991)	Vijayakumar et al,[17] 2006
Depression (n = 5)	Brief Beck Depression Inventory (Beck & Beck,[44] 1972)	Berger & Gelkopf,[10] 2009 Gelkopf & Berger,[7] 2009
	Children's Depression Inventory (CDI, Kovacs,[45] 1985)	Brown et al,[4] 2006
	Depression Self-Rating Scale (DSRS, Asarnow & Carlson,[46] 1985)	Goenjian et al,[11] 1997 Goenjian et al,[12] 2005
Functioning (n = 5)	Diagnostic Interview Schedule or Children/ Diagnosis Predictive Scale (DISC/DPS, Lucas et al,[47] 2001)	Berger et al,[5] 2007 Berger et al,[6] 2012 Berger & Gelkopf,[10] 2009 Gelkopf & Berger,[7] 2009
	Instrument devised by study authors	Wolmer et al,[19] 2005
Somatic complaints (n = 5)	Diagnostic Interview Schedule or Children/ Diagnosis Predictive Scale (DISC/DPS, Lucas et al,[47] 2001)	Berger et al,[5] 2007 Berger et al,[6] 2012 Berger & Gelkopf,[10] 2009 Gelkopf & Berger,[7] 2009
	Youth Self-Rating scale (YSR, Achenbach,[43] 1991)	Vijayakumar et al,[17] 2006

and enhanced peer support. For example, Brown and colleagues[4] attributed the improvement in depression with a September 11 classroom intervention in part to the social component of the intervention. Group interventions must be designed and implemented to avoid the potential for children to be overwhelmed by the experiences and reactions of other group participants, however.

Universal disaster interventions rely heavily on various cognitive behavioral techniques similar to those described for traumatized children in general.[32] **Table 4** displays summary data on the components used in the reviewed interventions based on author descriptions. Except for an emergency management preparedness intervention[8] and a psychoeducation intervention,[15] the interventions used a variety of multimodal approaches (see **Table 4**).

The summary data presented in **Table 4** reveal the prominence of coping skill development (n = 15, 88.2%), affect processing techniques (n = 14, 82.4%), social support (n = 13, 76.5%), psychoeducation (n = 12, 70.6%), and stress management (n = 12,

Table 4
Components included in the universal interventions reviewed

Component	Preparedness Interventions (n = 5)	Postdisaster Interventions (n = 12)	Total n = 17 (%)
Psychoeducation	4	8	12 (70.6)
Exposure/narrative	3	6	9 (52.9)
Relaxation skills	3	2	5 (29.4)
Stress management	4	8	12 (70.6)
Affect awareness/modulation	5	9	14 (82.4)
Coping	5	10	15 (88.2)
Social support	4	9	13 (76.5)
Future safety and/or future plans	5	6	11 (64.7)
Parent	4	6	10 (58.8)

70.6%) in universal disaster and terrorism mental health interventions. Parents were included in more than one-half of the interventions (n = 10, 58.8%). In some interventions, parents provided assessments of their children[8,19,20]; in others, parents received psychoeducation[5–7,15,18] and/or participated in other intervention activities. For example, several studies included parents in homework assignments,[5,6,8,10] and one delivered family intervention to students and parents when indicated.[12] The studies did not examine or compare the relative benefit of various intervention components.

FUTURE DIRECTIONS

Despite increased attention to the disaster-related needs of children and a growing evidence base for disaster mental health interventions, several areas warrant attention. To unite universal preparedness and postdisaster interventions, it would be helpful for all studies to include assessments of disaster knowledge and preparedness as well as emotional and behavioral indicators. Although the theory links preinterventions and postinterventions as stepped processes in community response and preparedness, the research literature evaluating these interventions does not use similar assessments.

The extant literature has not clarified which, if any, specific intervention approach or component is responsible for benefit. In fact, only one of the studies in this review compared 2 interventions, finding no significant difference in outcome using the two.[14] It is possible that some common factor, or factors, among interventions (eg, the therapeutic relationship, the expectation of therapeutic success, acknowledgment of difficulties, the process of facing the trauma, the opportunity to ventilate and/or gain mastery over the problem)[48] is, or are, responsible for the success of the various approaches used in the interventions studied. Thus, future studies will need to compare intervention approaches, dismantle multimodal interventions to identify the elements that are responsible for benefit, and address the effects of natural recovery. Future studies must also be methodologically rigorous using control groups and other elements of well-designed studies, such as clearly defined target symptoms, reliable and valid measures, blinded evaluators, assessor training, replicable interventions, random assignment, and treatment-adherence measures.[49] Studies with longer follow-up assessments are important, and preparedness interventions should be evaluated after the incident.

The next generation of studies should identify and examine various child, intervention, and situational factors that may influence intervention delivery and outcomes. For example, culture is rarely discussed, though it should be a consideration in intervention development and delivery. Berger and Gelkopf[10] described in some detail the steps they took to adapt their intervention, which had been administered to Israeli children exposed to the chronic threat of terrorism, to the cultural differences in Sri Lankan children exposed to the 2004 Indian Ocean tsunami. The adaptation required the investigators to explore emotional expression and processing in the Sri Lankan population and to modify intervention activities to better represent and incorporate the social and spiritual beliefs and practices of this population.

While the science of universal intervention evaluation advances, so must attention to service delivery issues. Many universal preventive interventions are administered in school settings where children are accessible in groups. Efforts to equip schools and other venues as well as personnel are essential. For example, the importance of models and materials for recruiting and training teachers and others to deliver these interventions cannot be overstated. Those planning services should consider adopting a stepped care approach whereby some services, such as universal public health interventions, are provided to all children in a disaster setting, with referral to selected and indicated services determined by children's clinical status and needs.

SUMMARY

As part of the public health component of the disaster system of care, universal preventive services are used for children in general populations who have a range of exposures, experiences, and needs. These services include screening and case finding as well as both preparedness and postevent interventions. Universal activities are typically administered in a group format in settings where children naturally convene, such as schools. Several instruments are available to screen children for a variety of outcomes, though these have not been well studied in the disaster context. Most predisaster and postdisaster interventions have addressed children's emotional and behavioral reactions, though some have focused on children's disaster knowledge and disaster management. Most interventions are multimodal, incorporating common elements to educate children, normalize their reactions, process their emotions and manage stress, enhance coping, and provide social support. The field awaits research on several key issues related to the relative efficacy of intervention approaches and components, the timing and setting of intervention delivery, and the preparation of providers. Also important will be closer attention to the interface of universal, selected, and indicated services.

REFERENCES

1. Kilmer RP, Gil-Rivas V, Macdonald J. Implications of major disaster for educators, administrators, and school-based mental health professionals: needs, actions, and the example of Mayfair elementary. In: Kilmer RP, Gil-Rivas V, Tedeschi RG, et al, editors. Helping families and communities recover from disaster: lessons learned from Hurricane Katrina and its aftermath. Washington, DC: American Psychological Press; 2010. p. 167–91.
2. National Research Council and Institute of the National Academies. Committee on the prevention of mental disorders and substance abuse among children, youth, and young adults: research advances and promising interventions. In: O'Connell ME, Boat T, Warner KE, editors. Preventing mental, emotional, and

behavioral disorders among young people. Progress and possibilities. Washington, DC: The National Academies Press; 2009. p. 1–562.

3. Ronan KR, Finnis K, Johnston DM. Interventions with youth and families: a prevention and stepped care model. In: Reyes G, Jacobs GA, editors. Handbook of international disaster psychology. volume 2: practices and programs. Westport (CT): Praeger Publishers; 2006. p. 13–35.

4. Brown EJ, McQuaid J, Farina L, et al. Matching interventions to children's mental health needs: feasibility and acceptability of a pilot school-based trauma intervention program. Educ Treat Children 2006;29(2):257–86.

5. Berger R, Pat-Horenczyk R, Gelkopf M. School-based intervention for prevention and treatment of elementary-students' terror-related distress in Israel: a quasi-randomized controlled trial. J Trauma Stress 2007;20(4):541–51.

6. Berger R, Gelkopf M, Heineberg Y. A teacher-delivered intervention for adolescents exposed to ongoing and intense traumatic war-related stress: a quasi-randomized controlled study. J Adolesc Health 2012;51(5):453–61.

7. Gelkopf M, Berger R. A school-based, teacher-mediated prevention program (ERASE-Stress) for reducing terror-related traumatic reactions in Israeli youth: a quasi-randomized controlled trial. J Child Psychol Psychiatry 2009;50(8): 962–71.

8. Ronan KR, Johnston DM. Hazards education for youth: a quasi-experimental investigation. Risk Anal 2003;23(5):1009–20.

9. Wolmer L, Hamiel D, Laor N. Preventing children's posttraumatic stress after disaster with teacher-based intervention: a controlled study. J Am Acad Child Adolesc Psychiatry 2011;50(4):340–8.

10. Berger R, Gelkopf M. School-based intervention for the treatment of tsunami-related distress in children: a quasi-randomized controlled trial. Psychother Psychosom 2009;78(6):364–71.

11. Goenjian AK, Karayan I, Pynoos RS, et al. Outcome of psychotherapy among early adolescents after trauma. Am J Psychiatry 1997;154(4):536–42.

12. Goenjian AK, Walling D, Steinberg AM, et al. Prospective study of posttraumatic stress and depressive reactions among treated and untreated adolescents 5 years after a catastrophic disaster. Am J Psychiatry 2005;162(12):2302–8.

13. Hardin SB, Weinrich S, Weinrich M, et al. Effects of a long-term psychosocial nursing intervention on adolescents exposed to catastrophic stress. Issues Ment Health Nurs 2002;23(6):537–51.

14. Ronan KR, Johnston DM. Behaviourally-based interventions for children following volcanic eruptions: an evaluation of effectiveness. Disaster Prev Manag 1999; 8(3):169–76.

15. Sahin NH, Yilmaz B, Batigun A. Psychoeducation for children and adults after the Marmara earthquake: an evaluation study. Traumatology 2011;17(1):41–9.

16. Stewart JB, Hardin SB, Weinrich S, et al. Group protocol to mitigate disaster stress and enhance social support in adolescents exposed to Hurricane Hugo. Issues Ment Health Nurs 1992;13(2):105–19.

17. Vijayakumar L, Kannan GK, Kumar BG, et al. Do all children need intervention after exposure to tsunami? Int Rev Psychiatry 2006;18(6):515–22.

18. Wolmer L, Laor N, Yazgan Y. School reactivation programs after disaster: could teachers serve as clinical mediators? Child Adolesc Psychiatr Clin N Am 2003; 12(2):363–81.

19. Wolmer L, Laor N, Dedeoglu C, et al. Teacher-mediated intervention after disaster: a controlled three-year follow-up of children's functioning. J Child Psychol Psychiatry 2005;46(11):1161–8.

20. Wolmer L, Hamiel D, Barchas JD, et al. Teacher-delivered resilience-focused intervention in schools with traumatized children following the second Lebanon war. J Trauma Stress 2011;24(3):309–16.
21. Ursano RJ, Friedman MJ. Mental health and behavioral interventions for victims of disasters and mass violence: systems, caring, planning, and needs. In: Ritchie EC, Watson PJ, Friedman MJ, editors. Interventions following mass violence and disasters: strategies for mental health practice. New York: Guilford Press; 2006. p. 405–14.
22. Rolfsnes ES, Idsoe T. School-based intervention programs for PTSD symptoms: a review and meta-analysis. J Trauma Stress 2011;24(2):155–65.
23. Pullins LG, McCammon SL, Lamson AS, et al. School-based post-flood screening and evaluation: findings and challenges in one community. Stress Trauma Crisis Int J 2005;8(4):229–49.
24. Dean KL, Langley AK, Kataoka SH, et al. School-based disaster mental health services: clinical, policy, and community challenges. Prof Psychol Res Pract 2008;39(1):52–7.
25. Gelkopf M, Ryan P, Cotton SJ, et al. The impact of "Training the Trainers Course" for helping tsunami-survivor children on Sri Lankan disaster volunteer workers. Int J Stress Manag 2008;15(2):117–35.
26. Abdeen Z, Qasrawi R, Nabil S, et al. Psychological reactions to Israeli occupation: findings from the national study of school-based screening in Palestine. Int J Behav Dev 2008;32(4):290–7.
27. Stallard P, Velleman R, Baldwin S. Psychological screening of children for post-traumatic stress disorder. J Child Psychol Psychiatry 1999;40(7):1075–82.
28. Cochrane AL, Holland WW. Validation of screening procedures. Br Med Bull 1971;27(1):3–8.
29. Pfefferbaum B, Jacobs AK, Houston JB. Children and disasters: a framework for mental health assessment. J Emerg Manag 2012;10(5):349–58.
30. McDermott BM, Palmer LJ. Post-disaster service provision following proactive identification of children with emotional distress and depression. Aust N Z J Psychiatry 1999;33(6):855–63.
31. Pfefferbaum B, North CS. Assessing children's disaster reactions and mental health needs: screening and clinical evaluation. Can J Psychiatry 2013;58(3):135–42.
32. Cohen JA, Bukstein O, Walter H, et al, American Academy of Child and Adolescent Psychiatry (AACAP). Practice parameter for the assessment and treatment of children and adolescents with posttraumatic stress disorder. J Am Acad Child Adolesc Psychiatry 2010;49(4):414–30.
33. Pfefferbaum B, Sconzo GM, Flynn BW, et al. Case finding and mental health services for children in the aftermath of the Oklahoma City bombing. J Behav Health Serv Res 2003;30(2):215–27.
34. Saylor C, Deroma V. Assessment of children and adolescents exposed to disaster. In: La Greca AM, Silverman WK, Vernberg EM, et al, editors. Helping children cope with disasters and terrorism. Washington, DC: American Psychological Association; 2002. p. 35–53.
35. Ohan JL, Myers K, Collett BR. Ten-year review of rating scales. IV. Scales assessing trauma and its effects. J Am Acad Child Adolesc Psychiatry 2002;41(12):1401–22.
36. Balaban VF, Steinberg AM, Brymer MJ, et al. Screening and assessment for children's psychosocial needs following war and terrorism. In: Friedman MJ, Mikus-Kos A, editors. Promoting the psychosocial well being of children following war and terrorism. Amsterdam: IOS Press, Inc; 2005. p. 121–61.

37. Liu A, Tan H, Zhou J, et al. Brief screening instrument of posttraumatic stress disorder for children and adolescents 7-15 years of age. Child Psychiatry Hum Dev 2007;38(3):195–202.
38. Ketumarn P, Sitdhiraksa N, Pithayaratsathien N, et al. Prevalence of posttraumatic stress disorder in students 23 months after tsunami. Asian J Psychiatr 2009;2(4):144–8.
39. Steinberg AM, Brymer MJ, Decker KB, et al. The University of California at Los Angeles post-traumatic stress disorder reaction index. Curr Psychiatry Rep 2004;6:96–100.
40. Foa EB, Johnson KM, Feeny NC, et al. The Child PTSD Symptom Scale: a preliminary examination of its psychometric properties. J Clin Child Psychol 2001;30(3): 376–84.
41. Birmaher B, Khetarpal S, Brent D, et al. The screen for child anxiety related emotional disorders (SCARED): scale construction and psychometric characteristics. J Am Acad Child Adolesc Psychiatry 1997;36(4):545–53.
42. March JS, Parker JD, Sullivan K, et al. The Multidimensional Anxiety Scale for Children (MASC): factor structure, reliability, and validity. J Am Acad Child Adolesc Psychiatry 1997;36(4):554–65.
43. Achenbach TM. Manual for the child behavioral checklist/4–18 and 1991 profile. Burlington (VT): University of Vermont, Department of Psychiatry; 1991.
44. Beck AT, Beck RW. Screening depressed patients in family practice. A rapid technic. Postgrad Med 1972;52(6):81–5.
45. Kovacs M. The Children's Depression Inventory (CDI). Psychopharmacol Bull 1985;21(4):995–8.
46. Asarnow JR, Carlson GA. Depression self-rating scale: utility with child psychiatric inpatients. J Consult Clin Psychol 1985;53(4):491–9.
47. Lucas CP, Zhang H, Fisher PW, et al. The DISC Predictive Scales (DPS): efficiently screening for diagnoses. J Am Acad Child Adolesc Psychiatry 2001; 40(4):443–9.
48. Weinberger J. Common factors aren't so common: the common factors dilemma. Clin Psychol Sci Pract 1995;2(1):45–69.
49. Foa EB, Meadows EA. Psychosocial treatments for posttraumatic stress disorder: a critical review. Annu Rev Psychol 1997;48(1):449–80.

Indicated and Selective Preventive Interventions

Meghan L. Marsac, PhD[a,b], Katharine Donlon, MS[c],
Steven Berkowitz, MD[b,*]

KEYWORDS

- Posttraumatic stress • Posttraumatic stress disorder • Preventive interventions
- Child trauma

KEY POINTS

- The number of children exposed to trauma each year necessitates intervention to prevent the onset and reduce the severity of emotional reactions to trauma.
- Current evidence on how to best prevent negative emotional reactions in children exposed to trauma suggests that interventions include psychoeducation, parent-child communication, skill building, and a family focus. However, a gold standard for selective and indicated preventive interventions has yet to be established.
- More research on preventive interventions is needed. To inform interventions, future research should aim to identify other factors and their interrelationships involved in the development of posttraumatic stress symptoms or other emotional reactions.

INTRODUCTION

Exposure to potentially traumatic events during childhood is an unavoidable fact of life for most children. A potentially traumatic event (PTE) can be defined as one in which an individual experiences or witnesses actual or threatened death or serious injury to one's self or others.[1] Epidemiologic research has indicated that many youth are exposed to 1 or more traumatic events in their lifetimes.[2] For example, each year millions of children are involved in family violence,[3] incur injuries,[4] battle severe and/or chronic illnesses,[5] or experience a natural disaster.[6] Many children subsequently develop significant posttraumatic stress symptoms (PTSS) or other negative emotional reactions following these traumatic experiences.[7–13] DSM-5 (*Diagnostic*

The authors have nothing to disclose.

[a] Department of Pediatrics, Center for Injury Research and Prevention, The Children's Hospital of Philadelphia, 3535 Market Street, Philadelphia, PA 19104, USA; [b] Department of Psychiatry, Perelman School of Medicine, University of Pennsylvania, 3451 Walnut Street, Philadelphia, PA 19104, USA; [c] Virginia Polytechnic Institute and State University, 109 Williams Hall, Blacksburg, VA 24060, USA
* Corresponding author.
E-mail address: steven.berkowitz@uphs.upenn.edu

Abbreviations	
ADAPT	After deployment: adaptive parenting tools
CFTSI	Child and family traumatic stress intervention
CISD	Critical incident stress debriefing
FOCUS	Families overcoming under stress
PTE	Potentially traumatic event
PTSD	Posttraumatic stress disorder
PTSS	Post-traumatic stress symptoms
RCT	Randomized controlled trial
SFSF	Strong families strong forces
SPR	Skills for psychological recovery

and Statistical Manual of Mental Disorders, 5th edition) criteria for posttraumatic stress disorder (PTSD) include symptoms of intrusion (eg, recurrent distressing memories, flashbacks), avoidance (eg, not thinking about the PTE), alterations in cognition and mood (eg, unrealistic thoughts about the cause of the trauma), and hyperarousal (eg, irritability, exaggerated startle response).[1] In addition to causing distress for children and families, PTSS are also related to worse functional outcomes.[14-16]

Early interventions for children exposed to a PTE can help prevent chronic PTSS/PTSD. Prevention refers to measures taken to prevent diseases or injuries rather than curing them or treating their symptoms. In this article, the discussion of preventive interventions refers to the prevention of PTSS and other negative emotional reactions (eg, depression, anxiety) following exposure to PTE. Preventive interventions can be categorized as universal, selective, or indicated. It should be noted that there are several ways to define these categories. This article uses Vernberg's (2002) definition,[17] whereby universal interventions are defined as those provided to all children following a large-scale trauma. (See the article by Pfefferbaum elsewhere in this issue for a review of universal interventions.) Selective prevention is designed for individuals with significant PTSS but without additional risk factors for long-term impairment of functioning. Here the authors consider selective prevention for all persons who have been exposed to a PTE and who are demonstrating distress or dysfunction. Indicated prevention is designed for individuals or groups who exhibit marked distress, early PTSS, and other comorbid symptoms, or other risk factors for poor long-term outcomes in regard to mental health.[17]

Although selective and indicated preventive interventions for children after trauma are in their infancy, several have promising results. Across these interventions, common elements include providing psychoeducation, involving the family, and encouraging child-parent communication. **Table 1** summarizes selective and indicated interventions.

REVIEW OF THE PERTINENT LITERATURE
Prevalence of PTE Exposure and PTSS in Children

Trauma exposure during childhood is an unfortunately common experience. In the United States alone, a nationally representative telephone survey indicated that 60% of children experienced or witnessed a PTE in the preceding year.[2] Worldwide, estimates suggest that millions more are exposed to PTE during childhood, including domestic and community violence,[3,18] severe and/or chronic illnesses and injuries,[5] and natural disasters.[6] Compared with other age groups, adolescents are more likely to be exposed to PTEs such as being victimized, being involved in incidents outside of the home, experiencing threat to life, and suffering physical injuries.[19] Anywhere from

Table 1
Summary of controlled preventive intervention studies with children

Authors,[Ref.] Year	Population	Age (y)	Intervention	Outcomes
Cox et al,[48] 2010	Unintentional injury	7–16	Information provision in the form of a booklet and a Web site	Decrease in anxiety for intervention group
Kassam-Adams et al,[60] 2011	Unintentional injury	8–17	Stepped preventive care model	No differences in PTSS between intervention and control groups
Kenardy et al,[35] 2008	Unintentional injury	7–15	Information provision in the form of booklets for parents and children	Decrease in anxiety for children in intervention group. Fewer PTSS for parents in intervention group
Marsac et al,[46] 2013	Unintentional injury	6–17	Psychoeducation and coping strategies via an interactive Web site for parents	No differences in parent knowledge or PTSS at follow-up
Nugent et al,[67] 2010	Unintentional injury	10–18	Administration of propranolol	No differences in PTSD between groups
Ponsford et al,[47] 2001	Mild traumatic brain injury	6–15	Psychoeducation with coping strategies via booklet	Intervention group reported fewer psychological symptoms and behavioral problems
Stallard et al,[52] 2006	Unintentional injury	7–18	Debriefing 4 wk after trauma	No differences in PTSS between intervention and control groups
Zehnder et al,[53] 2010	Unintentional injury	7–16	Single-session manualized intervention consisting of psychoeducation, drawings, and accident-related toys	No differences in PTSS between overall groups. Preadolescent children in the intervention group had lower levels of depression and fewer behavioral problems
Berkowitz et al,[69] 2011	Exposed to multiple PTE types	7–17	Four-session caregiver-child early intervention designed to enhance social support and coping skills	Fewer PTSS and anxiety symptoms for children in the intervention group

Table includes studies designed to evaluate early intervention strategies, and does not include information pertaining to studies using retroactive chart reviews to evaluate the effectiveness of specific intervention strategies.

Abbreviations: PTE, potentially traumatic event; PTSD, posttraumatic stress disorder; PTSS, posttraumatic stress symptoms.

12% to 50% of children develop significant PTSS and/or other negative emotional reactions following exposure to PTE, depending on the type and level of exposure in addition to the presence of risk factors.[11,20]

Risk and Protective Factors in PTSS Development

As mentioned previously, children who are exposed to a PTE and demonstrate significant distress or dysfunction may benefit from both selective and indicated intervention. In addition to the factors associated with the event, individual, familial, and community-ecological risk and protective factors have been more recently studied and well categorized for adults and youth.[21,22] The cumulative epidemiologic evidence indicates that the adverse effects of traumatic stress experienced from infancy through adolescence may extend well into adulthood, increasing the risk for lifelong problems such as depression, PTSD, substance abuse, marital discord, low occupational attainment, and poor physical and mental health.[23]

To determine whether a child should receive a more intensive intervention (ie, one with more indicated components), several risk factors can be assessed. In conceptualizing factors associated with PTSS risk, it is helpful to categorize them within the pre-, peri-, and posttrauma periods. Research has suggested a role for pretrauma variables of child sex, child age, trauma history, and psychological symptoms,[20,24–27] peritrauma variables of appraisals and physiologic indicators,[20,24,27–33] and posttrauma variables of parental PTSS, social support, and cognitive strategies in predicting PTSS in children following PTE.[24,34,36–39]

Specific to pretrauma factors, children who are female are at higher risk for PTSS.[24] It remains unclear as to how a child's age at the time of exposure to a traumatic event affects the onset or severity of PTSD, as there have been mixed findings.[24–26] Youth exposed to multiple traumas are particularly vulnerable to a range of psychological, behavioral, and emotional problems,[40] social maladjustment,[41] and academic failure.[42] In addition, children who present with symptoms of anxiety, depression, dissociation, and/or acute stress before a PTE are more likely to later develop PTSD.[20,24,27]

During the peritrauma period, appraising the PTE as more threatening is consistently related to the development of PTSS.[20,24,27] In particular, children's strong sense of fear, life threat, and loss of control during or after PTEs places them at higher risk for PTSS, in comparison with children who reported a lesser degree of subjective threat.[28–30] In addition, physiologic reactions, such as elevated heart rate and cortisol levels, can arise from neurobiological stress responses to trauma that are activated when children are faced with threatening situations (ie, fight-or-flight response). In children with injury, elevated heart rate and cortisol levels in the early aftermath of injury predict subsequent PTSS.[31–33]

Following trauma, the child's use of avoidant cognitive strategies (eg, thought suppression) has been associated with PTSS.[24] In addition, parental reactions to the event affect the child's adjustment.[34] Parents commonly experience PTSS following a child's exposure to a PTE in part from feelings of guilt and witnessing the event, or because of events preceding the PTE.[36,37] Parental PTSS is also linked to poorer postinjury adjustment in children.[39] A low level of social support is another factor associated with an increased risk of PTSS in children after trauma. In general, individuals who have high levels of social support are more prepared to manage stressors. Parents, peers, and teachers all play important roles in providing social support to children after trauma, and evidence indicates that children may be at risk for negative psychological outcomes after trauma when they report inadequate social support.[38]

Recent studies have discovered and explicated many protective factors, the most significant of which appear to be social and family support, a sense of self-efficacy, and a positive family environment.[43] In ongoing threat situations such as war, strategies such as actively seeking information, diversion (reframing, humor, acceptance), concentrating only on the valid threat rather than generalizing, having realistic expectations, developing routines to obtain necessities, and working to live have been linked to better outcomes.[44] Many of the findings from studies of risk, vulnerability, and resilience factors have informed monitoring and identification of high-risk individuals as well as particular early interventions. Whereas nonmalleable risk factors (eg, child gender, physiologic indicators) may be useful in screening for the risk for PTSS, malleable variables (eg, cognitive appraisals, social support) offer an opportunity to use preventive efforts to reduce the risk of developing PTSS.

Preventive Interventions

Early interventions for PTSD/PTSS in youth may be delivered under various public health models that include universal, selective, and indicated preventive interventions. In consideration of the universal, selective, and indicated model, many preventive interventions have components spanning each of these classifications. Universal prevention targets typically the broadest population category in which no specific individual has been identified to be at risk but has been exposed to a PTE (see the article by Pfefferbaum elsewhere in this issue for a detailed description of universal interventions). Selective and indicated strategies fall under the larger rubric of targeted intervention strategies. Here the authors consider selective prevention for all those who have been exposed to a PTE with some distressing PTSS, but no other known risk factors. Indicated preventive interventions target individuals who have multiple risk factors for poor long-term outcomes (eg, early PTSS with other preexisting psychopathology). Interventions that include universal, selective, and indicated intervention pathways are often called stepped models, as they typically provide general education about traumatic reactions to all, but screen for signs or symptoms and provide an early intervention for those who are at risk.

Although there are many approaches to preventive interventions, a recent meta-analysis identified several common components found in most selective and indicated interventions: psychoeducation about typical posttraumatic reactions; promotion of coping strategies; and safe exposure to trauma triggers.[45]

Given the overlapping components and goals of selective and indicated interventions, they are not distinguished herein. Rather, the authors present a summary of the evidence-based or informed preventive interventions to date that target children in either category. These interventions include programs with components of psychoeducation, debriefing, psychological first aid, family-child communication, promotion of safe exposure, and, possibly, pharmacology.

Intervention Outcomes

Psychoeducation

Psychoeducational interventions serve to normalize emotional reactions to trauma, and can provide the foundation for the development of coping skills. Providing psychoeducational information to children and parents allows them to control the degree of their participation in the intervention, which is appropriate for most children who only require minimal assistance with their reactions. Some psychoeducational interventions have been proved to increase knowledge and are rated as helpful to families,[46] while others have also shown promising results in decreasing children's distress. For example, in 2001 Ponsford and colleagues[47] provided parents of children who sustained a head injury with an information booklet about common symptoms of head injury and the expected course of these symptoms. Parents reported fewer neuropsychological symptoms and behavioral difficulties in their children 3 months after the intervention. Another example is information-based intervention for children and their parents after pediatric injury, as described by Kenardy and colleagues[35] in 2008. Their research indicated that the intervention was effective in reducing children's anxiety symptoms. When they added a combined Web-based component (booklet plus Web site), results indicated that children had less anxiety. A trend also emerged for decreased symptoms of anger, depression, and PTSS.[48] When effective, psychoeducation is an appealing intervention because it is cost-effective and does not require a trained professional to implement.

Debriefing

The use of debriefing interventions has had mixed results.[49] Psychological debriefing is a preventive intervention designed to be delivered very soon after the PTE, with the intentions of normalizing children's reactions to trauma and promoting emotional processing of the event. One form of debriefing is a structured intervention known as critical incident stress debriefing (CISD), which was initially developed in 1983[50] and later modified for use with children.[51] CISD consists of multiple components, including factual reconstruction of the traumatic event, discussion of trauma-related cognitions and trauma-related emotions, normalizing reactions, and providing information about coping. Two randomized controlled trials (RCTs) have been conducted to evaluate the efficacy of psychological debriefing as a preventive intervention after pediatric trauma. Stallard and colleagues[52] used a debriefing intervention with children 4 weeks after they experienced a road traffic accident, but found no differences in PTSS between the intervention group and the control group. These children reported that early contact after a trauma was therapeutic because it validated their experience and provided an opportunity to discuss possible reactions, symptoms, and feelings. Zehnder and colleagues[53] similarly used a debriefing approach with children aged 7 to 16 years who experienced a road traffic accident. This study differed in that the intervention was implemented 10 days after the trauma, and included drawing and playing with toys as intervention components. Although no overall significant group differences emerged regarding symptoms of acute stress, PTSS, depression, and behavioral problems, outcomes for a subgroup of younger children who received the debriefing intervention reported a decrease in depressive symptoms and behavioral problems. More research is needed to better understand psychological debriefing as a preventive intervention, but initial evidence suggests that when delivered correctly, these types of interventions have the potential to be an efficacious intervention after pediatric trauma.

Psychological first aid

Although no intervention model has been proved to be efficacious for those individuals who encounter mass trauma (eg, natural disaster, terrorist attacks), in most part attributable to the difficulty evaluating interventions in the immediate postdisaster context, the use of psychological first aid may be beneficial. In applying psychological first aid, experts recommend inclusion of the following evidence-informed intervention components: (1) promoting a sense of safety, (2) use of techniques to promote calming, (3) capitalizing on a sense of self-efficacy and community efficacy, (4) encouraging connectedness, and (5) encouraging hope.[54] Experts note the limitation in empirical evidence supporting the implementation of these principles of psychological first aid, but suggest including these principles based on a review of current evidence on the prevention and treatment of trauma.[54]

Intervention for residual symptoms post disaster
Skills for Psychological Recovery (SPR) is an evidence-informed intervention designed to be used in the weeks and months after trauma with individuals who experience residual symptoms. SPR relies on skill-based instruction to promote recovery and prevent maladaptive behaviors in the aftermath of trauma and disaster. The core skills of SPR include building problem-solving skills, promoting positive activities, managing reactions, promoting helpful thinking, and rebuilding healthy social connections. By working with individuals to identify specific areas of need and teaching targeted skills, intervention providers can foster a sense of efficacy in survivors while navigating their psychological recoveries.[55] Although it has not undergone a rigorous empirical evaluation, health providers have perceived SPR to be an acceptable and useful intervention after receiving a brief training on its implementation.[56]

Intervention for at-risk military families
Although an RCT has not yet been conducted to evaluate its effectiveness, Families OverComing Under Stress (FOCUS) is a promising intervention designed for at-risk military families facing deployment, which uses a strength-based and family-centered approach to promote resilience. The FOCUS intervention comprises components from existing evidence-based interventions, and includes parent, child, and family sessions. The intervention involves the creation of a family narrative, provision of psychoeducation, and skill building in the areas of emotional regulation, communication, problem solving, goal setting, managing trauma and loss reminders, and family communication.[57]

Preliminary evidence suggests that After Deployment: Adaptive Parenting Tools (ADAPT) and Strong Families Strong Forces (SFSF) are promising interventions for families with a parent who is reintegrating into life after deployment. The Web-enhanced parenting program teaches core parenting skills (skills encouragement, positive involvement, limit setting, problem solving, and monitoring), integrates aspects of emotion socialization training depending on family needs, emphasizes the importance of a united-parenting front, and incorporates military culture and values.[58] SFSF is a multisession reintegration program designed to support veterans and their families during the deployment cycle. Based on the idea that young children experience numerous emotional and behavioral difficulties during and following a parent's deployment, the home-based intervention seeks to reduce the impact of deployment (including separation, combat stress, or other mental health concerns) on parenting, coparenting, and the parent-child relationship.[59]

Stepped preventive care models
Preventive interventions using stepped preventive care models have mixed results. Kassam-Adams and colleagues[60] implemented a stepped preventive care model (including selective and indicated components) for children hospitalized for injury and their parents. The intervention is evidence-informed and tailored to children's identified needs. Children were screened and placed into either a low-risk or an at-risk group. Those identified as at risk were randomized into either usual care or intervention care. All children in the intervention group were provided with psychoeducation and 2 sessions during which the interventionists conducted assessments to identify additional needs. Children with identified needs were then offered services such as more contact from the interventionist, assistance in communicating with medical providers for care coordination, assistance with medical adherence, a brief parent-child intervention to improve communication and coping, an evaluation by

a mental health provider, and/or trauma-focused cognitive-behavioral therapy. However, no differences emerged between the usual-care group and the intervention group, suggesting that there is room for improvement of the intervention.[60]

To the authors' knowledge, the Child and Family Traumatic Stress Intervention (CFTSI)[61] is the only prevention model for children and adolescents at risk of developing PTSD that has effectiveness demonstrated through an RCT. In this model, which spans selective and indicated prevention, youth are screened for new traumatic stress symptoms in the aftermath of a PTE, and are treated only if they have one new distressing symptom. CFTSI is a 4- to 6-session caregiver(s)-child intervention for children aged 7 years and older, and is delivered within 45 days of experiencing a PTE. The CFTSI focuses on 2 key risk factors of poor social or familial support and poor coping skills in its effort to prevent chronic PTSD. CFTSI addresses these issues by: (1) increasing communication between the affected child and his or her caregivers about feelings, symptoms, and behaviors, with the goal of increasing the caregivers' support of the child; (2) facilitating communication between caregivers and child, which serves to aid in processing the experience; and (3) providing specific behavioral skills to the caregivers and child to assist in coping with symptoms.

To evaluate CFTSI, 106 youth aged 8 to 17 years participated in an RCT and were randomized to either CFTSI (n = 53) or to a 4-session psychoeducational and supportive intervention (n = 53). Youth participants were recruited from a pediatric emergency department, a forensic sexual abuse program, and a police department's victim services department, and had experienced a wide range of events including exposure to violence, assaults, sexual trauma, intentional and unintentional injury, and so forth. Youth who participated in CFTSI were 65% less likely to develop chronic PTSD at the 3-month follow-up than youth who participated in the comparison condition. In addition, CFTSI recipients were 73% less likely to present significant PTSS. CFTSI recipients also reported significantly fewer PTSS and anxiety symptoms after treatment, which remained lower at 3 months.[61]

Pharmacologic interventions

There have been increasing numbers of trials using several different pharmacologic agents to prevent PTSD for adults and, increasingly, for youth who are hospitalized following physical injury. Psychopharmacologic trials attempting to prevent the onset of PTSD agents are typically initiated soon after the PTE (often within hours). It is hypothesized that administering pharmacologic interventions may inhibit the full encoding of the extreme negative emotional response with the traumatic memory. The first medication shown to effectively prevent PTSD in youth was morphine used on a burns unit[62]; subsequent evaluations of morphine in both injured children and adults have similarly effectively prevented PTSD.[63] For example, children who were admitted to hospital for acute burn injuries and who received higher doses of morphine had lower levels of PTSD symptoms at 6-month follow-up.[64] Another nonrandomized investigation of 48 youth recruited from the emergency department also demonstrated a similar association. Although acute morphine administration showed no association with PTSD at 4 weeks after PTE, it was associated with lower PTSD symptoms at 6 months and with a reduction of symptoms between 1-month and 6-month follow-ups.[64] Stoddard and colleagues[65] evaluated the correlation between PTSD symptoms at 3 and 6 months after PTE and morphine administration during medical care in 70 very young (12- to 48-month-old) children with burns. Findings demonstrated a significant decrease in PTSD symptoms in correlation with morphine dose. Putative mechanisms have included the inhibition of emotional memory and pain control. It is also possible that these mechanisms are synergistic.[65]

Following a study by Pitman and colleagues (2002)[66] demonstrating the effectiveness of acute propranolol administration in adults, propranolol has been evaluated for its potential to prevent PTSD in children. Subsequent studies of adolescents have failed to demonstrate efficacy.[67] A caveat for the conflicting findings may pertain to the timing of propranolol administration. It seems there may be a small window after the injury within which the medication needs to be initiated in order for it to be effective.[68] Other medications, such as prazosin, have similar mechanisms of action but with more selective receptor activity, and warrant future study of their effectiveness when administered acutely. In addition, current trials are using acute administration of nasal oxytocin in adults, and have already documented positive responses in animal models.[28] Although early pharmacologic interventions are promising, it is unclear as to whether they will be applicable beyond the hospital setting given the timing of administration and the potential need for close monitoring. However, the use of medications in combination with psychosocial interventions may be an important future direction of study.

Challenges to Effective Implementation Strategies for Early Preventive Interventions

Numerous complications regarding the provision of early preventive interventions for youth make research on the effectiveness of early interventions especially difficult. For example, there may be an optimal time at which to deliver either a medication or a psychosocial intervention after a traumatic exposure. As previously mentioned regarding propranolol, it may be possible that only very early administration is effective. Moreover, how long after a traumatic exposure is an intervention considered early? For indicated interventions, are there specific signs or symptoms that should prompt an intervention? Many risk factors for the development of PTSD such as trauma history and parental/family functioning seem to have predictive value.[69] Therefore, should screening include these variables and, if so, how?

Probably the most common early preventive intervention is a crisis response that occurs any time within minutes to several days after exposure to a PTE. For children and adolescents, crisis response may most often occur in schools (eg, after a threat from outside, or after a death or violent event in the school community, such as a serious fight, student suicide, or otherwise).[70] Although the term crisis response seems to imply a one-time contact, most models recognize the need for further interaction, and view the first contact as an opportunity to provide psychoeducation and safety planning. Research has clearly shown that one-time interventions have minimal effect on longer-term outcomes for exposed individuals.[71] However, perhaps the most important function of a crisis response is the identification of individuals who may require ongoing monitoring and/or further intervention. Addressing this lack of identification of at-risk youth may be the most readily reparable issue with early interventions. Child-serving programs including emergency departments, primary care, child welfare, and law enforcement routinely come into contact with children who have experienced a PTE. Many of these settings are well positioned to identify and even screen these children, or refer them to organizations that can screen and intervene. Regardless of the growing recognition of predictive factors for the development of PTSD, clinicians are still unable to unequivocally forecast who will develop long-term posttraumatic difficulties. Ideally, all individuals exposed to a PTE would be monitored temporarily for signs or symptoms, much as one might monitor a physical injury. Effective collaborations between organizations that meet, support, or treat children soon after PTEs and trauma-informed behavioral health or victim service agencies that can monitor and provide interventions is crucial.

The typical pathway after traumatic exposure has been well described, with initial symptoms and distress resolving over time. However, it is not clear when screening during the traumatic period is most accurate, and resources are insufficient to monitor all children exposed to a PTE. Thus, recognizing the individual child's risk and protective factors are essential in effectively making use of limited resources to monitor the children at highest risk.

Benefits of Early Preventive Interventions for Children, Families, and Health Care

Early interventions are rooted in the assumption that they could potentially prevent future psychological symptoms. Any decrease in distress, symptoms, or posttrauma-related disorders benefits children, families, and health care, as well as cost benefits arising from the decreased cost of later treatment. In addition, positive emotional recovery is linked to positive functional recovery, highlighting the important interplay between the two separate areas of well-being.[14–16]

Although the primary aim of early interventions is to promote recovery and resilience to future PTEs, they also can serve the function of identifying youth at increased risk for a range of psychopathologies. Providers may have the opportunity to assess youth's reactions, history of exposure, pre-event functioning and family functioning, and relationships. Youth that seem to be at risk based on the initial assessment can be monitored by providers and family members or, if necessary, may be referred for more specific interventions or treatment.[69]

Clinical Practice Application

Given the sheer number of children exposed to PTEs, all those who are in direct contact with children should be aware of the likelihood of working with some children with emotional reactions related to trauma. Educators, child carers, medical staff, behavioral health providers, emergency responders, and the police force can play a role in identifying children at risk, and make an effort to prevent PTSS and other emotional reactions. Although as yet there is no gold standard of prevention of PTSS, implementing key elements such as education and family involvement should be standard practice.

SUMMARY

Current evidence suggests promising avenues for preventing PTSS in children exposed to PTEs. However, more empirical evidence to support the effectiveness of early preventive interventions is needed; specifically, identifying the most potent intervention components and determining how to best translate these components for real-world applications is necessary for sustainable resources. Efforts to embed interventions in child-serving programs (eg, Community Advisory Committee, Education Department, Primary Care, Child Welfare, schools) may help to reach more children than delivery of preventive interventions in behavioral health settings alone. Advances in training pediatric medical providers may be particularly helpful. Based on research to date, training should include awareness of potential trauma histories and symptoms, how to screen for PTSS, how to provide support to families, and when to refer children for additional services.[72]

REFERENCES

1. American Psychiatric Association. Diagnostic and statistical manual of mental disorders. 5th edition. Arlington (VA): American Psychiatric Publishing; 2013.

2. Finkelhor D, Ormrod RK, Turner HA. Lifetime assessment of poly-victimization in a national sample of children and youth. Child Abuse Negl 2009;33:403–11.

3. McDonald R, Jouriles EN, Ramisetty-Mikler S, et al. Estimating the number of American children living in partner-violent families. J Fam Psychol 2006;20: 137–42.

4. Grossman DC. The history of injury control and the epidemiology of child and adolescent injuries. The Future of Children 2000;10(1):23–52.

5. Murray C, Lopez A. The global burden of disease: a comprehensive assessment of mortality and disability from diseases, injuries, and risk factors in 1990 and projected to 2020. Cambridge (MA): Harvard University Press; 1996.

6. Pronczuk J, Surdu S. Children's environmental health in the twenty-first century. Ann N Y Acad Sci 2008;1140(1):143–54.

7. Balluffi A, Kassam-Adams N, Kazak A, et al. Traumatic stress in parents of children admitted to the pediatric intensive care unit. Pediatr Crit Care Med 2004;5: 547–53.

8. Kean E, Kelsay K, Wamboldt F, et al. Posttraumatic stress in adolescents with asthma and their parents. J Am Acad Child Adolesc Psychiatry 2006;45:78–86.

9. Mintzer L, Stuber M, Seacord D, et al. Traumatic stress symptoms in adolescent organ transplant recipients. Pediatrics 2005;115(6):1640–9.

10. Walker A, Harris G, Baker A, et al. Posttraumatic stress responses following liver transplantation in older children. J Child Psychol Psychiatry 1999;40(3): 363–74.

11. La Greca AM, Silverman WK, Lai B, et al. Hurricane-related exposure experiences and stressors, other life events, and social support: concurrent and prospective impact on children's persistent posttraumatic stress symptoms. J Consult Clin Psychol 2010;78(6):794–805.

12. Margolin G, Vickerman KA. Posttraumatic stress in children and adolescents exposed to family violence: I. Overview and Issues. Prof Psychol Res Pr 2007; 38(6):613–9.

13. Rossman BB, Hughes HM, Rosenberg MS. Children and interparental violence: the impact of exposure. Philadelphia (PA): Brunner/Mazel; 2000.

14. Holbrook T, Hoyt D, Coimbra R, et al. Long-term posttraumatic stress disorder persists after major trauma in adolescents: new data on risk factors and functional outcome. J Trauma 2005;58(4):764–9.

15. Landolt MA, Vollrath M, Gnehm H, et al. Post-traumatic stress impacts on quality of life in children after road traffic accidents: prospective study. Aust N Z J Psychiatry 2009;43(8):746–53.

16. Zatzick D, Jurkovich G, Fan M, et al. Association between posttraumatic stress and depressive symptoms and functional outcomes in adolescents followed up longitudinally after injury hospitalization. Arch Pediatr Adolesc Med 2008;162(7): 642–8.

17. Vernberg EM. Intervention approaches following disasters. In: La Greca AM, Silverman WK, Vernberg EM, et al, editors. Helping children cope with disasters and terrorism. Washington, DC: American Psychological Association; 2002. p. 55–72.

18. Klasen F, Gehrke J, Metzner F, et al. Complex trauma symptoms in former Ugandan child soldiers. J Aggress Maltreat Trauma 2013;22(7):698–713.

19. Harpaz-Rotem I, Murphy RA, Berkowitz S, et al. Clinical epidemiology of urban violence responding to children exposed to violence in ten communities. J Interpers Violence 2007;22(11):1479–90.

20. Kahana SY, Feeny NC, Youngstrom EA, et al. Posttraumatic stress in youth experiencing illnesses and injuries: an exploratory meta-analysis. Traumatology 2006;12(2):148–61.
21. Brymer MJ, Steinberg AM, Watson PJ, et al. Prevention and early intervention programs for children and adolescents. In: Beck JG, Sloan DM, editors. The Oxford handbook of traumatic stress disorders. New York (NY): Oxford University Press; 2012. p. 381–92.
22. Litz BT, Maguen S. Early intervention for trauma. In: Friedman MJ, Keane TM, Resick PA, editors. Handbook of PTSD: science and practice. New York (NY): The Guilford Press; 2007. p. 306–29.
23. Felitti MD, Vincent J, Anda MD, et al. Relationship of childhood abuse and household dysfunction to many of the leading causes of death in adults: the Adverse Childhood Experiences (ACE) Study. Am J Prev Med 1998;14(4):245–58.
24. Trickey D, Siddaway AP, Meiser-Stedman R, et al. A meta-analysis of risk factors for post-traumatic stress disorder in children and adolescents. Clin Psychol Rev 2012;32(2):122–38.
25. Fairbank JA, Putnam FW, Harris WW. The prevalence and impact of child traumatic stress. In: Friedman MJ, Keane TM, Resick PA, editors. Handbook of PTSD: science and practice. New York (NY): The Guilford Press; 2007. p. 229–51.
26. Cohen JA, Bukstein O, Walter H, et al. Practice parameter for the assessment and treatment of children and adolescents with posttraumatic stress disorder. J Am Acad Child Adolesc Psychiatry 2010;49(4):414–30.
27. Werba BE, Kazak AE. Commentary: life threat, risk, and resilience in pediatric medical traumatic stress. J Pediatr Psychol 2009;34(1):27–9.
28. Langeland W, Olff M. Psychobiology of posttraumatic stress disorder in pediatric injury patients: a review of the literature. Neurosci Biobehav Rev 2008;32(1):161–74.
29. Ehlers A, Mayou RA, Bryant B. Cognitive predictors of posttraumatic stress disorder in children: results of a prospective longitudinal study. Behav Res Ther 2003;41(1):1–10.
30. Meiser-Stedman R, Dalgleish T, Glucksman E, et al. Maladaptive cognitive appraisals mediate the evolution of posttraumatic stress reactions: a 6-month follow-up of child and adolescent assault and motor vehicle accident survivors. J Abnorm Psychol 2009;118(4):778.
31. Kassam-Adams N, Garcia-España JF, Fein JA, et al. Heart rate and posttraumatic stress in injured children. Arch Gen Psychiatry 2005;62(3):335.
32. Nugent NR, Christopher NC, Delahanty DL. Emergency medical service and in-hospital vital signs as predictors of subsequent PTSD symptom severity in pediatric injury patients. J Child Psychol Psychiatry 2006;47(9):919–26.
33. Delahanty DL, Nugent NR, Christopher NC, et al. Initial urinary epinephrine and cortisol levels predict acute PTSD symptoms in child trauma victims. Psychoneuroendocrinology 2005;30(2):121–8.
34. Layne CM, Warren JS, Saltzman WR, et al. Contextual influences on posttraumatic adjustment: retraumatization and the roles of revictimization, posttraumatic adversities, and distressing reminders. In: Schein LA, Spitz HI, Burlingame GM, et al, editors. Psychological effects of catastrophic disasters: group approaches to treatment. London: Haworth Press; 2006. p. 235–86.
35. Kenardy J, Thompson K, Le Brocque R, et al. Information provision intervention for children and their parents following pediatric accidental injury. Eur Child and Adolesc Psychiatry 2008;17(5):316–25.

36. Cox CM, Kenardy JA, Hendrikz JK. A meta-analysis of risk factors that predict psychopathology following accidental trauma. J Spec Pediatr Nurs 2008; 13(2):98–110.

37. Landolt MA, Vollrath M, Ribi K, et al. Incidence and associations of parental and child posttraumatic stress symptoms in pediatric patients. J Child Psychol Psychiatry 2003;44(8):1199–207.

38. Vernberg EM, La Greca AM, Silverman WK, et al. Prediction of posttraumatic stress symptoms in children after Hurricane Andrew. J Abnorm Psychol 1996; 105(2):237.

39. Nugent NR, Ostrowski S, Christopher NC, et al. Parental symptoms of PTSD as a moderator of child's acute biological response and subsequent symptoms of PTSD in pediatric trauma patients. J Pediatr Psychol 2007;32:309–18.

40. Paolucci EO, Genuis ML, Violato C. A meta-analysis of the published research on the effects of child sexual abuse. J Psychol 2001;135(1):17–36.

41. Schwartz D, Proctor LJ. Community violence exposure and children's social adjustment in the school peer group: the mediating roles of emotion regulation and social cognition. J Consult Clin Psychol 2000;68(4):670.

42. Delaney-Black V, Covington C, Ondersma SJ, et al. Violence exposure, trauma, and IQ and/or reading deficits among urban children. Arch Pediatr Adolesc Med 2002;156(3):280.

43. Graham-Bermann SA, DeVoe ER, Mattis JS, et al. Ecological predictors of traumatic stress symptoms in Caucasian and ethnic minority children exposed to intimate partner violence. Violence Against Women 2006;12(7): 662–92.

44. Shalev AY, Adessky R, Boker R, et al. Clinical intervention for survivors of prolonged adversities. In: Ursano RJ, Fullerton C, Norwood A, editors. Terrorism and disaster, individual and community mental health interventions. New York (NY): Cambridge University Press; 2003. p. 162–86.

45. Kramer DN, Landolt MA. Characteristics and efficacy of early psychological interventions in children and adolescents after single trauma: a meta-analysis. Eur J Psychotraumatol [Online] 2011;2. Available at: http://www.ejpt.net/index.php/ejpt/article/view/7858. Accessed September 12, 2013.

46. Marsac ML, Hildenbrand AK, Kohser KL, et al. Preventing posttraumatic stress following pediatric injury: a randomized controlled trial of a web-based psycho-educational intervention for parents. J Pediatr Psychol 2013; 38(10):1101–11.

47. Ponsford J, Willmott C, Rothwell A, et al. Impact of early intervention on outcome after mild traumatic brain injury in children. Pediatrics 2001;108(6):1297–303.

48. Cox CM, Kenardy JA, Hendrikz JK. A randomized controlled trial of a web-based early intervention for children and their parents following unintentional injury. J Pediatr Psychol 2010;35(6):581–92.

49. Pender DA, Prichard KK. ASGW best practice guidelines as a research tool: a comprehensive examination of the Critical Incident Stress Debriefing. J Sp Group Work 2009;34(2):175–92.

50. Mitchell JT. When disaster strikes: the Critical Incident Stress Debriefing process. JEMS 1983;8(1):36–9.

51. Dyregrov A. Grief in children: a handbook for adults. Philadelphia (PA): Jessica Kingsley Publishers; 2008.

52. Stallard P, Velleman R, Salter E, et al. A randomised controlled trial to determine the effectiveness of an early psychological intervention with children involved in road traffic accidents. J Child Psychol Psychiatry 2006;47(2):127–34.

53. Zehnder D, Meuli M, Landolt MA. Effectiveness of a single-session early psychological intervention for children after road traffic accidents: a randomised controlled trial. Child Adolesc Psychiatry Ment Health 2010;4(7):1–10.

54. Hobfoll SE, Watson P, Bell CC, et al. Five essential elements of immediate and mid-term mass trauma intervention: empirical evidence. Psychiatry 2007; 70(4):283–315 [discussion: 316–9].

55. Berkowitz S, Bryant R, Brymer M, et al. Skills for psychological recovery: field operations guide. The National Center for PTSD & the National Child Traumatic Stress Network; 2010. Available at: http://www.psychiatry.org/File%20Library/Practice/Professional%20Interests/Disaster%20Psychiatry/NCTSN-Skills-for-Psychological-Recovery.pdf. Accessed October 20, 2013.

56. Forbes D, Fletcher S, Wolfgang B, et al. Practitioner perceptions of skills for psychological recovery: a training programme for health practitioners in the aftermath of the Victorian bushfires. Aust N Z J Psychiatry 2010;44(12): 1105–11.

57. Lester P, Mogil C, Saltzman W, et al. Families Overcoming Under Stress: implementing family-centered prevention for military families facing wartime deployments and combat operational stress. Mil Med 2011;176(1):19–25.

58. Hanson SH, Brockberg D, Gerwitz A. Development and evaluation of web-enhanced parenting program for reintegrating National Guard and Reserve families: after deployment, adaptive parenting tools/ADAPT. CYF News. 2013. Available at: https://www.apa.org/pi/families/resources/newsletter/2013/. Accessed October 19, 2013.

59. DeVoe E, Ross AM. Engaging and retaining National Guard/Reserve families with very young children in treatment: the Strong Families Strong Forces Program. CYF News. 2013. Available at: https://www.apa.org/pi/families/resources/newsletter/2013/. Accessed October 19, 2013.

60. Kassam-Adams N, Garcia-Espana JF, Marsac ML, et al. A pilot randomized controlled trial assessing secondary prevention of traumatic stress integrated into pediatric trauma care. J Trauma Stress 2011;24(3):252–9.

61. Berkowitz SJ, Stover CS, Marans SR. The Child and Family Traumatic Stress Intervention: secondary prevention for youth at risk of developing PTSD. J Child Psychol Psychiatry 2011;52(6):676–85.

62. Saxe G, Stoddard F, Courtney D, et al. Relationship between acute morphine and the course of PTSD in children with burns. J Am Acad Child Adolesc Psychiatry 2001;40(8):915–21.

63. Bryant RA, Creamer M, O'Donnell M, et al. A study of the protective function of acute morphine administration on subsequent posttraumatic stress disorder. Biol Psychiatry 2009;65(5):438–40.

64. Nixon RD, Nehmy TJ, Ellis AA, et al. Predictors of posttraumatic stress in children following injury: the influence of appraisals, heart rate, and morphine use. Behav Res Ther 2010;48(8):810–5.

65. Stoddard FJ Jr, Sorrentino EA, Ceranoglu TA, et al. Preliminary evidence for the effects of morphine on posttraumatic stress disorder symptoms in one- to four-year-olds with burns. J Burn Care Res 2009;30(5):836–43.

66. Pittman RK, Sanders KM, Zusman RM, et al. Pilot study of secondary prevention of posttraumatic stress disorder with propranolol. Biol Psychiatry 2002;51(2): 189–92.

67. Nugent NR, Christopher NC, Crow JP, et al. The efficacy of early propranolol administration at reducing PTSD symptoms in pediatric injury patients: a pilot study. J Trauma Stress 2010;23(2):282–7.

68. Davydow DS, Katon WJ, Zatzick DF. Psychiatric morbidity and functional impairments in survivors of burns, traumatic injuries, and ICU stays for other critical illnesses: a review of the literature. Int Rev Psychiatry 2009;21(6):531–8.
69. Berkowitz SJ, Watson PJ, Brymer MJ. Early preventive interventions for adolescents exposed to a potentially traumatic event. Minerva Pediatr 2011;63(3):201.
70. Brock SE, Nickerson AB, Reeves MA, et al. Development, evaluation, and future directions of the PREP a RE school crisis prevention and intervention training curriculum. J Sch Violence 2011;10(1):34–52.
71. Mayou RA, Ehlers A, Hobbs M. Psychological debriefing for road traffic accident victims. Three-year follow-up of a randomised controlled trial. Br J Psychiatry 2000;176(6):589–93.
72. Cohen JA, Kelleher KJ, Mannarino AP. Identifying, treating, and referring traumatized children: the role of pediatric providers. Arch Pediatr Adolesc Med 2008;162(5):447–52.

Psychological and Pharmacologic Treatment of Youth with Posttraumatic Stress Disorder
An Evidence-based Review

Brooks R. Keeshin, MD[a,b,*], Jeffrey R. Strawn, MD[b,c]

KEYWORDS

- Posttraumatic stress disorder
- Trauma-focused cognitive behavior therapy (TF-CBT)
- Selective serotonin reuptake inhibitor (SSRI, SRI) • Trauma • Prevention

KEY POINTS

- Posttraumatic stress disorder (PTSD), in children and adolescents, is a constellation of symptoms that likely represent multiple pathophysiologic responses to stress.
- Psychotherapy is the mainstay of treatment of pediatric PTSD, with the greatest evidence supporting the use of trauma-focused psychotherapies.
- Pharmacotherapy should be used in conjunction with ongoing psychotherapy when prolonged and severe symptoms (including comorbid conditions such as depression and anxiety disorders) warrant additional intervention.

EVIDENCE FOR PSYCHOTHERAPEUTIC TREATMENT OF YOUTH WITH PTSD

Children exposed to violence and abuse experience a wide range of psychological sequelae, including attention disorders, mood disorders, and anxiety disorders.[1] Many children, especially those who are exposed to child abuse and neglect, as

Disclosures: B.R. Keeshin has received research support from the American Academy of Child and Adolescent Psychiatry and the Doris Duke Foundation. J.R. Strawn has received research support from Eli Lilly, Shire, Forest Research Laboratories, and from the American Academy of Child and Adolescent Psychiatry.

[a] Department of Pediatrics, Mayerson Center for Safe and Healthy Children, Cincinnati Children's Hospital Medical Center, 3333 Burnet Avenue, Cincinnati, OH 45229, USA; [b] Division of Child and Adolescent Psychiatry, Department of Pediatrics, Cincinnati Children's Hospital Medical Center, 3333 Burnet Avenue, Cincinnati, OH 45219, USA; [c] Department of Psychiatry and Behavioral Neuroscience, College of Medicine, University of Cincinnati, 260 Stetson Street, Cincinnati, OH 45219, USA
* Corresponding author. Mayerson Center for Safe and Healthy Children, Cincinnati Children's Hospital, Cincinnati, Ohio.
E-mail address: brooks.keeshin@cchmc.org

Child Adolesc Psychiatric Clin N Am 23 (2014) 399–411
http://dx.doi.org/10.1016/j.chc.2013.12.002
1056-4993/14/$ – see front matter © 2014 Elsevier Inc. All rights reserved.

Acronyms	
CAPS	Clinician-Administered PTSD Scale
CBITS	Cognitive Behavioral Interventions for Trauma in Schools
CFTSI	Child and Family Traumatic Stress Intervention
CGI	Clinical global impression scale
CPP	Child Parent Psychotherapy
DSM-5	Diagnostic Statistical Manual of Mental Disorders
EMDR	Eye Movement Desensitization and Reprocessing
PE-A	Prolonged Exposure for Adolescents
SRI	Serotonin reuptake inhibitor
SSRI	Selective serotonin reuptake inhibitor
TGCT	Trauma and grief component therapy
TSCC	Traumatic Symptom Checklist for Children

well as a variety of disasters and noninterpersonal forms of trauma, may experience stress disorders, including posttraumatic stress disorder (PTSD).[1] In the recently released *Diagnostic Statistical Manual of Mental Disorders, Fifth Edition* (DSM-5),[2] the criteria for PTSD has been revised and new, developmentally sensitive criteria for children who experience trauma before the age of 6 years is available to guide clinicians in diagnosis of both young and older children. The revision of these criteria from the *Diagnostic Statistical Manual of Mental Disorders, Fourth Edition, Text Revision* (DSM-IV-TR) criteria includes the separation of avoidance and negative alterations in mood into separate categories, as well as the categorization of dissociative experiences as a qualifier. Because PTSD has various neuroendocrine and neuroanatomic correlates that predict specific phenomenologic characteristics (reviewed by De Bellis elsewhere in this issue), it is likely that this new classification will help clinicians design treatment strategies based on specific impairing symptoms rather than on the broad, often heterogenous symptoms of PTSD.

Psychotherapeutic interventions are the mainstay of treatment of traumatized children with symptoms of traumatic stress, including those with PTSD, regardless of the cause. Although there are many permutations of these psychotherapeutic interventions, including adaptation to specific target populations (eg, individual, dyadic, group) and foundational theory (eg, cognitive behavioral, psychodynamic, and so forth), there are several core unifying concepts that characterize most evidence-based psychotherapies for traumatized youth. These include: (1) ensuring safety from continued trauma; (2) providing psychoeducation regarding the potential effects from, and responses to, trauma; (3) providing effective coping/behavior management strategies; (4) assisting children in mastering trauma avoidance, typically through trauma narration and/or exposure activities; and (5) engaging parents or other caregivers in treatment and enhancing the parent-child relationship. These concepts crosscut psychotherapeutic modalities with an emphasis on different components often depending on the specific therapy model and the child's most debilitating symptoms.[3] For example, increased focus on self-calming coping strategies are key in an adolescent with extreme hyperarousal, whereas the parent-child relationship and behavior management are areas of focus in a young child who is reexperiencing symptoms that are born out through aggressive and assaultive play. This article reviews the primary components, target populations, and effectiveness of the most studied and commonly available evidence-based trauma treatments for children.

COGNITIVE BEHAVIOR THERAPY–BASED THERAPIES
Trauma-focused Cognitive Behavior Therapy

Trauma-focused cognitive behavior therapy (TF-CBT; www.musc.edu/tfcbt) is the most studied treatment of symptomatic children exposed to trauma,[1] with 13 randomized controlled trials showing its efficacy both in waitlist and head-to-head therapeutic trials for children aged 3 to 17 years (**Fig. 1**). Benefits of TF-CBT include reduction of PTSD symptoms and remission of PTSD, improvement of a variety of other mental health symptoms, as well as enhanced parental capacity to meet the child's emotional and behavioral needs.[1] TF-CBT has been used in a myriad of treatment settings in children exposed to a wide range of abusive and traumatic experiences, some of whom continued to experience trauma or the threat of trauma during treatment.[4] Moreover, cognitive behavior therapy (CBT)–based therapies for trauma have shown gains that continue long after treatment, with trauma symptom reduction effect sizes greater than 2 when measured at more than 6 months.[5]

The first 3 components of TF-CBT (psychoeducation, parenting skills, and relaxation skills) stabilize trauma-related physiologic and behavioral dysregulation and prepare the child and family for the therapeutic work ahead. Additional components such as affect modulation and cognitive processing give the child the capacity to better modulate dysregulated emotions and understand the interconnectedness between thoughts, feeling, and behaviors. Once the child has practiced self-regulation and has an increased capacity to modulate behavioral, cognitive, and affective states, the child and therapist begin to construct the trauma narrative. Developing the trauma narrative is a collaborative therapeutic process during which the therapist encourages the child to describe even those details about traumatic experiences that the child thinks are unspeakable, thus overcoming shame, stigma, and avoidance, and gaining mastery of the content in session. Maladaptive trauma-related cognitions are processed using cognitive processing techniques learned earlier in treatment. If the child

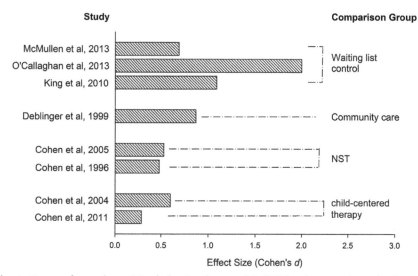

Fig. 1. Trauma-focused cognitive behavior therapy (TF-CBT) has been evaluated relative to several comparison treatments as well as waiting list comparison groups. In general, effect sizes are robust, although they depend on the comparison group, with lower effect sizes typically being observed when TF-CBT is compared with an active treatment. NST, non-directive supportive therapy.

becomes distressed while recalling aspects of the narrative, the therapist assists the child in using previously taught self-relaxation and coping techniques and then returns to the narrative, thus reinforcing mastery. Children develop mastery over generalized fears through the use of in vivo exposure hierarchies. The final TF-CBT sessions are spent in conjoint parent-child sessions. The parent typically participates with the child to share the child's narrative, to engage in safety planning, and to discuss the continued effective use of the CBT skills once TF-CBT is terminated.

Several Cognitive Behavior Therapies Have at Least One Randomized Controlled Trial Showing Efficacy with Traumatized Youth

Prolonged exposure for adolescents (PE-A) includes the development of an exposure hierarchy, practiced in vivo exposure during sessions, and assigning in vivo exposures such as listening to taped recordings by the patient recounting the trauma. Compared with a manualized, conflict-based, psychodynamic intervention, adolescents who received PE-A showed a greater reduction in symptoms of posttraumatic stress and improved rate of PTSD remission both at the end of treatment and at follow-up[6]; however, study limitations complicate a head-to-head comparison, including differences in the frequency of treatment and experience of therapists between the groups receiving psychodynamic psychotherapy and PE-A.

A 10-week CBT trial for children with single-incident traumatic exposure and PTSD maintained for a 4-week lead-in period showed significant improvement compared with a waitlist comparison group, with only 10% in the active arm meeting criteria for PTSD at the end of treatment compared with 60% in the waitlist group.[7] In contrast with TF-CBT, there was no relaxation-training component and parent-child sessions were not part of the manual but were used when deemed clinically necessary. Of primary focus was exposure to the traumatic memory through writing, talking, or drawing, with cognitive restructuring designed to modify cognitive distortions of the trauma and related symptoms.

Narrative exposure therapy (KIDNET) is an 8-week, narrative-driven individual therapy designed specifically for pediatric refugee populations.[8] During the course of therapy, a therapist uses a variety of child-friendly recall assistance techniques to enable the child to develop a coherent narrative of the child's life, with special focus given to traumatic events, both remote and recent. The development of the narrative offers the opportunity for habituation to traumatic memories. Reductions in posttraumatic symptoms were significant in the active treatment arm of the study and were maintained at both 6-month and 12-month follow-ups.[8]

NON-CBT THERAPIES
Child-Parent Psychotherapy

Child-parent psychotherapy (CPP) is a dyadic, attachment-based therapy intended for traumatized children aged 3 to 5 years. Through both joint sessions and individual sessions with the mother (or caregiver), CPP promotes affect regulation and improved behavior for the child and caregiver, and assists the dyad in producing a joint trauma narrative that resolves interdyad conflict and improves the mother-child relationship.[9] Compared with case management with community provider therapy, CPP significantly improved children's trauma-related symptoms and overall behavior problems, as well as maternal avoidance symptoms. A 6-month follow-up study with two-thirds of the original mother-child dyads observed continued improvement in children's behavior problems and maternal distress in dyads who received CPP.[10] Other attachment-based models include preschooler-parent psychotherapy, which improves maladaptive maternal representations and mother-child relationship expectations in families with maltreated children.[11] At this time, there are few studies that have directly compared cognitive behavior and attachment/dynamic-based therapies in terms of efficacy and long-term outcomes.

Other therapies have been proposed and are often used in clinical practice to treat traumatized children, whether or not they meet criteria for PTSD. Such therapies include eye movement desensitization and reprocessing therapy (EMDR). In a meta-analysis on the use of EMDR in traumatized pediatric populations, EMDR had a medium effect size (d = .56, $P<.001$).[12] However, of the 7 pediatric studies included for analysis, only 2 had a standardized treatment comparison (CBT), and most participants completed 4 or fewer total sessions, making meaningful comparisons on the effectiveness of EMDR compared with full doses of CBT or other community treatments difficult to assess. Play therapy has also been suggested to be of value to young children exposed to traumatic events. One meta-analysis[5] showed improved social functioning with the use of play therapy techniques, whereas a later review of play therapy studies in children with and without a history of maltreatment showed improvements in both groups, suggesting that play therapy likely improves play and social skills in children, regardless of trauma history.[13]

SCHOOL-BASED/GROUP THERAPIES

The nature of large-scale disasters or widespread community violence results in increased symptoms of posttraumatic stress in children at a time of compromised resources. Therefore, using nontraditional methods of mental health care delivery, such as schools, has been investigated as a way to treat large numbers of children with available resources.

Cognitive behavioral interventions for trauma in schools (CBITS) is an example of a school-based trauma intervention.[1] CBITS includes components of psychoeducation, parent sessions, relaxation skills, affect modulation skills, cognitive coping skills, individual breakout sessions for developing and processing a trauma narrative, in vivo mastery of trauma reminders, and wrap-up sessions enhancing safety. CBITS has been shown to be effective in both natural disasters and community violence settings.[14] In addition to demonstrated efficacy, school-based programs likely improve completion rates of treatment in traumatized children. One study that compared the completion rates of CBITS with clinic-based TF-CBT in New Orleans approximately 18 months after Hurricane Katrina showed that, for every 6 children who completed CBITS, only 1 child completed TF-CBT, suggesting that school-based therapies increase access to treatment of traumatized children, especially after a disaster damages community infrastructure.[15] Trauma and grief component therapy for adolescents (TGCT) is a classroom-based group intervention, and has been evaluated in several settings in which children have been exposed to natural or man-made disasters.[16] TGCT is different than CBITS in that it includes the active promotion of beneficial grieving as a core module of the program. One randomized controlled trial showed efficacy of TGCT compared with a school-based psychoeducation program. The area of greatest improvement was grief, which was significantly better in children who received TGCT compared with the control group.[16]

PSYCHOPHARMACOLOGIC TREATMENTS

Over the last several decades, the evidence base for psychopharmacologic interventions in youth has increased, although only within the last decade have these treatments been subjected to randomized clinical trials. In general, the development of these psychopharmacologic interventions has been largely based on data from medication trials in adults with PTSD.

ANTIDEPRESSANTS
Tricyclic Antidepressants

To date, 1 randomized, double-blind, controlled trial suggests that ultrabrief treatment with imipramine may reduce some PTSD symptoms in youth.[17] A second study of the tricyclic antidepressant imipramine and the selective serotonin reuptake inhibitor (SSRI) fluoxetine (as well as a placebo arm)[18] failed to observe differences between the treatment groups. However, this study should be interpreted cautiously given that this is a 7-day trial. The American Academy of Child and Adolescent Psychiatry recommends routine electrocardiogram monitoring in pediatric patients treated with tricyclic antidepressants.

SSRIs

There are now several studies of SSRIs in pediatric patients with PTSD. In the first study of the SSRI sertraline, Cohen and colleagues[19] compared adjunctive sertraline (mean dose 150 mg/d, range 50–200 mg/d) with placebo in pediatric patients with PTSD who were also receiving TF-CBT. No statistically significant differences were observed in the Child Global Assessment Scale scores between patients treated with sertraline compared with those receiving placebo.[19] As a caveat, it is important to recognize that, in this trial, the treatment being compared was adjunctive to a highly effective treatment (TF-CBT), which likely made the detection of any potential sertraline-related improvement difficult. A second study of sertraline in pediatric patients with PTSD evaluated flexibly dosed sertraline using similar dosing in children with PTSD (n = 131, duration 10 weeks) and did not observe differences in the University of California at Los Angeles (UCLA) PTSD-I 17-item total score between sertraline-treated patients and those receiving placebo.[20] In addition, 1 open-label trial evaluated the safety and tolerability of citalopram over the course of an 8-week treatment period. In this study, Clinician-administered PTSD Scale (CAPS) total and symptom cluster scores as well as the Clinical Global Impression Scale (CGI) score improved over the course of treatment.[21]

ANTIADRENERGIC AGENTS

Over the last several years, several reports have documented noradrenergic hyperactivity in pediatric patients with both motor vehicle accident–related PTSD[22] and in adolescents with sexual abuse–related PTSD.[23] These observations parallel similar findings in adults with sexual abuse–related PTSD and combat-related PTSD (see Strawn and Geracioti,[24] 2008, for review). Given these neuroendocrine data suggesting noradrenergic hyperactivity, antiadrenergic interventions have received increased attention over the last several years in the pediatric population.

Guanfacine and Clonidine

An open-label study recently evaluated extended-release guanfacine (1–4 mg daily) in pediatric patients with attention-deficit/hyperactivity disorder (ADHD) and co-occurring posttraumatic stress symptoms (n = 19).[25] In this 8-week open-label trial, guanfacine XR was well tolerated (mean dose, 1.2 mg ± 0.4 mg) and UCLA PTSD RI (Reaction Index) scores decreased over the course of treatment for re-experiencing, avoidant, and hyperarousal symptoms. In addition, guanfacine XR was well tolerated. To date, case series–level evidence also suggests that immediate-release guanfacine may be effective in the treatment of nightmares associated with PTSD in youth.[26]

The nonselective alpha-2 agonist clonidine has also been shown to attenuate reenactment symptoms in children.[27,28] In addition, an interesting case report of a child with PTSD suggested that clonidine treatment may be associated with increased ratios of n-acetylaspartate to creatine in the anterior cingulate cortex, suggesting increased neuronal integrity within this region.[29]

Prazosin

Despite multiple placebo-controlled trials of the alpha-1 antagonist prazosin in adults, there are only a few reports of the use of this agent in youth. To date, case reports suggest that it may be effective as an adjunctive treatment,[30,31] as well as monotherapy in children[32] and adolescents[33,34] with PTSD. However, to date, there are no open-label trials or double-blind, placebo-controlled trials of prazosin in youth with PTSD.

Propranolol

The centrally acting β-blocker propranolol was evaluated by Famularo and colleagues[35] in 11 children with childhood abuse–related PTSD. In this study, significantly fewer symptoms were observed during the course of propranolol treatment. This agent has been also evaluated in several secondary prevention trials in traumatized youth at risk for PTSD (eg, those who have experienced burn trauma or motor vehicle accident trauma).[36,37] Additional information on these trials is given by Berkowitz elsewhere in this issue.

SECOND-GENERATION ANTIPSYCHOTICS

Several second-generation antipsychotics (SGAs) have been evaluated in adults with PTSD and these medications have been subjected to randomized controlled trials. In addition, retrospective studies suggest that exposure to trauma or abuse in pediatric patients is associated with higher rates of SGA prescribing.[38] However, the extant data for the use of PTSD are limited.

Risperidone

The SGA risperidone has been evaluated in 1 open-label trial of pediatric patients with PTSD and in several case reports. In a group of preschool-aged children (n = 3) with serious thermal burns and acute stress disorder, improvement was observed in intrusive, hyperarousal, and avoidance symptoms.[39] In addition, an open-label treatment of youth resulted in remission of PTSD symptoms in 13 of 18 youth, although many of the patients in this sample had comorbid mood disorders and thus it remains possible that some of the improvement may have been the result of improvement in symptoms that syndromically overlapped with PTSD.[40] In addition, case report–level evidence suggests that adjunctive risperidone treatment may be associated with symptomatic improvement.[41]

Quetiapine

The low-potency, SGA quetiapine has been evaluated in an open-label study of adolescents aged 15 to 17 years (n = 6). In this study, patients received flexibly dosed quetiapine (50–200 mg/d) over the course of 6 weeks and improvements were observed in Traumatic Symptom Checklist for Children posttraumatic stress t scores and in symptoms of anxiety, depression, and anger.[42] Moreover, quetiapine was well tolerated in this small study.

MOOD STABILIZERS AND OTHER MEDICATIONS

Although mood stabilizers/antiepileptic agents have been extensively evaluated in adults with PTSD, there are few data regarding these agents in traumatized youth with PTSD. To date, carbamazepine has been evaluated in pediatric patients with sexual abuse–related PTSD[43] and in this study, involving youth who were in residential treatment (n = 28), carbamazepine was titrated to achieve serum levels of 10 to 11.5 μg/mL. Most patients (79%) were asymptomatic at the end point.[43] In addition, open-label treatment with divalproex in youth with PTSD was associated with clinical improvement and good tolerability.[44] Boys (n = 12) aged 16 ± 1 years with comorbid conduct disorder and PTSD received either high-dose or low-dose divalproex. Youth who were randomized to the high-dose treatment had improvements in CGI score over the course of the trial.[44] In addition to the mood stabilizers, the serotonin and H_1 receptor antagonist cyproheptadine has been observed, in a retrospective chart review, to reduce nightmares associated with PTSD.[45]

CLINICAL PRACTICE APPLICATION

Several factors should be considered when choosing the appropriate therapeutic approach, including the experience of the practitioner and the availability of different treatment modalities in the community. Therefore advocacy and education of community providers is of the utmost importance in developing and maintaining an adequate mental health infrastructure, capable of providing evidence-based trauma therapies to address the effects of trauma in the community. In addition to availability and resources, the other factors to consider are discussed later.

Timing of Trauma

Whether or not the trauma and development of symptoms is remote or recent not only affects diagnosis, it can also direct different interventions. Recent traumatic events or recent disclosures of past traumatic events with symptoms of posttraumatic stress may benefit from a brief intervention such as Child and Family Traumatic Stress Intervention (CFTSI) (Discussed by Berkowitz elsewhere in this issue). This PTSD prevention therapy uses many of the core concepts of psychoeducation/symptom identification, enhanced parent-child relationship through improved communication, and adoption of healthy coping strategies that are advocated by other evidence-based modalities. In CFTSI, there is no exposure component such as a trauma narrative. However, in more chronic manifestations, an exposure component found in other trauma therapies such as TF-CBT, CPP, and PE-A likely assists in improving core symptoms of PTSD.

Single Versus Repeated/Multiple Traumas

One of the greatest lessons from the large body of the Adverse Childhood Experiences Study and similar research is that the effects of trauma are cumulative,[46] and that individuals with multiple exposures likely carry a greater symptom burden. Although the literature does not support the use of any particular modality for PTSD in the setting of complex or repeated trauma, it is important to recognize and prepare families for the realization that children who have experienced severe and chronic adversity may require lengthy treatment or may need to return for an additional course of treatment at subsequent developmental stages. In addition, chronic child abuse and neglect are associated with developmental and cognitive impairment,[47] and assessment, recognition, and intervention for cognitive and developmental issues (eg, individualized educational plans, 504 plans) in maltreated children may be of great clinical usefulness.

Comorbid Symptoms

Children who experience child abuse are at increased risk for both medical and psychiatric comorbidity that may affect PTSD-targeted interventions.[38,48] Clinicians, in consultation with families, are faced with the task of determining which symptoms or diagnosis results in the greatest amount of distress and functional impairment for the child, and then to develop a logical, stepwise treatment approach. For example, a 10-year-old child in foster care with a history of sexual abuse 6 months ago meets criteria for both PTSD and generalized anxiety disorder. It is possible that the anxiety disorder preceded the abuse, but there is no history or collateral information to support or refute this. As such, clinicians could proceed with a therapy such as TF-CBT and, at the end of therapy, reassess for any persistent symptoms of anxiety and treat appropriately. In contrast, if a child with PTSD also has severe, untreated ADHD that preceded the trauma, clinicians might choose to address the ADHD pharmacologically so that the patient could function better at school as well as in the trauma therapy.

Age of the Child

A child's developmental and chronologic age is of critical importance when choosing the appropriate therapy, and although some modalities (such as TF-CBT) can be performed in a wide range of ages, certain considerations need to be taken with younger or developmentally delayed children. In general, younger children are likely to benefit from dyadic approaches in which their behaviors (eg, parent-child interaction therapy) as well as relational and attachment issues (CPP) can be addressed in the therapeutic setting. Many of these families seek help for aggression or behavioral issues rather than PTSD, and require education regarding the connection of trauma and behaviors as part of a trauma-informed behavioral or dyadic intervention. In contrast, older children, especially those in foster care or those who have been emancipated, may benefit from developing a therapeutic alliance with the therapist in the individual setting, or learning from and engaging in therapy with their peers in a group setting. In addition, older children with a history of trauma are at greater risk for several sequelae such as self-harm/suicidal behaviors[38] and substance use disorders,[49] requiring escalated levels of care or specific and targeted therapies to address those symptoms (dialectical behavioral therapy, motivational enhancement therapy, and so forth) concurrent with or before trauma therapy.

Safety Concerns

Appropriate and comprehensive safety assessments are critical before and throughout treatment. For many children, especially those who experience interpersonal violence in the family, school, or community, the threat of violence continues while in treatment. In some settings, hypervigilance and avoidance are protective and adaptive rather than symptoms of PTSD. In settings in which there are persistent, ongoing threats of violence, and in which a clear understanding of the safety issues is lacking, it is impossible to make critical clinical assessments of the severity of the patient's symptoms. In addition, in settings in which some of the safety concerns are modifiable, appropriate case management to address housing, school, or legal issues that decrease the threat of continued violence may be of equal or greater benefit than evidence-based trauma treatments. Provided appropriate consent, open communication with children's services, law enforcement, and prosecutors may provide additional information and support that enhances the capacity of the system and family to provide a safe and nurturing environment for the child.

FUTURE DIRECTIONS

Accumulating data suggest that both biological and behavioral components contribute to the deleterious health effects of exposure to childhood adversity in adults[46] and children.[48] The publication of DSM-5, in conjunction with accumulating data regarding the underlying pathophysiology of stress response systems, in the face of repeated and chronic adversity,[50] provides ample opportunity for the incorporation of biomarkers into pediatric PTSD treatment studies and for investigations directed at identifying Hypothalamic Pituitary Adrenal axis (HPA) and sympathetic nervous system biomarkers of treatment response. For example, pretreatment levels of cortisol and/or norepinephrine might be useful in determining which patients may respond to specific treatments known to directly affect these stress response systems.[51] Research examining the relationship between treatment of pediatric PTSD and the resultant long-term physical and mental health is urgently needed.

SUMMARY

Strong evidence supports the efficacy of trauma-focused psychotherapies for the treatment of pediatric PTSD. In addition, a small body of literature suggests efficacy of several psychopharmacologic interventions as monotherapy for pediatric PTSD (eg, alpha-2 agonists, alpha-1 antagonists, several SGAs, and several antiepileptic agents), although double-blind, placebo-controlled trials of SSRIs do not suggest a benefit for PTSD symptoms in youth. Clinicians should tailor treatment based on the individual child's most distressing and functionally impairing symptoms in a developmentally sensitive manner.

REFERENCES

1. Cohen JA, Bukstein O, Walter H, et al. Practice parameter for the assessment and treatment of children and adolescents with posttraumatic stress disorder. J Am Acad Child Adolesc Psychiatry 2010;49(4):414–30.
2. American Psychiatric Association. Diagnostic and statistical manual of mental disorders. (DSM-5). 5th edition. Washington, DC: American Psychiatric Association; 2013.
3. Plakun EM, Sudak DM, Goldberg D. The Y model: an integrated, evidence-based approach to teaching psychotherapy competencies. J Psychiatr Pract 2009;15(1):5–11.
4. Cohen JA, Mannarino AP, Murray LK. Trauma-focused CBT for youth who experience ongoing traumas. Child Abuse Negl 2011;35(8):637–46.
5. Hetzel-Riggin MD, Brausch AM, Montgomery BS. A meta-analytic investigation of therapy modality outcomes for sexually abused children and adolescents: an exploratory study. Child Abuse Negl 2007;31(2):125–41.
6. Gilboa-Schechtman E, Foa EB, Shafran N, et al. Prolonged exposure versus dynamic therapy for adolescent PTSD: a pilot randomized controlled trial. J Am Acad Child Adolesc Psychiatry 2010;49(10):1034–42.
7. Smith P, Yule W, Perrin S, et al. Cognitive-behavioral therapy for PTSD in children and adolescents: a preliminary randomized controlled trial. J Am Acad Child Adolesc Psychiatry 2007;46(8):1051–61.
8. Ruf M, Schauer M, Neurner F, et al. Narrative exposure therapy for 7 to 16 year olds: a randomized controlled trial with traumatized refugee children. J Trauma Stress 2010;23(4):437–45.

9. Lieberman AF, Van Horn P, Ippen CG. Toward evidence-based treatment: child-parent psychotherapy with preschoolers exposed to marital violence. J Am Acad Child Adolesc Psychiatry 2005;44(12):1241–8. http://dx.doi.org/10.1097/01.chi.0000181047.59702.58.

10. Lieberman AF, Ghosh Ippen C, Van Horn P. Child-parent psychotherapy: 6-month follow-up of a randomized controlled trial. J Am Acad Child Adolesc Psychiatry 2006;45(8):913–8. http://dx.doi.org/10.1097/01.chi.0000222784.03735.92.

11. Toth SL, Maughan A, Manly JT, et al. The relative efficacy of two interventions in altering maltreated preschool children's representational models: implications for attachment theory. Dev Psychopathol 2002;14(4):877–908.

12. Rodenburg R, Benjamin A, de Roos C, et al. Efficacy of EMDR in children: a meta-analysis. Clin Psychol Rev 2009;29(7):599–606. http://dx.doi.org/10.1016/j.cpr.2009.06.008.

13. Silverman WK, Ortiz CD, Viswesvaran C, et al. Evidence-based psychosocial treatments for children and adolescents exposed to traumatic events. J Clin Child Adolesc Psychol 2008;37(1):156–83. http://dx.doi.org/10.1080/15374410701818293.

14. Rolfsnes ES, Idsoe T. School-based intervention programs for PTSD symptoms: a review and meta-analysis. J Trauma Stress 2011;24(2):155–65. http://dx.doi.org/10.1002/jts.20622.

15. Jaycox LH, Cohen JA, Mannarino AP, et al. Children's mental health care following Hurricane Katrina: a field trial of trauma-focused psychotherapies. J Trauma Stress 2010;23(2):223–31. http://dx.doi.org/10.1002/jts.20518.

16. Layne CM, Saltzman WR, Poppleton L, et al. Effectiveness of a school-based group psychotherapy program for war-exposed adolescents: a randomized controlled trial. J Am Acad Child Adolesc Psychiatry 2008;47(9):1048–62.

17. Robert R, Blakeney PE, Villarreal C, et al. Imipramine treatment in pediatric burn patients with symptoms of acute stress disorder: a pilot study. J Am Acad Child Adolesc Psychiatry 1999;38(7):873–82. http://dx.doi.org/10.1097/00004583-199907000-00018.

18. Robert R, Tcheung WJ, Rosenberg L, et al. Treating thermally injured children suffering symptoms of acute stress with imipramine and fluoxetine: a randomized, double-blind study. Burns 2008;34(7):919–28. http://dx.doi.org/10.1016/j.burns.2008.04.009.

19. Cohen JA, Mannarino AP, Perel JM, et al. A pilot randomized controlled trial of combined trauma-focused CBT and sertraline for childhood PTSD symptoms. J Am Acad Child Adolesc Psychiatry 2007;46(7):811–9. http://dx.doi.org/10.1097/chi.0b013e3180547105.

20. Robb AS, Cueva JE, Sporn J, et al. Sertraline treatment of children and adolescents with posttraumatic stress disorder: a double-blind, placebo-controlled trial. J Child Adolesc Psychopharmacol 2010;20(6):463–71. http://dx.doi.org/10.1089/cap.2009.0115.

21. Seedat S, Stein DJ, Ziervogel C, et al. Comparison of response to a selective serotonin reuptake inhibitor in children, adolescents, and adults with posttraumatic stress disorder. J Child Adolesc Psychopharmacol 2002;12(1):37–46. http://dx.doi.org/10.1089/10445460252943551.

22. Pervanidou P, Kolaitis G, Charitaki S, et al. The natural history of neuroendocrine changes in pediatric posttraumatic stress disorder (PTSD) after motor vehicle accidents: progressive divergence of noradrenaline and cortisol concentrations over time. Biol Psychiatry 2007;62(10):1095–102. http://dx.doi.org/10.1016/j.biopsych.2007.02.008.

23. Keeshin BR, Strawn JR, Out D, et al. Elevations in salivary alpha amylase in acute posttraumatic stress disorder. Poster session presented at the Annual Meeting of the American Academy of Child and Adolescent Psychiatry in Orlando, October 22–27, 2013.

24. Strawn JR, Geracioti TD. Noradrenergic dysfunction and the psychopharmacology of posttraumatic stress disorder. Depress Anxiety 2008;25(3):260–71. http://dx.doi.org/10.1002/da.20292.

25. Connor DF, Grasso DJ, Slivinsky MD, et al. An open-label study of guanfacine extended release for traumatic stress related symptoms in children and adolescents. J Child Adolesc Psychopharmacol 2013;23(4):244–51. http://dx.doi.org/10.1089/cap.2012.0119.

26. Horrigan JP. Guanfacine for PTSD nightmares. J Am Acad Child Adolesc Psychiatry 1996;35(8):975–6. http://dx.doi.org/10.1097/00004583-199608000-00006.

27. Harmon RJ, Riggs PD. Clonidine for posttraumatic stress disorder in preschool children. J Am Acad Child Adolesc Psychiatry 1996;35(9):1247–9. http://dx.doi.org/10.1097/00004583-199609000-00022.

28. Porter DM, Bell CC. The use of clonidine in post-traumatic stress disorder. J Natl Med Assoc 1999;91(8):475–7.

29. De Bellis MD, Keshavan MS, Harenski KA. Anterior cingulate N-acetylaspartate/creatine ratios during clonidine treatment in a maltreated child with posttraumatic stress disorder. J Child Adolesc Psychopharmacol 2001;11(3):311–6. http://dx.doi.org/10.1089/10445460152595649.

30. Brkanac Z, Pastor JF, Storck M. Prazosin in PTSD. J Am Acad Child Adolesc Psychiatry 2003;42(4):384–5. http://dx.doi.org/10.1097/01.CHI.0000052509.98293.97.

31. Fraleigh LA, Hendratta VD, Ford JD, et al. Prazosin for the treatment of posttraumatic stress disorder-related nightmares in an adolescent male. J Child Adolesc Psychopharmacol 2009;19(4):475–6. http://dx.doi.org/10.1089/cap.2009.0002.

32. Strawn JR, Keeshin BR. Successful treatment of posttraumatic stress disorder with prazosin in a young child. Ann Pharmacother 2011;45(12):1590–1. http://dx.doi.org/10.1345/aph.1Q548.

33. Strawn JR, Delbello MP, Geracioti TD. Prazosin treatment of an adolescent with posttraumatic stress disorder. J Child Adolesc Psychopharmacol 2009;19(5):599–600. http://dx.doi.org/10.1089/cap.2009.0043.

34. Oluwabusi OO, Sedky K, Bennett DS. Prazosin treatment of nightmares and sleep disturbances associated with posttraumatic stress disorder: two adolescent cases. J Child Adolesc Psychopharmacol 2012;22(5):399–402. http://dx.doi.org/10.1089/cap.2012.0035.

35. Famularo R, Kinscherff R, Fenton T. Propranolol treatment for childhood posttraumatic stress disorder, acute type. A pilot study. Am J Dis Child 1988;142(11):1244–7.

36. Nugent NR, Christopher NC, Crow JP, et al. The efficacy of early propranolol administration at reducing PTSD symptoms in pediatric injury patients: a pilot study. J Trauma Stress 2010;23(2):282–7. http://dx.doi.org/10.1002/jts.20517.

37. Pitman RK, Delahanty DL. Conceptually driven pharmacologic approaches to acute trauma. CNS Spectr 2005;10(2):99–106.

38. Keeshin BR, Strawn JR, Luebbe AM, et al. Hospitalized youth and child abuse: a systematic examination of psychiatric morbidity and clinical severity. Child Abuse Negl 2013. http://dx.doi.org/10.1016/j.chiabu.2013.08.013.

39. Meighen KG, Hines LA, Lagges AM. Risperidone treatment of preschool children with thermal burns and acute stress disorder. J Child Adolesc Psychopharmacol 2007;17(2):223–32. http://dx.doi.org/10.1089/cap.2007.0121.

40. Horrigan JP, Barnhill LJ. Risperidone and PTSD in boys. J Neuropsychiatry Clin Neurosci 1999;11:126–7.

41. Keeshin BR, Strawn JR. Risperidone treatment of an adolescent with severe posttraumatic stress disorder. Ann Pharmacother 2009;43(7):1374. http://dx.doi.org/10.1345/aph.1M219.

42. Stathis S, Martin G, McKenna JG. A preliminary case series on the use of quetiapine for posttraumatic stress disorder in juveniles within a youth detention center. J Clin Psychopharmacol 2005;25(6):539–44.

43. Looff D, Grimley P, Kuller F, et al. Carbamazepine for PTSD. J Am Acad Child Adolesc Psychiatry 1995;34(6):703–4.

44. Steiner H, Saxena KS, Carrion V, et al. Divalproex sodium for the treatment of PTSD and conduct disordered youth: a pilot randomized controlled clinical trial. Child Psychiatry Hum Dev 2007;38(3):183–93. http://dx.doi.org/10.1007/s10578-007-0055-8.

45. Gupta S, Austin R, Cali LA, et al. Nightmares treated with cyproheptadine. J Am Acad Child Adolesc Psychiatry 1998;37(6):570–2. http://dx.doi.org/10.1097/00004583-199806000-00003.

46. Felitti VJ, Anda RF, Nordenberg D, et al. Relationship of childhood abuse and household dysfunction to many of the leading causes of death in adults. The Adverse Childhood Experiences (ACE) Study. Am J Prev Med 1998;14(4):245–58.

47. De Bellis MD, Woolley DP, Hooper SR. Neuropsychological findings in pediatric maltreatment: relationship of PTSD, dissociative symptoms, and abuse/neglect indices to neurocognitive outcomes. Child Maltreat 2013;18(3):171–83. http://dx.doi.org/10.1177/1077559513497420.

48. Flaherty EG, Thompson R, Litrownik AJ, et al. Adverse childhood exposures and reported child health at age 12. Acad Pediatr 2009;9(3):150–6. http://dx.doi.org/10.1016/j.acap.2008.11.003.

49. Ford JD, Elhai JD, Connor DF, et al. Poly-victimization and risk of posttraumatic, depressive, and substance use disorders and involvement in delinquency in a national sample of adolescents. J Adolesc Health 2010;46(6):545–52. http://dx.doi.org/10.1016/j.jadohealth.2009.11.212.

50. Johnson SB, Riley AW, Granger DA, et al. The science of early life toxic stress for pediatric practice and advocacy. Pediatrics 2013;131(2):319–27. http://dx.doi.org/10.1542/peds.2012-0469.

51. De Bellis MD. Developmental traumatology: the psychobiological development of maltreated children and its implications for research, treatment, and policy. Dev Psychopathol 2001;13(3):539–64.

Index

Note: Page numbers of article titles are in **boldface** type.

Child Adolesc Psychiatric Clin N Am 23 (2014) 413–425
http://dx.doi.org/10.1016/S1056-4993(14)00014-5
1056-4993/14/$ – see front matter © 2014 Elsevier Inc. All rights reserved.

childpsych.theclinics.com

Moving?

Make sure your subscription moves with you!

To notify us of your new address, find your **Clinics Account Number** (located on your mailing label above your name), and contact customer service at:

Email: journalscustomerservice-usa@elsevier.com

800-654-2452 (subscribers in the U.S. & Canada)
314-447-8871 (subscribers outside of the U.S. & Canada)

Fax number: 314-447-8029

Elsevier Health Sciences Division
Subscription Customer Service
3251 Riverport Lane
Maryland Heights, MO 63043

*To ensure uninterrupted delivery of your subscription, please notify us at least 4 weeks in advance of move.

ELSEVIER

Printed and bound by CPI Group (UK) Ltd, Croydon, CR0 4YY

03/10/2024

01040497-0007